BRAHMASTRA
for
PGI DENTAL MDS ENTRANCE EXAMS

Authentic and Largest Collection of PGI MDS Recall Papers of Last 22 Years (1995 to 2016)

Varun Chopra
Radhika Chopra
Pankaj

PEEPEE
PUBLISHERS AND DISTRIBUTORS (P) LTD.

BRAHMASTRA
For PGI Dental MDS Entrance Exams

Published by
Pawaninder P. Vij and Anupam Vij
Peepee Publishers and Distributors (P) Ltd.
Head Office: 160, Shakti Vihar, Pitam Pura
Delhi-110 034 (India)

Correspondence Address:
7/31, First Floor, Ansari Road, Daryaganj
New Delhi-110 002 (India)

Ph: 41512412, 23246245, 9811156083

e-mail: peepee160@yahoo.co.in

e-mail: peepee160@rediffmail.com

e-mail: peepee160@gmail.com

www.peepeepub.com

First Edition: 2017

ISBN : 978-81-8445-219-8

This book is dedicated to
My Parents
Dr. V.K. Chopra
(Chief Medical Officer, Rtd. GMSH-16, Chandigarh)
Mrs. Ritu Chopra
My Mentors
Dr. Zora Singh
(Chairman, Desh Bhagat Group of Institutes, Mandi, Gobindgarh)
Dr. Ravi Gupta
(Professor, Orthopaedics, GMCH-32, Chandigarh)
My Teachers and Students

Foreword

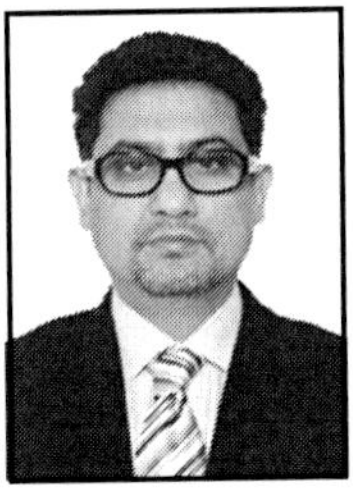

I am writing foreword of this book with a lot of pride and delight and there is a reason for that. I have known the author. Dr. Varun for a long time. His joining the dental profession and his gradual journey to the present have given me a great deal of satisfaction. That he has gone ahead to write yet another informative book, is another milestone in his journey.

While preparing for MDS entrance exams and thereafter getting selected in PGI as a resident I always felt the lacuna of a book which gave the students a feel of the PGIMER question bank. I hope with this book, the long wait for PG aspirants to get access to a comprehensive review of this highly reputed institute will be over.

Writing a book is not merely a matter of technical competence, it is also a matter of sensitivity towards the readers which is appropriately presented in the book Dr. Varun has imbibed the values from his illustrious and highly reputed parents who have contributed to the society through their medical profession. It, therefore, deems fit that Dr. Varun Chopra has dedicated his book to his distinguished parents. I wish him all the very best in this endeavour.

Dr. Sachin Passi
Principal, HOD, Department of Conservative Dentistry
Sukhmani Dental College, Derabassi

Foreword

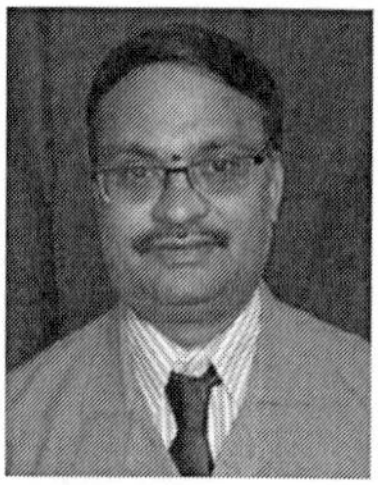

It gives me immense pleasure in writing a foreword to this book titled **"Brahmastra"** by **Dr. Varun Chopra**. I am very happy for more than one reason. I have seen Dr. Varun as an ardent student preparing for Entrance preparation and maturing himself as Guide for the students seeking various Dental entrances. He has been my co-author and contributed a major chunk to the **"Dental Bytes"** book. Now this young enthusiastic author has come out on his own, with a splendid book covering the previous year papers of ORAL HEALTH CENTRE of Post Graduate Institute of Medical Sciences, Chandigarh. It is a mammoth question bank covering the question papers for the last 22 years. I am confident that this book meets the expectation of the students and gives insight into the details and analysis of questions category-wise and subject-wise. Wish this series heralds the dawn of a new era in PG Dental entrance preparation. I wish Dr. Varun Chopra all the best in his future endeavours.

Dr. S. Gowri Sankar
Professor of Orthodontics
Narayana Dental College
Nellore

Preface

Dear friends,

As a PG aspirant I always felt a lacuna of a good book which could give me an idea about the pattern of PGI MDS/House job exam, though there are some books available in the market at present which might give an idea about the exam, but there is no comprehensive book covering the entire question bank of PGI. With this idea in mind I have ventured out with this project. Remember PGI CHD exam is a difficult ball game altogether we can't compare it with NEET/AIPG as the question bank and pattern is different. In the present scenario PGI being the last exam of the session after NEET and AIIMS is like a 'salvage' attempt for any aspirant for coveted PG seat. **Brahmastra** as mentioned in ancient epics and Vedas was a weapon to be used as a last resort, on a similar philosophy this book is an honest attempt to read and revise the entire question bank of PGI which remains an enigma to even the brightest of students so aspire and dream. The golden points given at the end are a useful tool for last minute revision of the PGI question bank.

Dr. Varun Chopra

"Dream is not that which you see while sleeping but that which does not let you sleep. Line your dreams."

Sh. A. P. J. Abdul Kalam

Acknowledgements

First of all I thank God Almighty who has bestowed upon the wisdom, strength and patience to take up this arduous task.

I express extreme gratitude to:

My Seniors and Teachers

Prof. Avtar Singh (Chairman, Sukhmani Group of Colleges)
Sh. Damanjit Singh (Director, Sukhmani Dental College, Derabassi)
Lt. Gen (Dr.) Paramjit Singh (Rayat and Bahra Dental College)
Dr. Rajeev Bali (Principal, DBDCH, Mandi, Gobindgarh)
Dr. Neeru Singh (Formerly, Principal, DBDCH, Muktsar)
Dr. Nandini Passi (Vice Principal, Sukhmani Dental College and Hospital, Derabassi)
Dr. Tarun Kalra (Principal, Rayat and Bahra Dental College, Sahauran, Mohali)
Dr. Kavipal Singh (Principal, SGRD Dental College, Sri Amritsar)
Dr. Gurvanit Lehl (Dean and HOD, Oral Health Centre, GMCH 32, CHD)
Dr. Manjit Talwar (Professor, Oral Health Centre, GMCH-32, CHD)
Dr. Rahul Dutta (Professor, Maxillofacial Surgery)
Dr. Rupinder Kaur (HOD, Maxillofacial Surgery, Sukhmani Dental College, Derabassi)
Dr. Rishi Bali (Professor, Maxillofacial Surgery, DAV Dental College, Yamunanagar)
Dr. Ramandeep Singh Bhullar (Professor, Maxillofacial Surgery, SGRD, Amritsar)
Dr. Anand Gupta (Consultant, Maxillofacial Surgery, GMCH-32, CHD)
Dr. Balveer Singh (HOD, Pharmacology, SSDCH)
Dr. Sandeep Mahajan (HOD, Pedodontics, SSDCH)
Dr. (Mrs.) Renu Dutta (HOD, Orthodontics, SSDCH)
Dr. Anup Kapoor (HOD, Periodontics, SSDCH)
Dr. Vinod Ratan (HOD, Biochemistry, SSDCH)
Dr. Monica (HOD, Microbiology, SSDCH)
Dr. Naresh Kumar (HOD, Maxillofacial Surgery, DBDCH)
Dr. Madhushankar Diwan (Professor, Maxillofacial Surgery)
Dr. Pankaj Gupta (HOD, Maxillofacial Surgery, Yamuna Dental College)
Dr. Amit Sood (Professor, Endodontics)
Dr. Ajitpal Singh (HOD, Anatomy, DBDCH, Mandi, Gobindgarh)
Dr. A.K. Singh (HOD, Biochemistry, SSDCH)
Dr. Nisha Garg (Professor, Endodontics, Dental College, Baddi)
Dr. Amit Garg (HOD, Maxillofacial Surgery, Rayat and Bahra Dental College)

Dr. Guljot Singh (Professor, Periodontics, Daswani Dental College, Kota)
Late Dr. Sumeet Sandhu (Formerly Principal, SGRD Dental College, Amritsar)
Dr. Amit Jain (Associate Professor, Pharmacology, GGS Medical College, Faridkot)
Shri J.S. Lamba and Mrs Jasbir Lamba
Mrs. Rajwinder Kaur (SSDCH)
Shri Vinay (SSDCH)

My Friends

Dr. Inderjot Singh (Professor, Maxillofacial Surgery, CMC, Ludhiana)
Dr. Devinder P.S. Ahluwalia (Professor, Orthodontics, HSJ Dental College, CHD)
Dr. Ramandeep Sohi (HOD, Department of Public Health, SSDCH, Derabassi)
Dr. Satnam Singh (Consultant, Oral Surgery, PGI, CHD)
Dr. Umesh Dharmani (Consultant, Endodontics, PGI, CHD)
Dr. Shivesh (Consultant, PGI Satellite Centre, Sangrur)
Dr. Gulshan Kumar (Reader, Prosthodontics, SSDCH, Formerly Resident, AIIMS, PGI, RML)
Dr. Sarthak Bhola (Reader, Periodontics, SSDCH, Derabassi)
Dr. Gaurav Malik (Director, Dental Centre Max Hospital)
Dr. Amol Bansal (Reader, Orthodontics, SSDCH)
Dr. Nisha Dua (Reader, OMDR, SSDCH)
Dr. Rohini Malik (Sr. Consultant, Max Hospital)
Dr. Deepti Dhingra (Reader, Endodontics, DBDCH, Mandi, Gobindgarh)
Dr. Poonam Bali (Reader, Prosthodontics, DIRDS, Faridkot)
Dr. Saurab Bither (Reader, Oral Surgery, LBDC, Patiala)
Dr. Samir Anand (Reader, Periodontics, Rayat and Bahra Dental College)
Dr. Shammi Kapoor (Reader, Prosthodontics)
Dr. Sanjeev Jindal (HOD, OMDR, Gian Sagar Dental College, Banur)
Dr. Shobha Nangrani (Consultant, Endodontics, Dental Wellness, Bangalore)
Dr. Deepika Gupta (Sr. Lecturer, Oral Surgery, SSDCH, Derabassi)
Dr. Malvika Goel (Sr. Lecturer, Pharmacology, SSDCH, Derabassi)
Dr. Gagandeep (Sr. Lecturer, Periodontics, DBDCH, Mandi, Gobindgarh)
Dr. Tanya Goyal (S. Lecturer, Pedodontics, DBDCH, Mandi, Gobindgarh)
Dr. Simarjeev Singh (Sr. Lecturer, OMDR, BRS Dental College, Sultanpur)
Dr. Gurinderbir Singh Thind (Consultant, Oral Surgery, SSDCH)
Dr. Arpit Sikri (Sr. Lecturer, Prosthodontics, Sudha Rustagi Dental College, Faridabad)
Dr. Ankur Sharma (Consultant, Endodontics, Chandigarh)
Dr. Kartesh Singla (Sr. Lecturer, Oral Pathology, SSDCH)
Dr. Sahil Chopra (Consultant, Orthodontist, Rajpura)

Dr. Pranav Nayyar (Reader, DBDCH, Mandi, Gobindgarh)
Dr. Eish Sethi (DBDCH, Muktsar OMFS)
Dr. Pallavi (Reader, Prosthodontics, DBDCH)
Dr. Hitesh Adya (Consultant, Ophthalmologist, Ludhiana)
Dr. Mukti (Sr. Lecturer, Biochemistry, SSDCH)
Dr. Yashmeet Kaur (Professor, Oral Surgery, SGRDI DS. Amritsar)
Dr. Anu Kaushal (BDS, Lecturer, SSDCH)
Sh. Major Mehta (Administrator, DBDCH, Mandi, Gobindgarh)
Sh. Charanjeet Singh (Administrator, SSDCH, Derabassi)
Dr. Minkal Arora (Consultant, Dental Surgeon, Sector 27, CHD)
Dr. Dipty (Lecturer, Prosthodontics, SSDCH)
Dr. Mukesh Dhameja (Reader, Oral Surgery, SSDCH)
Dr. Umang Jagga (Sr. Lecturer, Pedodontics, SSDCH)
Dr. Ramneet Kataria (Reader, Oral Surgery, Rayat and Bahra Dental College)
Dr. Gaganjot Kaur, MDS (PGI) (Consultant, Orthodontist)
Dr. Rajeshwar Chawla (HOD, Oral Pathology, JCD, Sirsa)
Dr. Sarika A Kapila (Professor, Oral Surgery, SGRD, Amritsar)
Dr. Amneet Kaur (Professor, OMFS, SGRD, Amritsar)
Dr. Jasmine Kaur (Professor, OMFS, SGRD, Amritsar)
Dr. Varun Pruthi (Consultant, Endodontist, Delhi)
Dr. Tanu Taneja (Reader, Oral Pathology, SSDCH)
Dr. Anupama Mahajan (HOD, Anatomy, SGRD, Amritsar)
Dr. Puneeta Salwan (Professor, Anatomy, SGRD, Amritsar)
Dr. Gaurav Agnihotri (Professor, Anatomy, GMC, Amritsar)
Dr. Poonamjit Kaur Kang (Demonstrator SSDCH, Oral Surgery)
Dr. Mehtab (BDS, BVP, Pune)

My Students

Dr. Namita Singh (Consultant, Prosthodontist)
Dr. Priya Malhotra (MDS, Perio Std., GDC, Patiala)
Dr. Jitender Banga (MDS, Prostho Std., GDC, Patiala)
Dr. Sudhanshu Shekhar (MDS, Prosthodontics)
Dr. Savy Arora (MDS, Prosthodontics)
Dr. Navdeep Kaur (Dental Surgeon)
Dr. Vinay Arora (BDS, DBDC, Muktsar)
Dr. Meetika Anand (BDS, LBDC, Patiala)
Dr. Meenakshi Kaundil (BDS, HIDS, Paonta Sahib)
Dr. Agami Mehta (BDS, HSJ, SEC 25, Chandigarh)
Dr. Priya Mukherjee (BDS, GDC, Patiala)

Dr. Mridha Sharma (BDS, SSDCH, Derabassi, Gold Medallist)
Dr. Kirandeep Kaur (BDS, SSDCH)
Dr. Mehak Sharma (BDS, SSDCH)
Dr. Nitika Sood (BDS, SSDCH, Derabassi)
Dr. Prabhjit Singh (BDS, Aadesh, Bhatinda)
Dr. Sepal Goyal (BDS, GDC, Patiala)
Dr. Vimlesh Kumari (BDS, GDC, Patiala)
Dr. Heena Sharma (BDS, DBDC, Muktsar)
Dr. Tanvi Singhmar (BDS, Rayat and Bahra Dental College)
Dr. Simrandeep Kaur (BDS, Rayat and Bahra Dental College)
Dr. Kawarpal Kaur (BDS, SSDCH, Derabassi)
Dr. Manpreet Kaur (BDS, SSDCH, Derabassi)
Dr. Sandeep Ghuman (SSDCH, Univ. Topper, Derabassi)
Dr. Shilpa (BDS, DBDC, Muktsar)
Dr. Komal (BDS, GDC, Patiala)
Dr. Milli Sahni (BDS, LBDC, Patiala)
Dr. Shiny (MDS Std., Oral Surgery, TMU)
Dr. Ankur Kumar Das (SSDCH, Derabassi)
Dr. Shina Jindal (MDS, Prosthodontics)
Dr. Sukhvir Singh (BDS Std., Aadesh, Bathinda)

Please convey your positive feedback at omfs2637@gmail.com

Special Thanks

This book would have been Impossible without you all....

Dr. Radhika Chopra (MBBS, MD, HCMS-I [Editor])
Dr. Pankajbir (MBBS, MD [Editor])
Dr. Harjot Kaur (Dental Surgeon, For Meticulous Proof Reading)
Dr. Ruchika Khanna (MDS, DMDR, Co-Editor)
Dr. Santokh Singh (Director, Dental Desk)
Dr. Vinay Arora (BDS, DBDCH, Muktsar)
Dr. Meetika Anand Popli (BDS, LBDC, Patiala)

Shri Pawanider P. Vij and his team
C/o Peepee Publishers and Distributors (P) Ltd.
DENTORICS INSTITUTE FOR DDS/MDS, CHANDIGARH

How to Prepare for PGI Chandigarh MDS Exams

Remember the lines by renowned motivator speaker and author Shri Shiv Khera "WINNERS DON'T DO DIFFERENT THINGS, THEY DO THINGS DIFFERENTLY"..... so what is required besides hard work and patience is SMART PREPRATION, meaning to say focusing on the important things more....

Dear friends, understanding how to prepare for PGI MDS/HOUSE SURGEON exam is no "rocket science" rather it's an accumulation of certain facts which one must remember at all times.

For PGIMER focus more on dental subjects, than on medical subjects. The subjects to be focused during the preparation and the books recommended are:

- ORTHODONTICS (JITENDER SHARAN, Kharbanda, ASHOK JENA, PROFITTs)
- ORAL SURGERY (ROWE AND WILLIAMS, PETERSON, FONSECA)
- COMMUNITY DENTISTRY (SOBEN PETER, CATALYST FOR PGI BOOK based on DR AMRIT TIWARI's compendium)
- Fluorides and indices though definitely a part of community dentistry occupies special importance for PGIMER EXAM (CATALYST FOR PGI)
- PEDODONTICS (Mc DONALDS, DR SHOBHA TANDON, CARIOLOGY FROM NEWBURN EARNEST, PRABHAKAR MCQs Clinical Vol Chapter on Cariology)
- ENDODONTICS AND CONSERVATIVE (COHEN AND STURDEVANT, NISHA GARG AND AMIT GARG)
- DENTAL MATERIALS (PHILIPS)
- ORAL PATHOLOGY (SHAFER'S AND NEVILLE)
- PROSTHODONTICS AND IMPLANTOLOGY (BOUCHER, SHILLINBURGH, STEWART, MISCH)
- GENERAL HUMAN ANATOMY (GRAYS, CHAURASIA, INDERBIR SINGH)

Repeats form an integral part of the PGI EXAM so reading and revising the previous year's question bank is of utmost importance.

Recommended MCQ books are Dental Pulse, Dentest, Dental Bytes, Ritu Duggal, Prabhakar, VP Singh (Prostho only), and National Board release papers.

Remember that PGI CHANDIGARH EXAM is a closely contested exam but at the same time it's quite predictable provided one is in the right direction, usually the expected cut-off is around 75% but may vary depending on difficulty of the paper. With the increase in number of PG seats and PGI CHD being the last exam and hope for the aspirants who missed NEET by a whisker, the importance of this exam in the present scenario need not be overemphasized. Persistence, Perseverance and Patience (3P's) is what is required to crack the exam.

"Great minds have purposes, others have wishes".

–WASHINGTON IRVING

So set your purpose (goal) today and toil hard and leave rest to God....

Wishing everyone good luck for their preparation...may the best win...

Dr. Varun Chopra
Associate Professor Maxillofacial Surgery
Director, Dentorics Institute for MDS/DDS Entrance
Chandigarh

Contents

PGI PAPERS

PGI Paper November 2016

1. **Burning pain after a nerve injury is known as:**
   A. Neuralgia
   B. Causalgia
   C. Hyperalgesia
   D. Allodynia

   Ans: B

2. **Which of the nerve is commonly injured following a fracture of angle of mandible?**
   A. Lingual nerve
   B. Inferior alveolar nerve
   C. Mental nerve
   D. Mylohyoid nerve

   Ans: B

Mandibular Angle Fracture and Nerve Injury

- Maxillofacial trauma frequently results in injuries to soft tissues and major skeletal components of the face. Facial injuries range from 3.2% to 8% of all injuries and 79.7% of all facial injuries involve mandible.Angle of the mandible is the weakest region and account for about 18%-30% of mandible fracture. Injury is 8 times more frequent in men than women and majority of angle fractures occur in the age range of 20-29 years.
- Fracture mandible is frequently associated with inferior alveolar nerve injury and altered neurosensory function. Inferior alveolar nerve lies in a bony canal called inferior dental canal which is enclosed within a tube of dense bone. It appears as two parallel radiopaque lines on panoramic radiograph one representing roof of canal and other the floor of canal. Fractures of the mandible are

associated with displacement and disruption of the continuity of inferior alveolar canal and damage to the nerve which can be neuropraxia, axontmesis or neurotmesis.

- It may present as paraesthesia, dysaesthesia and anesthesia. It results either from direct traumatic injury, edema causing compression, or compression, traction and dislocation of nerve bundle by displaced or comminuted fracture. Depending upon the type and degree of anatomic injury, loss of sensation can be permanent or temporary severe or moderate, partial or complete. Inferior alveolar nerve injury leads to abnormal sensory and functional consequences like numbness of ipsilateral lower lip, chin and lower teeth, difficulty in performing daily activities such as speech, mastication, shaving, tooth brushing, playing of wind instruments, and inability to maintain lip competence for retention and swallowing of liquid, foods and sometimes allodynia.
- It also affects psycho-emotional status of the patient. Different methods used for neurosensory evaluation are static touch, two point discrimination, brush stroke direction and sharp blunt differentiation.

3. True about new strategy for Tuberculosis control i.e., DOTS is:

A. Long course chemotherapy
B. Short course chemotherapy
C. No medication only observation

Ans: B

4. Calculus more common in Mandibular anterior region:

A. Brushite
B. Octa-calcium phosphate
C. Magnesium whitlockite
D. Hydroxyapatite

Ans: A

5. Common site for Branchial cyst:

A. Lower 1/3 of sternomastoid on anterior border
B. Lower 1/3 of sternomastoid on posterior border
C. Upper 1/3 of sternomastoid on anterior border
D. Upper 1/3 of sternomastoid on posterior border

Ans: C

Branchial Cleft Cyst

- Branchial cleft cyst is a congenital epithelial cyst that arises on the lateral part of the neck usually due to failure of obliteration of the second branchial cleft (or failure of fusion of the second and third branchial arches) in embryonic development. Less commonly, the cysts can develop from the first, third, or fourth clefts.
- Most branchial cleft fistulae are asymptomatic, but they may become infected. The cyst, however, usually presents as a smooth, slowly enlarging lateral neck mass that may increase in size after an upper respiratory tract infection.
- Branchial cleft cysts are remnants of embryonic development and result from a failure of obliteration of one of the branchial clefts, which are homologous to the structures in fish that develop into gills.
- Conservative (i.e., no treatment), or surgical excision. With surgical excision, recurrence is common, usually due to incomplete excision. Often, the tracts of the cyst will pass near important structures, such as the internal jugular vein, carotid artery, or facial nerve, making complete excision impractical.

6. **Burning feet syndrome is caused due to deficiency of:**

A. Vit B1
B. Vit B5
C. Vit B3
D. Vit B12

Ans: B. Vitamin B5, i.e., pantothenic acid or Chick anti-dermatitis factor

Structure Damaged During Tracheostomy

- **Surgical Anatomy:** The superior thyroid notch, cricoid and suprasternal notch usually can be easily palpated through the skin. The cricothyroid space can be identified by palpating a slight indentation immediately below the inferior edge of the thyroid cartilage. Cricothyroid arteries traverse the superior aspect of this space on each side and anastomose near the midline.
  The innominate artery crosses from left to right anterior to the trachea at the superior thoracic inlet. Its pulsations can be palpated and occasionally seen in the suprasternal

notch especially in case of a high riding vessel, representing a contraindication for a bedside percutaneous or open tracheostomy.
The isthmus of the thyroid gland lies across the 2nd to 4th tracheal rings and must be dealt with in any procedure at or around the upper trachea.

- **Complications and Risks of Tracheostomy**
  As with any surgery, there are some risks associated with tracheostomies. However, serious infections are rare.
  Early Complications that may arise during the tracheostomy procedure or soon thereafter include:
  - Bleeding.
  - Air trapped around the lungs (pneumothorax).
  - Air trapped in the deeper layers of the chest (pneumomediastinum).
  - Air trapped underneath the skin around the tracheostomy (subcutaneous emphysema).
  - Damage to the swallowing tube (esophagus).
  - Injury to the nerve that moves the vocal cords (recurrent laryngeal nerve).
  - Tracheostomy tube can be blocked by blood clots, mucus or pressure of the airway walls. Blockages can be prevented by suctioning, humidifying the air, and selecting the appropriate tracheostomy tube.
  - Many of these early complications can be avoided or dealt with appropriately with our experienced surgeons in a hospital setting.
  - Over time, other complications may arise from the surgery.

  Later complications that may occur while the tracheostomy tube is in place include:
  - Accidental removal of the tracheostomy tube (accidental decannulation).
  - Infection in the trachea and around the tracheostomy tube.
  - Windpipe itself may become damaged for a number of reasons, including pressure from the tube; bacteria that cause infections and form scar tissue; or friction from a tube that moves too much.

- These complications can usually be prevented or quickly dealt with if the caregiver has proper knowledge of how to care for the tracheostomy site.

Delayed Complications that may result after longer-term presence of a tracheostomy include:

- Thinning (erosion) of the trachea from the tube rubbing against it (tracheomalacia).
- Development of a small connection from the trachea (windpipe) to the esophagus (swallowing tube) which is called a tracheo-esophageal fistula.
- Development of bumps (granulation tissue) that may need to be surgically removed before decannulation (removal of trach tube) can occur
- Narrowing or collapse of the airway above the site of the tracheostomy, possibly requiring an additional surgical procedure to repair it.
- Once the tracheostomy tube is removed, the opening may not close on its own. Tubes remaining in place for 16 weeks or longer are more at risk for needing surgical closure.
- A clean tracheostomy site, good tracheostomy tube care and regular examination of the airway by an otolaryngologist should minimize the occurrence of any of these complications.

High-risk groups: The risks associated with tracheostomies are higher in the following groups of patients:

- Children, especially newborns and infants.
- Smokers.
- Alcohol abusers.
- Diabetics.
- Immunocompromised patients.
- Persons with chronic diseases or respiratory infections.
- Persons taking steroids or cortisone.

7. Sterilization of heat sensitve material is best done by:

A. Ethylene oxide
B. Autoclave
C. Hot air oven
D. Glutaraldehyde

Ans: A

Sterilization of Heat Sensitive Materials

- Ethylene oxide (also known as EO or EtO) processing is widely used for the sterilization of healthcare devices and instruments.
- It is an excellent sterilizer for heat sensitive items and ideal for electric instruments, flexible endoscopes and photographic instruments.
- The process involves exposing products to ethylene oxide gas under vacuum in a sealed chamber EO sterilization assures that a safe and sterile product will be delivered to the market each and every time.
- Ethylene oxide sterilization is a chemical process consisting of four primary variables: gas concentration, humidity, temperature and time. EO is an alkylating agent that disrupts the DNA of microorganisms, which prevents them from reproducing. The EO penetrates the breathable packaging and sterilizes all accessible surfaces of the product to render products sterile by alkylation of proteins essential for cell reproduction.
- Ethylene oxide can penetrate multiple layers of breathable packaging, making it suitable for the sterilization of a wide range of materials not compatible with other methods of sterilization:
  - Assembled complex devices.
  - Catheters.
  - Custom procedure packs.
  - Equipment with integrated-electronics.
  - Multi-lumen tubing products.
  - Stents.
  - Wound care dressings.
  - When selecting a sterilization partner, manufacturers need to choose a contractor who has the flexibility and technical capability to meet the demands of the specific devices.

8. Extracted teeth are discarded in which coloured bag:

A. Red
B. Yellow
C. Black
D. Blue

Ans: B

Waste Management

Yellow Bags	Red Bags	Blue Bags	Black Carboy
Infectious waste, bandages, gauze, cotton or any other objects in contact with body fuids, human body parts, placenta, etc.	Plastic waste such as catheters, injection syringes, tubings, IV bottles	All types of glass bottles and broken glass articles, outdated and discarded medicines	Needles without syringes, blades, sharps and all metal articles.

Intraoral Vertical Ramus Osteotomy (IVRO)

First described by Winstanley in 1968

- Indications
  - Primary indication for IVRO is patients with Horizontal mandibular excess in whom a good profile, arch and dental relationship can be obtained by retruding, the intact mandibular arch.
  - Mandibular asymmetry.
  - Correction of skeletal occlusal cant- two-jaw surgery
  - Minor occlusal discrepancy after isolated Le Fort-losteotomy.
  - Patients with significant TMJ complaints.

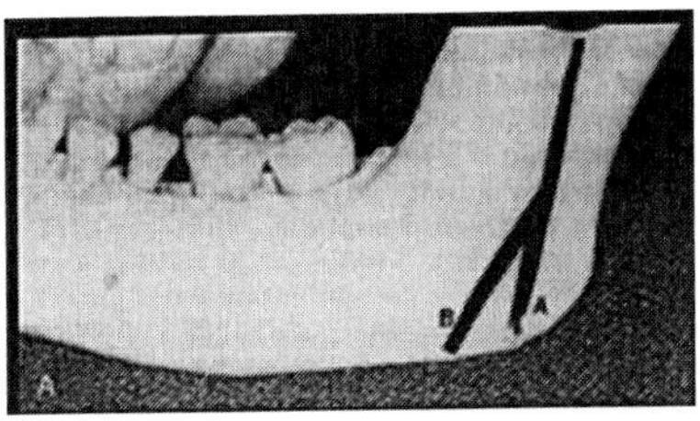

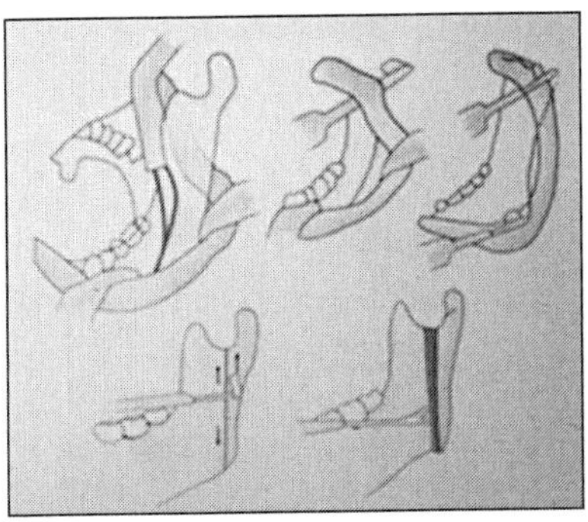

- Mainly for setback procedures and mandibular asymmetries.
- Not recommended for correction of anterior open bites.
- Contraindications:
  - Advancement of distal, tooth-bearing mandibular segment.
  - Recent condylar fractures.

Bilateral Sagittal Split Ramus Osteotomy (BSSRO)

- Most versatile mandibular osteotomy.
- An indispensable surgical procedure for correction of lower jaw deformities.
- Originally described by *Schuchardt* in 1942.
- Described by *Trauner and Hugo Obwegeser* in 1957.
- Indications:
  - Horizontal mandibular excess, deficiency and asymmetry.
  - Procedure of choice for mandibular advancement (when advancing beyond 10-12 mm should give consideration to extraoral proceed because of minimal overlap between proximal and the distal segments.
  - Mandibular setback of small to moderate magnitude (beyond 7 mm – inverted L or IVRO).
  - Correction of mandibular asymmetries.
- Contraindications:
  - Severe decreased posterior mandibular body height.
  - Extremely thin medial-later width of ramus.
  - Severe ramus hypoplasia; and
  - Severe asymmetries.

9. **Desquamative gingivitis can be found in all, *except*:**

A. Lichen planus　　B. Pemphigoid
C. Pemphigus　　D. Herpes simplex

Ans: D

Desquamative Gingivitis

- Gingival desquamation is a clinical sign in which the gingiva appears reddish, glazed and friable with destruction of the epithelium.
- Chronic desquamative gingivitis was first described by Tomes and Tomes in 1894. “Desquamative gingivitis” is a

descriptive term, first introduced by Prinz in 1932 that is synonymous with the presence of erythema, desquamation, erosion, and blistering of attached and marginal gingiva. Glickman and Smulow stated that desquamative gingivitis may be a clinical feature common to a wide number of disorders. A classification was proposed based on etiologic considerations, together with histologic and immunologic findings.

- Dermatological diseases.
- Cicatricial pemphigoid.
- Lichen planus.
- Pemphigus.
- Psoriasis.
- Bullous pemphigoid.
- Epidermolysis bullosa acquisita.
- Contact stomatitis.
- Endocrine disturbances.
- Estrogen deficiencies following oophorectomy and in postmenopausal stages.
- Testosterone imbalance.
- Hypothyroidism.
- Aging.
- Abnormal response to bacterial plaque.
- Idiopathic.
- Chronic infections.
- Tuberculosis.
- Chronic candidiasis.
- Histoplasmosis.

Overall, mucous membrane pemphigoid (MMP), oral lichen planus and pemphigus vulgaris have emerged as the most common causes of desquamative gingivitis, with the first two accounting for about 80% of cases.

Trigemino-Cardiac Reflex (TCR)

- The trigemino-cardiac reflex (TCR) is defined as the sudden onset of parasympathetic dysrhythmia, sympathetic hypotension, apnea or gastric hypermotility during stimulation of any of the sensory branches of the trigeminal nerve. The sensory nerve endings of the trigeminal nerve send neuronal signals via the Gasserian ganglion to the sensory nucleus of the trigeminal nerve, forming the afferent pathway of the reflex arc. This afferent pathway continues along the short internuncial nerve fibers in the reticular formation to connect with the efferent pathway in the motor nucleus of the vagus nerve. Clinically the trigemino-cardiac reflex has been reported to occur during craniofacial surgery, balloon-compression rhizolysis of the trigeminal ganglion, and tumor resection in the cerebellopontine angle. Apart from the few clinical reports, the physiological function of this brainstem-reflex has not yet been fully explored. From experimental findings, it may be suggested that the trigemino-cardiac reflex represents an expression of a central neurogenic reflex leading to rapid cerebrovascular vasodilatation generated from excitation of oxygen-sensitive neurons in the rostral ventrolateral medulla oblongata. By this physiological response, the adjustments of the systemic and cerebral circulations are initiated to divert blood to the brain or to increase blood flow within it. As it is generally accepted that the diving reflex and ischemic tolerance appear to involve at least partially similar physiological mechanisms, the existence of such endogenous neuroprotective strategies may extend the actually known clinical appearance of the TCR and include the prevention of other potentially brain injury states as well. This may be in line with the suggestion that the TCR is a physiological, but not a pathophysiological entity.

10. Reverse Bevel in Class 2 cavity is made on:

A. Mesio-facial wall
B. Mesio-lingual wall
C. Disto-facial wall
D. Disto-lingual wall

Ans: A

11. Filler size of 0.01-0.010 is classified under:

A. Hybrid
B. Microfilled
C. Nanofilled
D. Macrofilled

Ans: C

Size of nano-filled composites

Composite Restorative Materials

Type of Composite	Size of Filler Particles	Type of Restorations	Advantages	Disadvantages
Microfilled	0.4 µm– 0.75 µm	Class I,II,III,V	Best esthetics, good finish and gloss, continued smoothness	High shrinkage, lacks strength
Hybrid	0.2 µm– 3.0 µm	Class I,II,III,IV V	Good esthetics and strength	Lacks long-term smoothness
Nanofilled	0.01 µm– 0.015 µm	Class I,II,III,IV V, VI	Best polish, low shrinkage, high strength, high wear resistance	
Packable	0.2 µm– 3.0 µm	Class I,II,VI	Low shrinkage	Decreased wear resistance
Flowable	0.6 µm– 3.0 µm	Pediatrics, Class I, cervical lesions	Low modulus of elasticity	Increased wear

12. According to WHO classification of tooth injuries 873.64 is:

A. Complicated fracture
B. Uncomplicated fracture
C. Luxation
D. Crown/root fracture

Ans: D

WHO classification of tooth fracture

Who Classification

• 873.60: Ename fracture • 873.61: Crown fracture without pulp exposure • 873.62: Crown fracture with pulp exposure • 873.64: Root fracture • 873.64: Crown/Root fracture • 873.66: Tooth luxation • 873.67: Intrusion and extrusion	• 873.68 Avulsion 873.69: Other injuries (Soft tissue) • 802.20: Fracture of the alveolar process of the mandible • 802.40: Fracture of the alveolar process of the maxilla • 802.21: Fracture of the body of the mandible • 802.41: Fracture of the body of the Maxilla

13. Which of the following diseases shows vascular involvement and thrombosis?

A. Aspergillosis
B. Oculomycosis
C. Coccidiomycosis
D. Mucormycosis

Ans: D

14. Which of the following hormone has the greatest effect on wound healing?

A. Estrogen
B. Cortisol
C. ADH
D. Growth hormone

Ans: B

- Glucocorticoids interfere with wound healing by its anti-inflammatory effects by inhibiting collagen synthesis.

15. The centre of resistance to move maxillary anterior six tooth lie above:

A. Root of first and second premolar
B. In between roots of 2 central
C. In between lateral incisors and canine on both side
D. At mid point of max central

Ans: A

16. Form and function concept of craniofacial structure was given by:

A. Leon Williams
B. Enlow and Bang
C. Moss
D. Petrovic

Ans: C

17. Maximum osmotic pressure is raised by:

A. Albumin
B. Normal saline
C. 5% dextrose
D. Ringer's lactate solution

Ans: A

Plasma Volume and Transfusion Products

- **Dextrose 5%:** Dextrose 5% is a 'Maintenance Fluid' (Dextrose is d-glucose). It is isosmotic as administered and does not cause haemolysis. The glucose is rapidly taken up by cells. The net effect is of administering pure water, so it is distributed throughout the total body water. Each compartment receives fluid in proportion to its contribution to the TBW (i.e., 2/3rd to ICF and 1/3rd to ECF; the ECF fluid is distributed one quarter to plasma and three quarters to ISF).
  The distribution of 1,000 mls of dextrose 5% is:
  - ICF 670 mls.
  - ECF 330 mls (with ISF 250 mls and plasma 80 mls).

  Intravascular volume increases from 5000 to 5080 mls. This volume increase of less than 2% which will not be sensed by the volume receptors (as it is below the 7-10% threshold).
  The osmolality of plasma (3,200 mls) will decrease by: [287 - (287 × 3.20 / 3.28)] which is about 7 mOsmoles/l or a 2.5% decrease. This is enough to be detected by the osmoreceptors. ADH release will be decreased and renal water excretion will rise. A delay will occur because the changes have to be detected centrally and then ADH levels need 3 half-lives to fall to a new steady state.
- **Normal Saline:** Normal saline is an 'ECF Replacement Fluid'. Its [Na+] is similar to that of the extracellular fluid and this effectively limits its distribution to the ECF (distributing between the ISF and the plasma in proportion to their volume i.e., 3:1).
  The ISF will increase in volume by 750 mls. The plasma volume will increase by 250 mls. This is why blood loss of 1,000 mls requires about 3 to 4 times the volume of IV replacement fluid to restore normal intravascular volume. Plasma osmolality and tonicity will be unchanged because normal saline is isosmotic. The osmoreceptors do not contribute anything to the excretion of normal saline. Blood volume increases to 5250 mls; an increase of 5%. This is below the sensitivity of the volume receptors. It seems that the body has no clear way of excreting this excess

fluid as neither osmoreceptors nor volume receptors are stimulated! However, experiments have shown that replacement fluids' are excreted the most rapidly of all these groups.

How does this happen?An additional mechanism is relevant here. Normal saline contains no protein so the oncotic pressure in the blood is slightly lowered following the saline infusion. This has two effects:

- Movement of fluid into the ISF is favoured (Starling's Hypothesis).
- Glomerulotubular imbalance occurs: the lowered oncotic pressure immediately leads to an increase in GFR and a smaller reabsorption of water in the proximal tubule. Urine flow increases. This is a strictly local effect without any hormonal intermediary. The urine flow increases immediately. Fluid then moves back into the intravascular compartment and the urine flow continues until all the transfused fluid is excreted.

- **Plasma Protein Solution:** Plasma protein solution is a colloid and is distributed only to the intravascular fluid. The tonicity is unaltered. The blood volume increases from 5,000 mls to 6,000 mls; an increase of 20%. This is above the 7 to 10% threshold for the volume receptors. The result is a fall in ADH levels and the excretion of the excess water commences.

  This water loss tends to increase the plasma oncotic pressure and water moves from the ISF to the IVFVascular reflexes are important also in causing venous pooling and a decrease in the 'effective' circulating volume. These mechanisms tend to slow the excretion of the water load. The albumin is partly slowly redistributed to the ISF and metabolised. These changes are slow so the effect of plasma protein infusion on blood volume is both more pronounced and more prolonged.

  The pressure-volume control mechanisms important in long term regulation of blood volume are slow in onset but become relevant here as the blood volume change is more significant and more prolonged and occurs without change in osmolality (or initially in plasma oncotic pressure either).

Overview

Dextrose 5% is essentially treated by the body as pure water and a significant percent moves intracellularly. It is a useful fluid to replenish intracellular fluid but does so at the expense of tonicity. It is inappropriate for intravascular volume replacement. It is excreted because ADH levels decline in response to the drop in plasma osmolality.

Normal saline is a 'replacement fluid' (meaning ECF replacement) because it adds only to the ECF volume. Only about a third remains intravascularly. To replace intravascular volume will require transfusion with about 3 times the volume of blood lost. It is cheap and readily available. It is excreted because the small drop in plasma oncotic pressure causes glomerulotubular imbalance. ADH is not affected.

Plasma protein solutions (e.g., 5% human albumin) are excellent for replacing intravascular volume. ISF and ICF will not be replenished. Albumin is slow to be excreted and the transfused volume is excreted much slower than with replacement solutions. Plasma protein solutions are expensive and supply is limited. The fluid is initially excreted because of a fall in ADH level falling stimulation of the volume receptors.

18. **Tattle Tooth Program** (Dear students the exact question and option is not recalled. So overview of topic is given.)

- **"Tattletooth Program"–Texas Statewide Preventive Dentistry Program**

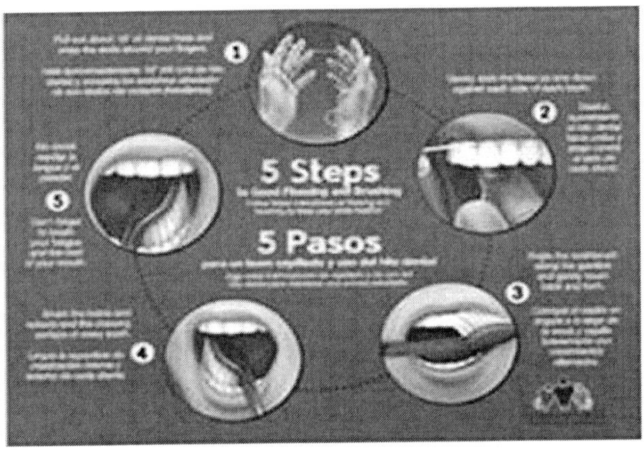

The Tattletooth program was developed in 1974-1976 as a cooperative effort between Texas DENTAL health professional organizations, the Texas Department of Health and the Texas Educational Agency through a grant from the Department of Health and Human Services to the Bureau of Dental Health. The program was pilot tested in 1975 and field tested in spring 1976 in schools within the states of Texas.

Separate lesson plans were developed for each grade and a systems approach was used to develop all educational material.

- Three videotapes were produced as part of the teacher-training package.
- The first videotape familiarizes the teacher with the lesson format and content.
- A second videotape, "Brushing and Flossing" was developed for the dual purpose of teacher training and as an educational unit to be used by the teacher with the students.
- A third videotape provides teachers with additional background information as a means of preparing them to teach the lessons.
- The materials that were developed to aid in the implementation of the program consisted of:
  - A bruchure that provides an overview of the program.
  - A school nurses brochure.

  A letter to school principals and nurses was sent out as part of a package distributed annually by the Bureau of Maternal and Child Health. A two hour training session using the materials in the new curriculum was televised to the schools via a video network.

Program Implementation

The Texas Department of health employs 16 hygienists in the eight public health regions to implement the Tattletooth program.

- The hygienist instructs teachers using videotapes designed for teacher training and provide them with a copy of the curriculum.
- Health promotion activities are encouraged and publicized within the school community.

- Teachers are encouraged to invite a dental professional to demonstrate brushing and flossing in the classroom.
- A field trip to a dental office is strongly recommended for kindergarten children.
- Bulletin board suggestions, a book list, films and videotapes are available on a free loan for appropriate grade leves.
- Other resources used are a list of companies providing supplementary classroom resources and a comprehensive glossary of vocabulary words written for the teacher in English that are used in all grades levels.

Program Evaluation

The students in grades 3,5,7,9 and 11 were given the Texas Assessment of Academic Skills (TAAS) by the Texas Education agency, to satisfy the legislative requirement that student performance be assessed.

- Dental health knowledge was significantly increased at all grades leves.
- Plaque levels were decreased by approximately 15% in a randomly selected sample of 2,142 children.
- Over 80% of the teachers judged the program to be helpful and effective, but evaluation questions suggested that they felt a need for additional technical help in brushing and flossing.

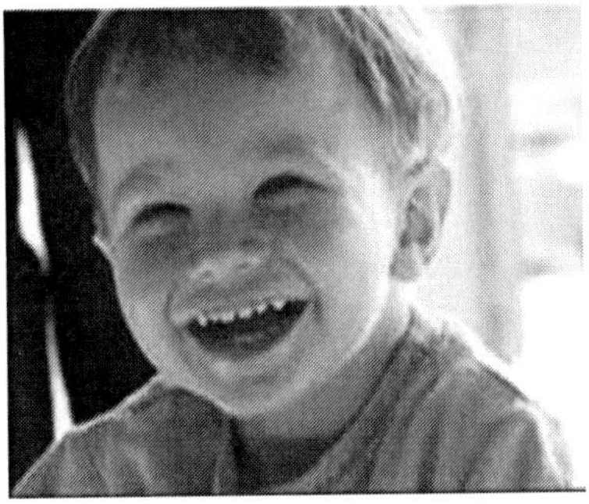

19. False about osseous craters:

A. 1/3 of all bony defects
B. 2/3 of Mandibular detects
C. Common in anterior segment
D. Twice in posterior segment as compared to anterior

Ans: C

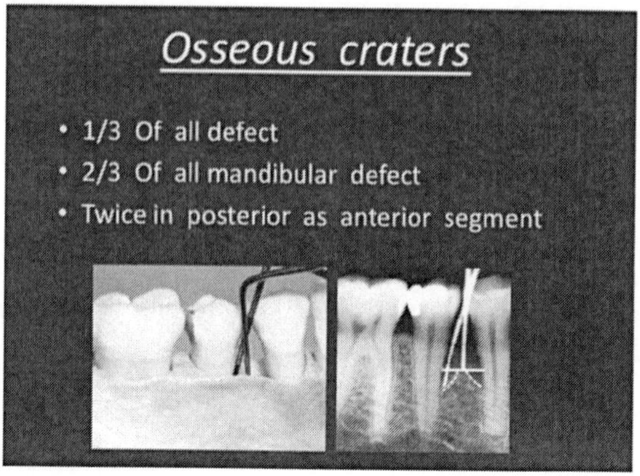

20. What is the most frequent cause of pulmonary embolism?

A. Congestive heart failure
B. Hemorrhagic fever
C. Deep vein thrombosis
D. Pneumonia

Ans: C

- Pulmonary embolism is caused by a blocked artery in the lungs. The most common cause of such a blockage is a blood clot that forms in a deep vein in the leg and travels to the lungs, where it becomes lodged in a smaller lung artery.

  Almost all blood clots that cause pulmonary embolism are formed in the deep leg veins. Clots also can form in the deep veins of the arms or pelvis.

  Sometimes blood clots develop in surface veins. But these clots rarely lead to pulmonary embolism.

  In rare cases, pulmonary embolism may be caused by other substances, including:
  - Small masses of infectious material.
  - Fat, which can be released into the bloodstream after some types of bone fractures, surgery , trauma, or severe burns.
  - Air bubbles or substances that get into the blood from trauma, surgery, or medical procedures.
  - Tumors caused by rapidly growing cancer cells.

21. True about sympathetic nervous system, *except*:

A. Heart rate increased
B. Decreased motility
C. Increased sweating
D. Increased salivary secretion

Ans: D

Sympathetic ad Parasympathetic Effects

Structure	Sympathetic	Parasympathetic
Eye (pupil)	Dilation	Constriction
Nasal Mucosa	Mucus reduction	Mucus increased
Salivary Gland	Saliva reduction	Saliva increased
Heart	Rate increased	Rate decreased
Arteries	Constriction	Dilation
Lung	Bronchial muscle relaxation	Bronchial muscle contraction
Gastrointestinal Tract	Decreased motility	Increased motility
Liver	Conversion of glycogen to glucose increased	Glycogen synthesis
Kidney	Decreased urine	Increased urine
Bladder	Contraction of Sphincter	Relaxation of sphincter
Sweat Glands	↑Sweating	No change

22. Eames technique is related to:

A. Glass ionomer cement
B. Class 2 cavity preparation
C. Silver amalgam alloy
D. Pin related silver amalgam restoration

Ans: C

Eames Technique

Irregular powder particles pack together relatively poorly and require a relatively large amount of mercury (50-60% by weight in the mixture) to fill in the spaces. After transfer of the mixture to the tooth preparation, it is possible to compact the mass and extrude some of the mercury-rich matrix. By eliminating the mercury-rich matrix as much as possible, the amount of reaction product matrix that forms is limited, improving the overall properties of the set amalgam. Mercury-rich mixtures, after trituration but before placement into the preparation, historically could be partially condensed by wringing the mass in a squeeze cloth. In the 1960s, Eames was the first to promote a low mercury-to-alloy mixng ratio (*Eames technique or no-squeeze-cloth technique*). Later, it was shown that by spheroidizing the alloy particles, the particles packed more efficiently and requied much less mercury to make a practical mixture. *Spherical particles* also increased the fluidity of the mixture by presenting less resistance to particle sliding. Using some or all spherical alloy particles, it is possible to reduce the mercury portion of the mixture to less than 50% by weight. The distinction between irregular (lathe-cut) and spherical particle geometries became the next major basis for classification of amalgam alloys. Most modern precapsulated amalgams are formulated with only 42% to 45% mercury by weight.

23. TMS stands for:

A. Threaded mate system
B. Transalveolar mandibular segment
C. Third molar surgery

Ans: A

Threaded Mate System

Self-Threaded Pins

- Developed by Dr. Going in 1966.
- Most popular type among all the different type of pins and extensively used.
- Made of stainless steel or titanium pins.
- Provide maximum retention among all types of pins.
- Cause craze lines.
- Used in vital teeth.

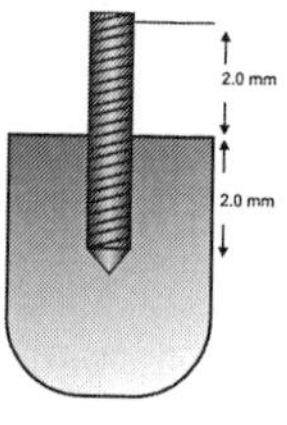

Self-threading pins

Types of pin sizes

Type of pin		Inches/mm
1. Minuta	–	0.015/0.38
2. Minikin	–	0.019/0.48
3. Minim	–	0.024/0.61
4. Regular	–	0.031/0.78

Advantages of TMS Pins

- Versatile design.
- Wide range of pin sizes.
- Color coding allows ease of use.
- Gold plating eliminates corrosion.
- Good retention.

TMS Link Series and Link Plus Pins

Name	Illustration (not to scale)	Color code
Link series Regular (single shear)	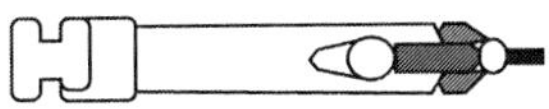	Gold
Regular (double shear)	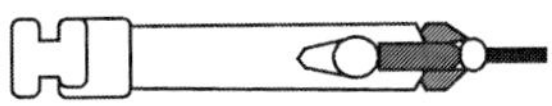	Gold
Minim (single shear)	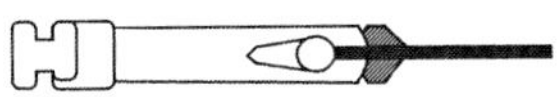	Silver
Minim (double shear)	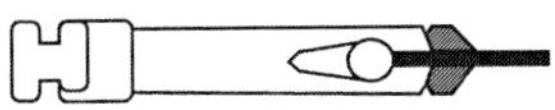	Silver
Minikin (single shear)	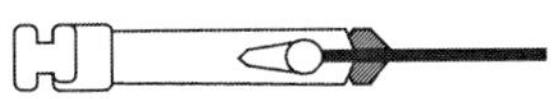	Red
Minuta (single shear)	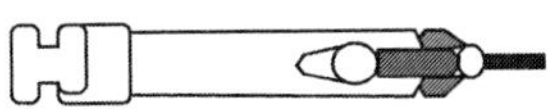	Pink
Link plus Minim (double shear)	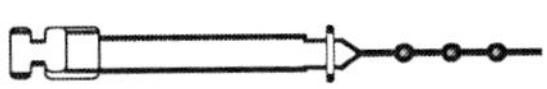	Silver

***Note: The PGI November 2016 paper was perceived as "tough" by majority of the aspirants as some of the options were too close. So as to preserve the originality, we have not fabricated any options, wherever options were not recalled the relevant theory text has been provided.**

24. Which nerve is near to mandibular third molar (medial aspect) and is likely to be damaged while removing 3rd molar?

A. Buccal nerve
B. Masseteric nerve
C. Lingual nerve
D. Inferior alveolar nerve

Ans: C

25. 9.6% Hydrofluoric acid:

Ans: Used to etch fluorosed teeth before bleaching.

26. Polishing agent for composite:

Ans: Polishing of composite restoration is done with very fine polishing disks, fine rubber points or cups, diamond impregnated polishers, or composite polishing pastes like aluminium oxide or diamond polishing paste. 12 fluted carbide finishing burs can be used to obtain excellent burs.

27. Syndrome of proxy:

Ans: Munchausen syndrome by proxy, mental health problem in which person with deep seated need for attention to fake sickness or injury. The term "by proxy" means "through substitute". In this, caretaker of child either makes up fake symptoms or cause real symptoms to make it appear as though child is injured or ill. Also considered a form of child abuse.

---

* Thanks to **Dr. Vinay Arora** (BDS, DBDC, Muktsar) and **Dr. Meetika Anand Popli** (BDS, LBDC, Patiala), students of Dentorics Institute, CHD for providing and solving the paper.

28. Why Bisphosphonates induced osteonecrosis found in jaws?

Ans: Bisphosphonates have a high affinity for hydroxyapatite and are rapidly absorbed in bone, especially in areas of high activity, this is the reason that bisphosphonates induced osteonecrosis only found in jaws. Bisphosphonate acts by inhibiting osteoclastic activity, which leads to less bone resorption. Bisphosphonate molecule incorporated into bone without being metabolised, during osteoclastic resorption the trapped bisphosphonates released and able to effect osteoclasts again.

29. Salivary reduction:

Ans: Reduction in saliva is not a disease, it is symptom. Reduction is saliva causes dry mouth known as Xerostomia. It may be due to any oral or systemic condition especially salivary gland dysfunction.

Unstimulated whole saliva flow rate: <0.1 ml/min.

Stimulated whole saliva flow rate: <0.7 ml/min.

30. Retention of saliva:

Ans: Mucocele is swelling caused by accumulation of saliva at the site of traumatized or obstructed salivary gland duct. It is of two types:

1. Mucous extravasation cyst–formed due to result of trauma to minor salivary gland excretory duct. Laceration of duct results in pooling of saliva in the adjacent submucosal tissue and results in swelling. More common than retention cyst. It does not have any epithelial lining.
2. Mucous retention cyst–retention mucocele is caused by obstruction of minor salivary gland duct by calculus or possibly by contraction of scar tissue around an injured minor salivary gland duct.

31. Minor connector:

Ans: Important points about minor connector:

- Rigid part of RPD.
- Minor connector should form a right angle with the major connector so that the gingival crossing is abrupt and cover little of gingival tissue.
- Only part of RPD that contacts the guiding plane of abutment.

Types of minor connector:

1. That join clasp assembly to major connector
2. That join indirect retainer or auxillary rests to major connectors.
3. That join the denture base to major connector
4. Servers as an approach arm for a bar clasp.

Functions:

1. To join other prosthesis such as clasp s, rests, indirect retainers and denture bases to major connector
2. Transfers functional stress to abutment teeth. This is a prosthesis to abutment function of the minor connector
3. Transfers the effect of the retainers, rests and stabilising components to the rest of the dentures. This is an abutment to prosthesis function of minor connector

32. First ossification centre of maxilla:

Ans: The primary ossification centre appears for each maxilla in the 7th week of uterine life. It has three ossification centres. One primary ossification centre is for maxilla proper and remaining two centres are for pre-maxilla.

33. Mandibular condylar growth occurs by:

A. Endochondral bone formation
B. Endosteal bone growth
C. Appositional growth
D. Subperiosteal surface addition

Ans: D

34. Immediate treatment for developing Class 2 malocclusion:

Ans: If patient is in mixed dentition phase, then wait and watch is choice, but if patient is in permanent dentition phase and canines have erupted then **MYOFUNCTIONAL APPLIANCE THERAPY.**

35. Class 3 relapse is not present in:

Ans: Pseudo class 3 malocclusion that occurs as a result of occlusal prematurity improves on removal of cause.

36. Chronic focal sclerosing Osteomyelitis:

Ans: Also known as Condensing Osteitis.

- Reaction to mild bacterial infection entering the bone through a carious tooth in persons who have a degree of tissue resistance and tissue reactivity.

- Arises most commonly in children and young adults.
- Tooth most commonly involved is mandibular first molar which presents a large carious lesion and there is mild pain associated with an infected pulp.
- Well circumscribed radiopaque mass of sclerotic bone surrounding and extending below the apex of one or both roots with intact lamina dura.
- Histologically examination reveals only a dense mass of bony trabeculae with little interstitial marrow tissue. Bony trabecule exhibit many reversal and resting lines giving pagetoid appearance. Osteoclastic activity may have completely subsided at the time of microscopic study.

37. Nasal floor best seen in:

Ans: Occlusal view of Maxilla > Water's view.

38. Bone pattern in anterior maxilla:

A. D1 B. D2
C. D3 D. D4

Ans: C

39. Treatment of AOT:

Ans: AOT (adenomatoid odontogenic tumor) is uncommon. Tumor associated with impacted maxillary cuspids. Treated by Excision also known as 2/3rd tumour.

40. Navy index:

Ans: Navy plaque index was developed by Grossman F.D. and Fedi P.F. in 1970. This index was designed to assess the plaque control status among naval personnels and to measure any subsequent changes using a disclosing solution. The index teeth are 16, 21, 24, 36, 41 and 44. The facial and lingual surfaces are divided into:

- Gingival (G)
- Mesial (M)
- Distal (D)
- A score of 3 is for mesial and disital, and score of 2 for gingival areas.

41. CAT in paediatric dentistry refers to:

A. Caries activity test
B. Caries risk assessment tool
C. Caries advancement tool
D. Child aptitude test

Ans: B

42. Activity test in survey:

Ans: Activity Survey: The Jenkins Activity Survey (JAS), is one of the most widely used methods of assessing Type A behaviour: The Jenkins Activity Survey is a psychometric survey of behavior and attitude designed to identify persons showing signs of Type A behavior. The test is multiple choice and self-administered. It was published in 1974 by C. David Jenkins, Stephen Zyzanski, and Ray Rosenman. The terms Type A and Type B personality were originally described in the work of Rosenman and Friedman in 1959.

43. Oral health survey was given by:

Ans: Dr. R.J . Baes

44. Term serial extraction was given by:

Ans: Serial extraction is the planned extraction of certain deciduous teeth and specific permanent teeth in an orderly sequence and pre-determined pattern to guide the erupting permanent teeth into a more favorable position. In 1929, Kjellgren of Sweden used the term "serial extraction" for the first time. In the 1940s the technique was popularised in the United States by Hayes Nance as "planned and progressive extraction". Nance is known as the father of serial extraction in the United States. In 1970 Hotz in Switzerland called it active "supervision of teeth by extraction".

45. Fluoride concentration of varnish:

Ans: Fluoride varnish is composed of a high concentration of fluoride as a salt or silane preparation in a fast drying,alcohol and resin-based solution. The concentration, form of fluoride, and dispensing method may vary depending on the manufacturer. While most fluoride varnishes contain 5% sodium fluoride at least one brand of fluoride varnish contains 1% difluorsilane in a polyurethane base and one brand contains 2.5% sodium fluoride that has been milled to perform similar to 5% sodium fluoride products in a shellac base.

46. Cul de sac is:

A. Grade 2 furcation B. Type of periodontitis
C. Grade 3 furcation D. Bone loss

Ans: A

47. **Type IV Gypsum material is:**
A. Impression plaster B. Model plaster
C. Dental stone D. Dental stone with high strength

Ans: D *(Ref. Phillips, 12th edn., p. 488)*

48. **Dentinogenesis imperfecta caused due to mutation of which chromosome?**
A. 4 B. 23
C. 1 D. 8

Ans: A

49. **Canine palatal eruption:**

Ans: Reason of Canine palatal eruption is due to retained deciduous teeth or it may be due less space for canine.

50. **Dentinogenesis imperfecta occurs due to disturbance in which stage during development?**
A. Morpho differentiation B. Histo differentiation
C. Initiation D. Apposition

Ans: B

51. **In submentovertex view, cantho meatus angulation is:**

Ans: In submentovertex view, image receptor is positioned parallel to patients' transverse plane and perpendicular to midsagittal and coronal planes. To achieve this position, the patient's neck is extended as far as backward as possible, with **canthomeatal line forming 10-degree angle with image receptor.**

52. **What is direction and angulation of central ray while taking bitewing:**
A. 10 degree above the horizontal plane
B. 10 degree below the horizontal plane
C. 10 degree to right
D. 10 degree to left

Ans: A

53. **Extraoral X-ray view used for fracture of mandible:**
A. Submentovertex view B. Posteroanterior view
C. Water's view D. Towne's view

Ans: B

PGI Paper

June 2016

1. **Nerve supply to ciliary muscles for accommodation of pupil is:**
   A. Red nucleus in mid brain
   B. Sympathetic
   C. Sympathetic
   D. Parasympathetic

2. **Which of the following is not a reason for increasing incidence of pulmonary tuberculosis in developing countries?**
   A. Population increase
   B. Human immunodeficiency virus infection
   C. Ineffective control programs
   D. Reduced priority for its control

3. **Which of the following is true about bisphosphonate?**
   A. Zoledronate is more potent because it has open nitrogen ring
   B. Risedronate is more potent because it has open nitrogen ring
   C. Zoledronate is more potent because of parenteral route of administration
   D. Risedronate is more potent because of parenteral route of administration

4. **Which is a side effect of Amlodipine?**
   A. Cough
   B. Fluid retention
   C. Renal impairment
   D. Postural hypotension and headache

5. **Which statement is not correct regarding systemic corticosteroid therapy?**
   A. The goal of therapy with corticosteroids is to induce remission in autoimmune diseases
   B. Dexamethasone, while more potent, is the drug of choice because it affects mostly the cellular phase of inflammation
   C. Systemic corticosteroids are the most predictable medications used to control autoimmune diseases and certain immune based inflammatory disorders
   D. The drug of choice is prednisone, an anti-inflammatory glucocorticoid that affects mostly the cellular phase of inflammation lymphocytes in particular

6. **Clindamycin is not active against:**
   A. Gram –ve aerobic rods
   B. Gram +ve aerobic cocci
   C. Gram –ve anaerobic rods
   D. Gram +ve anaerobic cocci

7. **Which broad antifungal agent is available only as a topical formulation due to its renal toxicity?**
   A. Clotrimazole B. Amphotericin B
   C. Nystatin D. Miconazole

8. **When blood pressure is 200-210/110-119, then the recommended action taken will be:**
   A. Wait for 3 weeks and measure again
   B. Wait for 1 month and re-evaluate
   C. Immediately start treatment
   D. Wait for 2 weeks and measure again

9. **What percentage of 3 canals is present in maxillary first premolar?**
   A. 2 to 8% B. 0.5 to 5%
   C. 10 to 15% D. 5 to 10%

10. **What is the overbite of the primary incisors?**
   A. 2.5 mm B. 2.0 mm
   C. 3.0 mm D. 1.5 mm

11. **Which of the following is required for the maturation of Cementoblast, Osteoblast and Fibroblast?**
   A. Osteogenin B. Osteocalcin
   C. Osteopontin D. Bone sialoprotein

12. **What is the difference in width of maxillary permanent and deciduous anterior teeth?**
    A. 7 mm B. 6 mm
    C. 6.5 mm D. 7.5 mm

13. **Which of the following is not a component of OMENS classification of hemifacial microsomia?**
    A. Eye B. Mandible
    C. Orbit D. Facial nerve

14. **Leutic glossitis is caused by:**
    A. Legionella B. M. Tuberculosis
    C. Streptococcus D. Treponema pallidum

15. **Which of the following is not a mixed radiolucent radio-opaque pericoronal lesion?**
    A. CEOT B. Cemento-ossifying fibroma
    C. AOT D. Compound odontoma

16. **Osteomas, intestinal polyposis, and sebaceous cysts are features of :**
    A. Hodgkin's disease
    B. Pierre Robin syndrome
    C. Gardner syndrome
    D. Goldenhar syndrome

17. **Popcorn cells are seen in:**
    A. Osteosarcoma
    B. Burkitt lymphoma
    C. Hodgkin lymphoma
    D. Non Hodgkin lymphoma

18. **Which of the following is also called as rodent ulcer?**
    A. Squamous cell carcinoma
    B. Basal cell carcinoma
    C. Ameloblastic carcinoma
    D. Intraepithelial carcinoma

19. **White sponge nevus of oral cavity:**
    A. Has tendency to transform into malignancy
    B. Is not a premalignant lesion
    C. Occurs in individual above 30 years of age
    D. Is associated with smoking habit

20. **Which statement is true about salivary gland tumours?**
    A. Mucoepidermoid carcinomas are well encapsulated tumours, therefore wide excision is not required

B. Adenocystic carcinoma are well encapsulated tumours therefore wide excision is not required
C. Mucoepidermoid carcinoma has tendency for perineural spread, therefore needs wide excision along course of nerve
D. Adenocystic carcinoma has no tendency for perineural spread, therefore needs wide excision along course of nerve

21. Occurrence of taurodontism is seen in children with:
A. Binder's syndrome
B. Papillon Lefevre syndrome
C. Klinefelter syndrome
D. Pierre Robin syndrome

22. The translucent brown-pigmented spots of the iris found in neurofibromatosis are called as:
A. Verocay bodies
B. Petechiae
C. Lisch nodules
D. Crow's sign

23. Which of the following is not a deep fungal infection involving maxillofacial region?
A. Aspergillosis
B. Cryptococcosis
C. Candidiasis
D. Mucormycosis

24. Heterotopic collections of sebaceous glands present in the oral cavity are known as:
A. Fordyce granules
B. Oral melanotic macule
C. Sulphur granules
D. Petechiae

25. Which of following statements is true regarding hemifacial atrophy and hemifacial microsomia?
A. Hemifacial microsomia is congenital
B. There is seizure activity on face in case of hemifacial microsomia
C. Hemifacial atrophy is congenital
D. There can be ear tags associated with hemifacial atrophy

26. In which of the following childhood syndromes is there presence of lower lip pits, alone or in combination with cleft lip and/or cleft palate?
A. Van der Woude syndrome
B. Treacher Collins syndrome

C. Fragile X syndrome
D. Williams syndrome

27. Oral lesions of tuberculosis:
A. Usually occur as primary lesion on tongue
B. Can be confirmed after taking biopsy
C. Show acid fast bacilli which appear blue or green on Ziehl-Neelsen staining
D. Can be easily differentiated from oral squamous cell carcinoma

28. Which of the following statement is true in context to the development of "The Goslon Yardstick", a system of assessing dental arch relationship in children with unilateral clefts of lip and palate?
A. The number of teeth in crossbite rather than degree of transverse arch narrowness is critical factor
B. Pre-existing dentoalveolar compensation in the presence of a reverse overjet was considered to be favourable
C. Canine crossbite of the smaller segment was considered worse than molar crossbite, which might be clinically acceptable
D. Reduced overbite was preferable to deep overbite

29. A quick way to decrease orbital pressure in emergency situation in a patient with post traumatic retrobulbar hematoma is:
A. Lateral tendon cantholysis
B. High dose corticosteroids
C. Intravenous acetazolamide
D. Surgical exploration to coagulate the bleeding vessels

30. A three-month-old baby reported to pediatric emergency with difficulty of feeding and bleeding from the anterior maxillary region. A rapidly growing mass, blackish in colour and starting two weeks after birth, was seen in the anterior maxilla. Computerized tomographic scan of face showed massive destruction of maxilla, plasma alpha-fetoprotein and urinary vanillyl mandelic acid levels were increased Immunocytochemistry showed positivity for cytokeratin, HMB- 45 and synaptophysin, but was negative for S-100. The most probable diagnosis is:
A. Prognoma
B. Congenital granular cell tumour

C. Neumann tumour
D. Abrikossoff's tumour

31. Which is not used as the pharmacological means of management of anaphylaxis?
A. Crystalloid fluid
B. 1: 1000 I.M. epinephrine
C. I.V. H1 blocker
D. 1:10000 I.V. epinephrine (pre-loaded)

32. Which of the following statement is false regarding lymph nodes?
A. Maximal diameter to minimal diameter ratio greater than 2 favours benign nodes and a ratio less than 2 favours malignancy
B. Nodal grouping can also help to identify pathologic nodes
C. Grouping refers to four or more nodes in continuity with each other, each measuring at least 4-5 mm in diameter
D. Malignant nodes typically show a rounded shape, with loss of the normal fatty hilum or focal cortical expansion

33. Classification of the craniofacial clefts was given by:
A. Boo Chai, 1887
B. AACPR, 1887
C. Morian, 1887
D. Karif, 1887

34. Which mandibular fracture is prone to facial widening?
A. Lefort fractures
B. Bilateral condyle and symphysis
C. Condyle fracture
D. Coronoid fracture

35. What is the minimum distance of osteotomy cuts from the tooth apex in orthognathic surgeries?
A. 1 mm
B. No need
C. 5 mm
D. 10-12 mm

36. Which of the following is not an indication for surgical exploration of orbital floor in zygomatic complex fractures?
A. Diplopia
B. Edema
C. Enophthalmos
D. Non resolving oculocardiac reflex

37. Which airway device provides protection against aspiration?
A. Nasopharyngeal airway
B. Laryngeal mask airway (LMA)

C. Oropharyngeal airway
D. Cuffed endotracheal tube

38. The site for chest compression during cardiopulmonary resuscitation is:
A. On the left nipple
B. Below the left nipple
C. Lower half of sternum
D. Upper half of sternum

39. According to American Heart Association (2010) guidelines, during adult two-rescuer cardiopulmonary resuscitation, chest compression are given at the rate of at least:
A. 30 per minute B. 50 per minute
C. 70 per minute D. 100 per minute

40. What is the second generation mandibular advancement appliance in sleep disordered breathing?
A. Appliances principally two piece in design and offering the potential for incremental advancement
B. Appliances permitting movements in all dimensions
C. One piece appliance with no ability to advance the mandible incrementally
D. Appliances permitting not only incremental advancement but also lateral movements of the mandible

41. The sharp pricking pain is picked up by which of the following nerve fibres in the pulp?
A. A-beta fibres B. A-delta fibres
C. A-gamma fibres D. A-alpha fibres

42. What is the most common cause of airway obstruction in unconscious patients?
A. Tongue B. Foreign body
C. Vomitus D. Removable denture

43. Bupivacaine is known to cause rapid and resistant cardiac toxicity when administered rapidly in high concentrations and volumes. What is the recent advancement to treat its cardiac toxicity?
A. Addition of mannitol to local anesthetic solution
B. Buffered local anethetics
C. Addition of another anesthetic to bupivacaine
D. Use of lipid emulsions to reverse the cardiotoxicity of local anesthetics

44. **A 50-year-old lady reported with a rapidly growing mass in left mandibular posterior region intraorally since two months. An orthopantomogram was done, which showed multiple radiolucent lesions in whole of mandible? Skull radiograph showed multiple punched out lesions. Serum calcium and haemoglobin were normal and renal function test were in the normal range. Parathormone level was increased. On histopathology the cells stained red with pyronin. The most probable diagnosis is:**
   A. Multiple myeloma
   B. Amyloidosis
   C. Hyperparathyroidism
   D. Hodgkin's lymphoma

45. **Which of the following statement is correct regarding the Belfast-Hamburg approach applied in the ortho-surgical management of over-retained deciduous teeth, non-eruption of permanent dentition, and presence of multiple supernumerary teeth in cleidocranial dysplasia?**
   A. The timing regarding the actual exposure of the permanent teeth is critical, and only two interventions are planned at distinct points in time, depending on the extent of root development
   B. Removal of all the supernumerary teeth only
   C. Extraction of all deciduous and supernumerary teeth and the exposure of all unerupted permanent teeth
   D. Surgical procedures are performed in a stage-by-stage series under general anesthesia, with the degree of root development of the permanent teeth dictating the timing of each stage

46. **According to Ellis and Davey's classification (1970) for traumatic injuries to teeth. 'Fracture of root with or without loss of crown structure' is included in:**
   A. Class VI B. Class V
   C. Class VIII D. Class VII

47. **Not a veneered stainless steel crown for primary teeth:**
   A. Pedostrip crown B. Nusmile
   C. Kinder crown D. White biter crown

48. Among the existing root canal filling materials for primary teeth, the most preferred one because of inherent advantage is:

A. $Ca(OH)_2$
B. $Ca(OH)_2$ + Iodoform
C. ZoE
D. Formocresol + Iodoform

49. Who proposed ferric sulphate as an alternative to formocresol as a pulpotomy agent?

A. John *et al.* in 1990
B. Torabinejad *et al.* in 1991
C. Jeng *et al.* in 1990
D. Fle *et al.* in 1991

50. Who introduced zygomatic ligatures as anchorage in partially edentulous patients for intrusion and retraction of the maxillary incisors?

A. Park, 1999
B. Lee, 2001
C. Melson, 1998
D. Sugawara, 1999

51. What is true regarding In-ovation-L?

A. Clear Aligner system
B. Computer control 3-D bracket
C. Not Recalled
D. Self ligating bracket system

52. Pitchfork analysis is given by:

A. Johnston in 1986
B. Panchenz in 1986
C. Pitchfork in 1986
D. Pitchfork in 1987

53. Retromolar pad contains all *except*:

A. Masseter
B. Buccinator
C. Temporalis
D. Superior constrictor

54. For balanced occlusion if incisal guidance is steep, then:

A. Decrease condylar guidance
B. Increase compensating curves
C. Increase condylar guidance
D. Decrease compensating curves

55. When selecting teeth for C.D., potentially dangerous and traumatic combination is:

A. Resin against resin
B. Porcelain against porcelain
C. Porcelain against resin
D. Porcelain against natural teeth

56. Which of the following is least rigid maxillary major connector?

A. Anterior posterior bar
B. U-shape
C. Complete palatal plate
D. Anterior posterior palatal strap

57. Failure to place a functional cusp bevel, while preparing a posterior tooth for full coverage restoration leads to:

A. Poor aesthetic
B. Weaker structure
C. Poor retention
D. Failure to produce accurate occlusion

58. Pontic having concave fitting surface is:

A. Saddle
B. Oval
C. Ridge lap
D. Sanitary

59. Criteria for infecting because of general flora on quantitative wound culture for bacteria is more than:

A. 10^2 bacteria/cm^3
B. 10^4 bacteria/cm^3
C. 10^3 bacteria/cm^3
D. 10^5 bacteria/cm^3

60. Splinting time for lateral luxation of a tooth with bone damage should be:

A. 1-2 weeks
B. 3-4 weeks
C. 2-3 weeks
D. 3-8 weeks

61. What is the traditionally recommended splinting protocol for management of root fracture?

A. 3-4 weeks semi rigid
B. 1-2 weeks semi rigid
C. 2-4 months rigid
D. 1-2 months rigid

62. The best pontic material in contact with ridge tissue is:

A. Polished resin
B. Polished noble metal alloy
C. Glazed porcelain
D. Polished nickel-chromium alloy

63. Where Zero degree teeth are indicated:

A. High well from ridge
B. Where balanced occlusion is not required
C. Resorbed ridge
D. Where greater cutting efficiency required

64. Which of the following statement is true regarding the relationship of incisal guidance and cuspal inclinations for creating balanced occlusion in complete denture?

A. There is no relationship
B. As the incisal guidance increases, the cuspal inclinations must decrease
C. As the incisal guidance increases, the cuspal inclinations must increase
D. The cuspal inclinations should not be selected based on incisal guidance

65. A pontic that has no contact with the edentulous ridge is:

A. Hygienic pontic
B. Modified ridge lap pontic
C. Orate pontic
D. Saddle pontic

66. Working length determination is done after initial coronal preparation in:

A. Crown down technique
B. Step back technique
C. Step down technique
D. Balanced force

67. Type II etching pattern of enamel surface is:

A. Dissolution of periphery first and of head later
B. Dissolution of Rods head first and of periphery later
C. Can be either of these
D. Dissolution of Rods head only

68. Which is most common tooth injury?

A. Luxation
B. Complicated crown fracture
C. Avulsion
D. Enamel fracture/uncomplicated crown fracture

69. Inhibitor in composite resin is:

A. Benzoyl peroxide
B. Phenyl propanedione
C. DMAEM
D. Butylated hydroxyl toluidine

70. Profile speed:

A. 150 to 300
B. 300 to 350
C. 250 to 350
D. 50 to 100

71. What is the compressive strength of microfilled composite?

A. 250 – 350 MPa
B. 250 – 400 MPa
C. 350 – 450 MPa
D. 200 – 250 MPa

72. What is the minimum requirement of fluoride for 6 months old baby, who is living in an area where fluoride concentration in water is less than 0.3 ppm?

A. 0.25 mg B. 0.5 mg
C. 1 mg D. 0 mg

73. Which of the following responses to root fracture is incorrect?

A. Healing with cementum
B. Healing with interproximal connective tissue
C. Healing with interproximal bone and connective tissue
D. Healing with calcified tissue

74. Magnifying loupes attached to eye glasses have a fixed magnification power of:

A. < 4 x B. < 10 x
C. < 2 x D. < 8 x

75. A marking file specially used intraorally to pillar file mark an archwire is:

A. Pillar file B. Mill Bastard file
C. Slim file D. Encapement file

76. According to WHO optimum concentration of fluoride in drinking water is:

A. 0.7 to 1.2 ppm B. 0.7 to 1 ppm
C. 0.5 to 0.7 ppm D. 0.2 to 0.5 ppm

77. The acronym HERO for HERO root canal preparation instruments stands for:

A. High elasticity in rotation
B. Heavy elasticity rotary instruments
C. High elasticity in revolution
D. Heavy elasticity rotational instruments

78. The daily recommended dosage of fluoride for humans (Farkas and Farkas, 1974) is:

A. 0.01-1.00 mg/kg body weight
B. 0.02-0.05 mg/kg body weight
C. 0.03-0.05 mg/kg body weight
D. 0.05-0.07 mg/kg body weight

79. The certainly lethal dose of fluoride has been put forth as:

A. 16-32 mg/kg body weight

B. 64-128 mg/kg body weight
C. 32-64 mg/kg body weight
D. 8-16 mg/kg body weight

80. In the milestone Kingston-Newburgh study of water fluoridation, the difference in DMFT scores in 12-14 years old children between control and experimental cities was:

A. 28% B. 48%
C. 55% D. 70%

81. Which topical fluoride should be applied on newly erupted teeth?

A. ApF B. Amino fluoride
C. SnF2 D. NaF

82. The largest pre-school program in United States of America is:

A. EPSDT program
B. Head start program
C. Medicated program
D. Lowa's Infant oral health program

83. In US, how much population is covered under community water fluoridation:

A. 50-60% B. 40-50%
C. 65-85% D. < 20%

84. Which of the following is not a common cause of atrial fibrillation?

A. Chest infection B. Pulmonary embolism
C. Hyperthyroidism D. Diabetes

85. Which dental cement release fluoride?

A. ZOE
B. Zinc phosphate
C. Zinc silicophosphate
D. Polycarboxylate

86. Not a component of INCONEL:

A. Silicon B. Titanium
C. Nickel D. Iron

87. Which of the following cement have maximum working time?

A. GIC B. Resin
C. ZnOE D. $ZnPO_4$

88. What is minimum level of anti HBS antibody for protection?

A. 12 mIU/ml B. 20 mIU/ml
C. 50 mIU/ml D. 10 mIU/ml

89. During submandibular incision, marginal mandibular branch of facial nerve lies in the:

A. Platysmal plane
B. Subplatysmal plane deep to facial vein
C. Subdermal fat plane
D. Subplatysmal plane superficial to facial vein

Answers

1.	D	2.	D	3.	A	4.	B
5.	B	6.	A	7.	B	8.	D
9.	A	10.	B	11.	B	12.	D
13.	A	14.	D	15.	B	16.	C
17.	C	18.	B	19.	B	20.	C
21.	C	22.	C	23.	C	24.	A
25.	A	26.	A	27.	B	28.	C
29.	A	30.	A	31.	A	32.	B
33.	C	34.	B	35.	C	36.	B
37.	D	38.	C	39.	A	40.	A
41.	B	42.	A	43.	D	44.	A
45.	C	46.	A	47.	A	48.	B
49.	D	50.	C	51.	D	52.	A
53.	A	54.	B	55.	C	56.	B
57.	B	58.	A	59.	D	60.	D
61.	A	62.	C	63.	C	64.	C
65.	A	66.	A	67.	A	68.	D
69.	D	70.	A	71.	A	72.	D
73.	A	74.	A	75.	D	76.	A
77.	A	78.	D	79.	C	80.	D
81.	D	82.	B	83.	C	84.	D
85.	C	86.	B	87.	D	88.	D
89.	D						

PGI Paper December 2015

1. In neural crest migration which rhombomere is responsible for 2nd arch development?

A. Rhombomere 1
B. Rhombomere 2
C. Rhombomere 3
D. Rhombomere 4

2. Circumpennate arrangement of which muscle?

A. Deltoid
B. Masseter
C. Temporalis
D. Tibialis anterior

3. Marginal mandibular nerve, a branch of facial nerve is present at:

A. Platysmal plane
B. Subplatysmal plane and deep to facial vein
C. Subdermal fat plane
D. Subplatysmal plane superficial to facial vein

4. Hypoxia causes:

A. It has no effects on the tissue
B. Tissue to become more radioresistant
C. Tissue to become more radiosensitive
D. None

5. In case of low oxygen saturation what happens?

A. Vasodilation of coronary artery
B. Vasoconstriction of coronary artery
C. Inhibition of chemoreceptors
D. Stimulation of chemoreceptors

6. Diarrhoea, Dermatitis and Dementia are associated with the deficiency of:

A. Riboflavin
B. Ascorbic acid
C. Niacin
D. Retinol

7. Which of the following is best fixative for the demonstration of enzymes?

A. Acetone
B. Osmium tetraoxide
C. Ethanol
D. Formalin

8. **Dye used in Synder test is:**
A. Bromocresol blue
B. Bromocresol purple
C. Bromocresol green
D. Formocresol green

9. **If 0.02% of NaF is used as mouthwash daily then ppm of fluoride is:**
A. 115 ppm
B. 90 ppm
C. 95 ppm
D. 250 ppm

10. **According to Farska and Farska, minimum daily requirement of fluoride:**
A. 0.15 mg/kg
B. 0.50 mg/kg
C. 0.05 mg/kg
D. 0.25 mg/kg

11. **Sodium monofluorophosphate discovered in the year:**
A. 1941
B. 1967
C. 1947
D. 1963

12. **Which of the following country have 100% artificially fluoridated water?**
A. Thailand and Polland
B. Thailand and Spain
C. Hong Kong and Singapore
D. Spain and France

13. **Prevention of initiation involves which mode of prevention?**
A. Tertiary
B. Primary
C. Primordial
D. Secondary

14. **Score 6 in gingival index indicates:**
A. Moderate gingivitis
B. Gingivitis with pocket formation
C. Mild gingivitis
D. Advanced destruction with loss of masticatory function

15. **In a 1000 population, normal SD 18.1 $\pm$ 1.9 microgm/dl.... approximately how much people will be below 20 microgm/dl?**
A. 831
B. 500
C. 683
D. 841

16. Sullage is:

A. Waste from garbage
B. Waste collected from human excreta
C. Waste of animals
D. Waste water from kitchen

17. Staghorn pattern is seen in:

A. Histioma
B. Hemangiopericytoma
C. Pericytoma
D. Hemangioma

18. Supra basilar split seen in:

A. Leukoplakia
B. Pemphigus vulgaris
C. Lichen planus
D. None

19. Restricted mouth opening is seen in all *except*:

A. Scleroderma
B. Infective endocarditis
C. Tetanus
D. Osmf

20. Which of the following statement is false regarding giant cell lesions?

A. Displacement of the teeth without resorption of tooth
B. Multilocular radiolucency with scalloped irregular border at the inferior border of mandible
C. Intralesional steroids can be the treatment provided
D. Rule out primary and secondary hyperparathyroidism

21. Goldenhar syndrome is:

A. Auricular abnormalities only
B. Facial and auricular abnormalities only
C. Facial deformity, auricular abnormalities, vertebral deformity and genital lesion
D. Facial deformity, auricular abnormalities and vertebral deformity

22. What is the difference between Hemifacial Microsomia and Hemifacial atrophy?

A. Seizures occur in hemifacial microsomia
B. Ear tags may be seen with hemifacial atrophy
C. Hemifacial atrophy is congenital
D. Hemifacial microsomia are congenital

23. What is not true about Sjörgen syndrome?

A. Parotid gland are not enlarged
B. Increased chances of B cell lymphoma due to B cell infiltration

C. Thick mucous secretion of Stenson duct are common
D. Dryness of eyes and mouth

24. Fordyces spots are seen in:
A. Buccal mucosa B. Skin/Palate
C. Corner of lip D. Nipple

25. Which of the following is true regarding salivary tumors?
A. Mucoepidermoid ca is encapsulated so doesn't require wide excision
B. Adenoid cystic ca shows perineural invasion thus requires wide excision
C. Mucoepidermoid ca shows perineural invasion thus requires wide excision
D. None of the above

26. New name of odontogenic keratocyst is:
A. Keratocyte ghost cell tumor
B. Odontogenic keratocyst ghost cell tumour
C. Keratocystic odontogenic tumour
D. None of the above

27. Gingival involvement is not seen in:
A. Pemphigus vulgaris
B. Lichen planus
C. Herpes simplex
D. Aphthous ulcer

28. Klein classified oral habits into:
A. Primary and secondary habits
B. Pressure and non-pressure habits
C. Intentional non-intentional
D. Compulsive non-compulsive

29. During face mask therapy forces are applied:
A. 15 degree downwards
B. Parallel to the occlusal plane
C. 30 degree downwards
D. 45 degree downward

30. Orthodontic tooth movement is inhibited by:
A. OPG B. OPG-FC
C. RANK D. RANKL

31. Which is true filling in orthodontics?
A. 3/4th filled B. Complete filled
C. 1/3rd filled D. Unfilled cavity

32. Meta positioning refers to:

A. Settling of undercorrected position
B. Relapse prevention
C. Overcorrected position
D. One portion superior and other inferior level of position

33. Which of the following statements with canine bonded retainer with segmental side involvement is true?

A. Extrusion of molar on balancing side
B. Both involvement of buccal left and right side with mesial inclination outwards
C. Both involvement of buccal left and right side with mesial inclination inwards
D. Intrusion of molars on working side

34. Turn over rate for junctional epithelium is:

A. 3 days B. 7 days
C. 10 days D. 14 days

35. Vitamin K is required for the growth of:

A. Streptococcus
B. Campylobacter
C. Treponema Pallidum
D. Prevotella and porphyromonas

36. Attachment of actinomycetemcomitans to the tooth surface can be prevented by:

A. Collagenase B. Lactoperoxidase
C. Myeloperoxidase D. None

37. What is required for the maturation of cementoblasts, osteoblasts and fibroblast?

A. Osteogen B. Osteopontin
C. Osteocin D. Bone sialoprotein

38. Free gingival graft is placed on:

A. PDL B. Periosteum
C. Cementum D. Bone

39. The bacteria which doesn't invade the cell?

A. Treponema denticola
B. Aa
C. P. Intermedia
D. Porphyromonas gingivalis

40. Sub antimicrobial dose of doxycycline in blood:

A. 0.2-0.5
B. 0.3-0.8
C. 0.7-0.9
D. 1.3-1.9

41. Microorganisms colonizing the gingival pocket utilize which of the following as energy source: in gingival sulcus?

A. High protein
B. Simple peptides
C. High carbohydrates
D. Saliva

42. Length of normal floss should be:

A. 12 inch
B. 10 cm
C. 18 inch
D. 18 cm

43. Maximum torque by hand for implantology:

A. 5-10 N cm
B. 10-20 N cm
C. 20-30 N cm
D. 60-70 N cm

44. Gene of P. Gingivalis fimbrae is:

A. Gene of Fimbrae c
B. Gene of Fimbrae b
C. Gene of Fimbrae d
D. Gene of Fimbrae a

45. When root is the pdl are very close together, what is the minimum distance between apex and mini implant for the root to resorb?

A. 0.6 mm
B. 0.5 mm
C. 0.8 mm
D. 1 mm

46. Which function as stromyelsin?

A. MMP9
B. MMP3
C. MMP1
D. MMP16

47. How much stress can a mini implant screw bear before fracture?

A. 300
B. 500
C. 700
D. 900

48. Reciprocal arm gives indirect retention when:

A. Arm on the supra bulge
B. Cast metal fabricated arm
C. Anterior to fulcrum line
D. Posterior to the fulcrum line

49. Can surveyor not used in:

A. Retentive wire
B. Intra coronal retainer placement
C. Guiding plane
D. Machining cast restoration

50. The relief is given under maxillary removable partial denture in:

A. Kennedy class I cases
B. Unlifted midline palatine suture cases
C. Kennedy class 4 cases
D. It is always given midline to prevent stress occurring palatally

51. Fluid wax technique, false is:

A. Open mouth technique functional movements done for recording non-functional movements border
B. Korrecta type 4 wax used
C. It corrects the distal extension edentulous ridges of the original master cast
D. Mainly used in closed mouth technique done for recording non-functional movements

52. In lingual retention case, rest seat function as:

A. Minor connector
B. Reciprocal arm
C. Indirect retainer
D. None

53. Which of the following statement regarding phonetics is not correct?

A. The sound are made with the tip of the tongue extending slightly between the upper and lower anterior teeth
B. If tip of tongue is more than 5 mm it indicates the teeth are lingual inclined
C. A patient with class I malocclusion, tip the tongue will be visible at distance of 3 mm
D. A patient with class II malocclusion, tip the tongue will be visible at distance more of 3 mm

54. Distance between incisive papilla and labial surface of tooth is:

A. Changes wide tooth size
B. Best guide in setting anterior teeth is the papilla incisor relationship
C. 8-10 mm
D. None

55. False about double lingual bar is:
A. Permanent direct transfer stress to abutment
B. Highly rigid structure
C. Features of lingual bar and lingual plate seen
D. Flexible connection between major connector and denture base

56. In incipient lesions, remineralization occurs in which of the following zone?
A. Body of lesion
B. Translucent zone
C. Surface layer
D. Dark zone

57. The night guard bleaching uses:
A. McInns solution
B. 10% carbamide peroxide
C. 30% H_2O_2
D. Superoxol and H_2O_2

58. Clinpro paste fuses which form of tri calcium phosphate?
A. Gamma
B. Delta
C. Alpha
D. Beta

59. Which of the following is disadvantage of minocycline in triple antibiotic paste?
A. Tooth staining
B. Hypoplastic defects are produced
C. Anaphylactic reactions are common side effects
D. Defective enamel formation

60. Magnification of microscope used in visualization of DENTINE surface of the tooth:
A. 5000 ×
B. 1000 ×
C. 100 × magnification
D. 10000 ×

61. Cavity varnish solution will not provide protection from:
A. Electrical
B. Pulp protection from microbial invasion
C. Thermal
D. Chemical

62. During intrusion of deciduous tooth, the root perforate the buccal plate; on radiograph appearance of the tooth:
A. Radiography is of no use
B. The roots appear elongated
C. The roots appear shortened
D. It may appear elongated or shortened

63. OPG invented by:

A. Knutson
B. Hofrath and Bent
C. Chestor F Carlson
D. Hudson Dickson

64. The disadvantage of digital radiography over conventional radiography is:

A. Time consuming
B. High cost
C. Processing defects
D. High radiation exposure

65. Limit of X-ray exposure annually for dentist should be less than:

A. 150 msv
B. 50 msv
C. 100 msv
D. 250 msv

66. Potter-Bucky diaphragm is used to:

A. To increase the kvp
B. To remove the scattered radiation
C. To decrease the exposure
D. To reduce the wavelength of radiations

67. In a 9-year-old child, fracture involves the parasymphyseal region and intracapsular sagittal fracture of condyle, possible treatment:

A. Rigid fixation of parasymphysis and condyle
B. Internal fixation of parasymphysis with elastics and achieve occlusion
C. Intermaxillary fixation done for 6 weeks
D. Intermaxillary fixation done for 3 weeks

68. A patient with crouzon syndrome and obstructive sleep apnoea, treatment shall be:

A. Maxillary distraction
B. CPAP
C. Tracheostomy
D. Rapid maxillary expansion

69. In subcondylar mandibular fracture:

A. Distal segment is the one containing condyle
B. Proximal segment is the one containing teeth
C. Proximal segment is the one containing condyle
D. Both proximal and distal segment may contain teeth

70. True about primary healing of bone:

A. Rigid fixation should be considered
B. Additional exogenous bone minerals have to be added
C. For healing there should be no gap left when compression forces are applied
D. For primary healing if 1mm gap is there the fragments still can be healed up

71. If carcinoma has occurred in the lower lip and it spread to upper lip then what is it called?

A. Contact cancer B. Transmissible cancer
C. Hug cancer D. Kiss cancer

72. While taking arterial blood gas sample which is most likely to be injured?

A. Radial artery B. Sternocleidomastoid
C. Ulnar artery D. Brachial artery

73. In dentin etching, superficially how much dissolution?

A. 0.1-0.3 mm B. 1.9-5.8 mm
C. 4.8-6 mm D. 0.3-0.7 mm

74. Maximum dentin bond strength is seen with:

A. 1st generation bonding agent
B. 2nd generation bonding agent
C. 4th generation bonding agent
D. 5th generation bonding agent

75. For liner/base under a restoration, false is:

A. Electrical protection
B. Mechanical protection
C. Chemical protection
D. Achieving adequate occlusal seal

76. For a material to be placed in cervical lesions, which property is most desirable?

A. Low elastic modulus
B. High wear resistance
C. High fluoride release
D. Low polymerization shrinkage

77. Chemically cured sealants/sealers are which generation?

A. 1st generation B. 2nd generation
C. 3rd generation D. 4th generation

78. After incipient caries, cavitation occurs in:

A. 10 $\pm$ 6 months
B. 5 years
C. 24 $\pm$ 6 months
D. 18.1 $\pm$ 6 months

79. C reactive protein secretion mediated by which interleukin?

A. IL-1
B. IL-6
C. IL-13
D. IL-10

80. In cariogram, yellow part represents:

A. Circumstances
B. Diet
C. Caries
D. Susceptibility

81. What is the amount of flush terminal in primary deciduous second molar?

A. 37%
B. 41%
C. 52%
D. 63%

82. Most common type of injury in primary teeth is:

A. Complicated crown fracture
B. Uncomplicated crown fracture
C. Alveolar fracture
D. Luxation

83. Splinting time for extrusive luxation is:

A. 2 weeks
B. 4 weeks
C. 2 months
D. 4 months

84. To decrease resorption of replanted tooth, immerse it in:

A. 1% NAF for 20 minutes
B. 1% NAF for 10 minutes
C. 2% NAF for 20 minutes
D. 2% NAF for 10 minutes

85. How much of midline diastema is seen in preschool children?

A. 10%
B. 20%
C. 30%
D. More than 50%

86. Chicken pox false is:

A. Herpes zoster is caused by herpes simplex virus
B. Water droplets is not the main mode of transmission
C. Chicken pox occurs after incubation of varicella zoster for 2 weeks
D. Dormant lesions of varicella zoster remain in the nerve ganglion and reappear as herpes zoster on decrease in immunity

87. High velocity injury causes thoracic disruption of arch of aorta causing traumatic aortic rupture. Which of that following is not true?

A. Systolic blood pressure increases more than 100 mmHg
B. Ligamentum arteriosum ruptured
C. Prognosis of such condition is poor
D. Blood, supply of upper and lower limb affected

88. In which of the following condition seizure is seen without aura?

A. Tonic clonic
B. Grand mal
C. Petit mal
D. Infantile epilepsy

89. Which of the following is not true about Proteus syndrome?

A. Mutation in AKT1 gene
B. Tumors of ovaries and testis seen
C. Overgrowth of skin and bones
D. Muscle mass is normally distributed

90. By rule of nine one limb burn will involve:

A. 18 percent
B. 8 percent
C. 36 percent
D. 56 percent

91. Minimum no. of microorganism required to infect a wound:

A. 10^3
B. 10^2
C. 10000
D. 100000

92. True about esophageal hiatus hernia is:

A. It is a pouch that knuckles and bifurcates below the level of the diaphragm
B. It is a pouch that is present on the lower portion of inferior constrictor
C. It is displaced proximally with esophagogastric junction displaced proximally into the thorax

93. Which of the following statement is true regarding parotid sialosis *except*?

A. Swelling is due to ductal sialectasia
B. Fatty infiltration of adipose tissue of parotid
C. Non inflammatory soft tissue swelling of parotid
D. No treatment, reassure patients saying its non neoplastic

94. Bisphosphonates are used in modification: Which is not true?

A. Have anticollagenase activity
B. Interfere with metabolism of osteoblast
C. Increase calcification
D. Increase bone density

95. Main components of self cure resin:

A. PMMA
B. UDMA
C. TEGDMA
D. Phosphoric acid

96. The fluoride flux is used in soldering of:

A. Gold with silver
B. Gold with Cr-Co
C. Silver with platinum
D. Gold with gold

97. Patient is called comatose if GCS is less than:

A. 1.5
B. 3.11
C. 2.10
D. 3.13

98. About Morsicatio Buccarum false is:

A. The lateral border of tongue resembles like hairy cell leukoplakia
B. No special treatment required and it can be completely curable
C. It is three times more common in females than in males
D. It is nothing but cheek bite

Answers

1.	D	2.	D	3.	D	4.	B
5.	D	6.	C	7.	A	8.	C
9.	A	10.	C	11.	A	12.	C
13.	B	14.	B	15.	D	16.	D
17.	B	18.	B	19.	B	20.	A
21.	D	22.	D	23.	A	24.	A
25.	B	26.	C	27.	D	28.	C
29.	A	30.	B	31.	A	32.	C
33.	C	34.	B	35.	D	36.	C
37.	B	38.	B	39.	C	40.	C
41.	A	42.	C	43.	C	44.	D
45.	A	46.	B	47.	B	48.	C
49.	A	50.	B	51.	D	52.	C
53.	A	54.	B	55.	D	56.	C
57.	B	58.	D	59.	A	60.	C
61.	C	62.	C	63.	D	64.	B
65.	B	66.	B	67.	D	68.	C
69.	B	70.	D	71.	D	72.	D
73.	B	74.	C	75.	D	76.	A
77.	B	78.	D	79.	B	80.	A
81.	A	82.	D	83.	A	84.	C
85.	D	86.	A	87.	A	88.	C
89.	D	90.	A	91.	D	92.	C
93.	A	94.	C	95.	A	96.	C
97.	A	98.	C				

PGI Paper

June 2015

---

1. **Fracture of the middle cranial fossa leads to hypo-secretion from eye caused by injury of:**
   A. Trigeminal ganglion
   B. Lesser petrosal nerve
   C. Greater petrosal nerve
   D. Optic nerve

2. **Large vein of Galen drains into:**
   A. EJV
   B. IJV
   C. Straight sinus
   D. Inferior sagittal sinus

3. **Muscle which does not originate from apex of orbit?**
   A. Inferior oblique
   B. Superior rectus
   C. Superior oblique
   D. Inferior rectus

4. **True about mucormycosis is all *except*:**
   A. May spread to orbit and brain
   B. Seen in immunocompetent patient
   C. Treated by third generation cephalosporin
   D. Does not cause palatal perforation

5. **In 80% cases of human infections due to candida species all of the following are captured histopathologically *except* one:**
   A. Candida albicans
   B. Candida glabrata
   C. Candida medicans
   D. Candida tropicalis

6. **C + file is:**
   A. Side cutting with square blank
   B. Side cutting with triangular blank
   C. End cutting with square blank
   D. End cutting with rhomboidal blank

7. Mohs micrographic surgery is used for:
A. Removal of basal cell carcinoma of eyelid
B. Wide excision of tissue
C. In ectodermal dysplasia
D. None

8. Resorption of femur head is seen in:
A. G6PD deficiency
B. Sickle cell anemia
C. Thalassemia
D. Aplastic anemia

9. Hurthle cell is seen in:
A. Thyroglossal cyst
B. Granulomatous thyroiditis
C. Hashimoto's thyroiditis
D. Papillary carcinoma of thyroid

10. Ann-Arbor staging system is used for:
A. OKC
B. Lichen planus
C. Osteosarcoma
D. Hodgkin lymphoma

11. Surgery should not be performed when neutrophil level is below:
A. $200/mm^3$
B. $400/mm^3$
C. $800/mm^3$
D. $1000/mm^3$

12. A patient taking bisphosphonate, comes to your clinic and has osteopenia. She is taking IV bisphosphonates continuously for 3 years. What would you do if you want to extract the tooth?
A. Stop bisphosphonates prior 3 weeks of extraction
B. No such treatment required you can extract
C. You are not advised to extract as she might develop osteoradionecrosis
D. Stop bisphosphonates prior 1 week of extraction

13. True about feature of giant cell arteritis:
A. It is due to the direct injury of the branch of external carotid artery
B. Biopsy of temporal artery is diagnostic
C. Involvement of temporal artery may lead to blindness
D. Mimics MPDs

14. Treatment of Ludwig's angina due to pericoronitis w.r.t. lower 3rd molar:

A. Intubation prior to surgery
B. I/D, antibiotics and removal of 3rd molar later on
C. Before any treatment tracheostomy should be done
D. I/D, antibiotics and removal of 3rd molar

15. Which of the following about luxators is correct?
A. Thin and fine rocking end that enters periodontal ligament
B. Thick rocking end help in easy removal of teeth
C. It uses fulcrum on adjacent teeth
D. None of the above

16. Patient has fracture of mandibular anterior symphysis and avulsion of mandibular incisor. During reduction of fracture which should be done?
A. Maintain the space in anterior mandible to prevent narrowing of mandible
B. Reduction of the space along with reduction and fixation
C. Acrylic prosthesis should be fabricated before the reduction of mandible
D. Place implant immediately in place of missing tooth at the time of reduction

17. During extraction of first molar, an opening into maxillary sinus has occurred. Treatment of choice:
A. Immediately close the opening
B. Remove tooth pieces and soft bone margins and close the opening
C. Immediately fill the opening with ribbon gauge
D. Suture immediately and definite surgery is performed later

18. Blood gas coefficient of nitrous oxide is:
A. 0.37 B. 0.57
C. 0.67 D. 0.47

19. When vertical load is supplied on incisor region in a patient with angle fracture, upward displacement is caused by:
A. Compressive force will lead to superior border flaring
B. Compressive force will lead to inferior border flaring
C. Tension force will lead to inferior border flaring
D. Tension force will lead to superior border flaring

20. Not true about couple:
A. Opposite in direction
B. Equal in magnitude

C. Forces are co-linear
D. Pure rotation can be achieved

21. In orthodontic treatment (early and late) the following treatment may not effect the treatment:
A. Ability of the patient to co-operate
B. Dental age
C. Severity of malocclusion
D. Chronological age of patient

22. Which of the following has highest stiffness?
A. Elgiloy wires B. Stainless steel
C. Titanium D. TMA wires

23. Not true about edgewise technique at bracket slot:
A. Tip and rotation is independent of torque
B. If torque is present at bracket slot, it causes tipping and rotation
C. If torque is present at bracket slot, it does not cause tipping and rotation
D. Torque is not present at bracket slot

24. Not true about couple:
A. It will always lead to tipping and torque when applied on edgewise
B. It will cause pure rotation at CR
C. It will not lead to change in centre of resistance
D. It will not always lead to tipping and torque when applied on edgewise

25. Not a stable landmark of mandible:
A. Contour of cortical plates
B. Contour of anterior surface of ramus
C. Contour of mandibular nerve canal
D. Contour of anterior portion of chin

26. Tip of nose on a lateral cephalograph:
A. SN B. TN
C. Prn (Pronasale) D. Point A/Po

27. Not true about lip bumper:
A. Buccal displacements of deciduous molars
B. Distolingual rotation of molar
C. Distalization of molar
D. Lingual tipping of incisors

28. Stanley and Kerber analysis is modification of which analysis?
- A. Total arch perimeter
- B. Tanaka Johnson
- C. Moyer's analysis
- D. Hixon and old father

29. Café-au-lait pigmentation seen in all *except*:
- A. Albright syndrome
- B. Peutz-Jeghers syndrome
- C. Noonan syndrome
- D. Neurofibromatosis type I

30. In osteochondroma, which of the following is involved?
- A. Involves coronoid only
- B. Involves both coronoid and condyle
- C. Involves condyle only
- D. Occurs in skull membranous bone

31. Xanthomas are:
- A. Granulomatous
- B. Neutrophils particulate
- C. True neoplasms
- D. Lipid laden macrophages

32. White sponge nevus:
- A. Can progress to neoplasm
- B. Associated with smokers only
- C. Not a precancerous lesion
- D. Not seen on buccal mucosa

33. Tuberculosis can be easily differentiated from squamous cell carcinoma by:
- A. Direct smear examination
- B. Biopsy can confirm the diagnosis
- C. Primary lesion occur on tongue
- D. Acid positive with Zeil Nelson stain

34. Specimen fixations is done with:
- A. Twenty percent neutral formalin
- B. Ten percent neutral formalin used
- C. Percent neutral formalin used
- D. Ammonium sulphate, N ethyl methyl in citrate buffer

35. Recurrent mouth ulcers, genital ulcers and ocular ulcers are manifestations of:
- A. Stevens-Johnson syndrome
- B. Erythema multiforme

C. Greenspan syndrome
D. Behcet syndrome

36. Dentinogenesis imperfecta incidence:
A. 1: 1000 B. 1: 4000
C. 1: 8000 D. 1: 10000

37. Gallbladder stone is influenced by all of following *except*:
A. Hyperalimentation
B. Primary biliary cirrhosis
C. Clofibrate
D. Hypercholestremia

38. Primary hyperthyroidism causes:
A. Hypermagnesia B. Hypercalcemia
C. Hypocalcemia D. Hyperphosphatemia

39. Which is not a feature of acute fluorosis?
A. Nausea, vomiting
B. CNS symptoms
C. Growth retardation
D. Acidosis

40. Primary hereditary syndrome is related to first degree relative:
A. 25% B. 50%
C. 75% D. 100%

41. Hour glass appearance is seen in:
A. Gastric carcinoma
B. Gastric lymphoma
C. Corrosive stricture
D. Gastric ulcer

42. Wide QT interval is seen in:
A. Digitalis toxicity
B. Pulmonary hypertension
C. Complete cardiac block
D. Acute myocardial infarction

43. Giant 'a' wave of JVP is not seen in:
A. Junctional arrhythmia
B. Tricuspid regurgitation
C. AV malformations
D. Complete cardiac block

44. First ECG finding seen in MI:
- A. Diminished R wave
- B. ST elevation
- C. ST depression
- D. Widening of QRS interval

45. Which of the following is not true about Wilson's disease?
- A. Increased ceruloplasmin
- B. Acute viral hepatitis
- C. HIV infection
- D. Increased copper in liver

46. Which is not seen in Lambert-Eaton syndrome?
- A. Associated with lung carcinoma
- B. 1st involves the pelvis muscle
- C. Proximal muscle weakness are usually involved
- D. It is seen more common in females

47. QT depressed in:
- A. Hypocalcemia
- B. Hypokalemia
- C. Hyperkalemia
- D. Hypercalcemia

48. Enamel biopsy given by:
- A. Murin
- B. Shakabh and Uruld
- C. Brudevold
- D. Shafer

49. Conservative adhesion restoration terms is given by:
- A. Simonson and Stallard in 1977
- B. Frankstein and Wellbeg in 1990
- C. Croll and Vinstein in 1992
- D. Wilklay and Murray in 2000

50. True about flasking of the denture:
- A. Cope will be the lower member
- B. Drag will hold the teeth and cope will hold the base
- C. Drag will hold the base and cope will hold the teeth
- D. Cope will cover the top of the flask

51. Which of the following is true?
- A. In classical immediate denture anteriors are extracted on the first appointment and posteriors are extracted on the final day of delivery
- B. Classical immediate denture later can be modified to serve as permanent prosthesis

C. Non-classical immediate denture later can be modified to serve as permanent prosthesis
D. In non-classical immediate denture both anteriors and posteriors are extracted on the day of prosthesis delivery

52. Incidence of implant fracture is reported in the:
A. 1 to 2%
B. 0.15 to 3.15%
C. 0.10 to 1.15%
D. 5 or more

53. Rugae are used as an indirect retention in:
A. Kennedy class 4
B. Do not provide retention
C. Horse-shoe shape connector
D. Complete palatal major connector

54. Disadvantage of plaster used for bite registration for occlusal correction:
A. Resistance to biting is very less
B. Irregular setting pattern of plaster
C. Distortion of the plaster during articulator transfer

55. Problem in underlying protrusive recording using POP is:
A. Recording material will be distorted
B. Setting of plaster in different steps
C. Difficulty in maintaining jaw in protruded position for long enough
D. Minimal resistance to biting force

56. True about Diagnodent:
A. 1992, 625 nm
B. 1998, 655 nm
C. 1994, 635 nm
D. 1996, 645 nm

57. In F2 protaper, rotation is done at:
A. 99 degree clockwise 45 degree anticlockwise
B. 45 degree clockwise, 90 degree anticlockwise
C. 180 degree clockwise rotation, 90 degree anticlockwise rotation
D. 144 degree clockwise rotation, 72 degree anticlockwise rotation

58. Iceberg of dental caries concept was given by:
A. Poulson
B. Heidmon
C. Pitts and Longbottom
D. Toudd

59. **Buccal approach of access opening is used in:**
 A. Calcified canals B. Crowding
 C. Multiple canals D. Buccaly tilted teeth

60. **Nd-Yag laser is used for all *except*:**
 A. Sterilization of tooth buccal surface
 B. Removal of intrinsic stains
 C. Removal of dental soft tissue
 D. For pit and fissure sealant

61. **Which of the following is disadvantage of minocycline in triple antibiotic paste?**
 A. Anaphylactic reactions are common side effects
 B. Defective enamel formation
 C. Tooth staining
 D. Hypoplastic defects are produced

62. **Which of the following is not true?**
 A. For soldering with base metal solder, fluoride flux is used
 B. Fluoride flux is used to solder gold with cobalt chromium
 C. Double gold solder are used
 D. For soldering of cast gold, boric acid flux is used

63. **Space control is most difficult to manage in:**
 A. Maxillary premolars
 B. Mandibular first molars
 C. Maxillary first molars
 D. Mandibular premolars

64. **Thiest experimental caries was given by:**
 A. Brathall B. Marsh
 C. Cuppenhoe D. Vonder Fehr

65. **Term Battered child was given by:**
 A. Helfer B. Henry
 C. Kempe D. Starkey

66. **Term incisor liability was given by:**
 A. Black B. Mayne
 C. Broadbent D. Baume

67. **Ectopically erupted molar treatment is:**
 A. Z spring B. Finger spring
 C. Coffin spring D. Kesling spring

68. True about amifostine:

A. Sialorrhea
B. Hypofunction of salivary gland
C. Xerostomia
D. Salivary gland infection

69. Pulp has:

A. Myelinated C fibers and unmyelinated A fibres
B. A fibres only
C. Unmyelinated C fibres and myelinated A fibres
D. C fibres only

70. Post with minimum tooth structure should be:

A. Rigid with high friction
B. Non rigid with high adhesion
C. Rigid with high adhesion
D. Non rigid with high friction

71. Mouse hole effect is due in:

A. Preparation extending through axial wall during access cavity preparation
B. Unable to locate multiple accessory canals in the apical region
C. Due to incomplete obturation
D. Access cavity is much enough large

72. Champagne bubble test is seen due to effect of:

A. Normal saline
B. Sodium hypochlorite
C. Chlorhexidine
D. H_2O_2

73. First systemic fluoride ion electrode is given by:

A. Frant and Ross (1966)
B. Shyler and Armstrong
C. Estrond (1970)
D. Duck and Morgan (1970)

74. Removable prosthodontics is given in:

A. Primary prevention
B. Tertiary prevention
C. Secondary prevention
D. Stabilize adjacent teeth with clasp

75. Study in which disease has already occurred?

A. Case control study
B. Randomized controlled trial
C. Cohort study
D. Descriptive study

76. Safely tolerated dose of fluoride is:
A. 8 to 16/kg body weight
B. 32 to 64 mg/kg body weight
C. 8 to 16 mg/kg body weight
D. 16 to 32 mg/kg body weight

77. Probable toxic dose of fluoride:
A. 5 mg/kg
B. 7 mg/kg
C. 8 mg/kg
D. 9 mg/kg

78. Fluoride level in food is best measured by:
A. Microdiffusion
B. Unable to collect
C. Passive diffusion
D. Ion electrode

79. Which of the following is not irreversible?
A. DMFT index
B. Bleeding index
C. Russel index
D. Gingival index

80. No tobacco day is:
A. 1st May
B. 31st May
C. 1st December
D. 31st July

81. Choking off is seen with:
A. SnF_2
B. Duraphat
C. NaF
D. APF

82. Term colorado stain was given by:
A. Dean
B. Mckay
C. Fejerkov
D. Kaithan

83. Gingival bleeding occur in AINAMO and BAY INDEX is considered positive within:
A. 10 sec
B. 30 sec
C. 20 sec
D. None

84. Primary defect in neutrophil adhesion is seen in which syndrome associated with aggressive periodontitis?
A. Papillon lefevre syndrome
B. Neutropenia
C. Chediak Higashi syndrome
D. Leukocyte adhesion deficiency syndrome

85. Most common cause of implant failure other than occlusal discrepancy is:
A. Operator error
B. Peri-implantitis with excess occlusal load
C. Horizontal bone loss
D. Peri-implantitis alone

86. Normal salivary flow per day is:

A. 200-400 ml
B. 800-1000 ml
C. 700-800 ml
D. 500-700 ml

87. Trauma from occlusion leads to change in periodontium:

A. Funnel shape in crest and angular defect in base with shallow pocket formation
B. Funnel shaped in base and angular at crest with deep pocket formation
C. Funnel shape in crest and angular defect in base without pocket formation
D. Funnel shape in base and angular at crest without pocket formation

88. Miller index is used in:

A. Furcation
B. Frenum attachment
C. Tooth mobility
D. Trauma from occlusion

89. Statement A: Patients infected with HIV have increased periodontal destruction due to immunocompromised state. Statement B: Patients infected with HIV are "not potential" candidates for implants and surgical procedure.

A. Both statements are true
B. Statement A is true, Statement B is false
C. Both statements are false
D. Statement A is false, Statement B is true

90. Ecological plaque hypothesis was given by:

A. Marsh
B. Listgartin
C. Soransky
D. Loesche

91. Atrophy of periodontium causes arrangement of PDL fibres:

A. Perpendicular to root
B. Arranged around the root surface
C. Parallel to root
D. Haphazard arrangement

92. Which increases in periodontium with age?

A. Increase in cellular activity
B. Increase in collagen fibres
C. Increase in keratinisation
D. Increase in elastic fibres

93. Gingival hyperplasia in children is not seen in person taking:

A. Amlodipine B. Nifedipine
C. Cyclosporine D. Phenobarbitone

94. Which of the following does not causes gingival enlargement in children/adults?

A. Amylodipine B. Phenobarbitone
C. Cyclosporine D. Nifedipine

95. Most aberrant resorption is shown by:

A. Primary maxillary incisors
B. Permanent canine and molars
C. Primary canine and molars
D. Deciduous molars

96. Cementum reaches same level in all canal walls in:

A. 1% B. 3%
C. 5% D. 7%

97. Which is true about hemotoxylin and eosin stain?

A. Hemotoxylin is acidic and stain nuclei blue
B. Eosin is acidic and stain nuclei blue
C. Hemotoxylin is basophilic and stain nuclei blue
D. Eosin is basophilic and stain nuclei blue

98. Chicken pox is caused by:

A. Cytomegalovirus B. Infectious mononucleosis
C. Varicella zoster D. Herpes simplex

99. ANUG cannot be differentiated from desquamative gingivitis by:

A. In ANUG lesion spreads to other oral structure, desquamative gingivitis involves only interdental gingiva
B. ANUG has crater like lesion, desquamative has diffuse lesion
C. ANUG involves marginal and papillary gingiva, desquamative gingivitis does not involve papillary gingiva
D. ANUG has no gender prediction, desquamative has gender prediction

100. Beta 2 microglobulin is marker of:

A. SLE B. AIDS
C. Multiple myeloma D. Chronic pancreatitis

Answers

1.	C	2.	C	3.	A	4.	C
5.	C	6.	C	7.	A	8.	B
9.	C	10.	D	11.	C	12.	A
13.	B	14.	C	15.	A	16.	A
17.	B	18.	D	19.	D	20.	C
21.	D	22.	A	23.	D	24.	C
25.	B	26.	C	27.	D	28.	D
29.	B	30.	B	31.	D	32.	C
33.	B	34.	B	35.	D	36.	C
37.	D	38.	B	39.	C	40.	A
41.	C	42.	D	43.	B	44.	B
45.	A	46.	D	47.	B	48.	C
49.	A	50.	C	51.	B	52.	A
53.	C	54.	B	55.	C	56.	B
57.	D	58.	C	59.	B	60.	B
61.	C	62.	C	63.	B	64.	D
65.	C	66.	B	67.	D	68.	C
69.	C	70.	C	71.	A	72.	B
73.	A	74.	B	75.	A	76.	C
77.	A	78.	A	79.	D	80.	B
81.	C	82.	B	83.	A	84.	D
85.	A	86.	B	87.	C	88.	C
89.	B	90.	A	91.	C	92.	D
93.	A	94.	A	95.	C	96.	C
97.	C	98.	C	99.	A	100.	C

PGI Paper December 2014

1. **Collagen fibers seen in cartilage is:**
   A. Type I B. Type II
   C. Type III D. Type IV

2. **Modiolus at the corner of the mouth is formed by all of the following muscles *except*:**
   A. Alaque Nasi B. Orbicularis oris
   C. Triangularis D. Buccinator

3. **Muller's muscle is seen in:**
   A. Lower eyelid B. Upper eyelid
   C. Medial canthus D. Nasal tip

4. **Least pH drop is shown by:**
   A. Lactose B. Glucose
   C. Fructose D. Maltose

5. **Average diameter of mammalian zygote is:**
   A. 10 mm B. 50 mm
   C. 100 mm D. 200 mm

6. **Mallory Weis tear is seen in:**
   A. Heart B. Stomach
   C. Esophagus D. Intestine

7. **Single most reliable diagnostic criteria for squamous cell carcinoma is:**
   A. Invasion B. Pleomorphism
   C. Degeneration D. Encapsulation

8. **In a 3-year-old child which of the following is the most common cyst located in the midline of neck?**
   A. Brachial cyst B. Thyroglossal cyst
   C. Cystic hygroma D. Lymphangioma

9. Complication of tracheostomy is all *except*:
A. Tracheal stenosis
B. Pneumothorax
C. Bronchoesophageal fistula
D. Tracheal artery fistula

10. Glasgow Coma score for flexion motor response is:
A. 1
B. 4
C. 3
D. 6

11. Hydropic degeneration of the basal cell of the stratum germinativum is a feature of:
A. Pemphigus
B. Lichen planus
C. Syphilis
D. Leukoplakia

12. The etiology of Mikulicz disease is:
A. Heredity
B. Autoimmunity
C. Inflammatory disease
D. Viral infection

13. Rumpel-Leede test is used to measure:
A. Factor IX deficiency
B. Capillary fragility
C. Blood pressure
D. Clotting time

14. Most common occurrence of cleft lip is:
A. Unilateral right
B. Unilateral left
C. Midline defect
D. Bilateral

15. Grinspan syndrome involves:
A. Pemphigus
B. Lichen planus
C. Pemphigoid
D. Leukoplakia

16. Which of the following is not a primary autoimmune blistering disease?
A. Bullous eczema
B. Epidermolysis bullosa acquisita
C. Pemphigus
D. Bullous pemphigoid

17. Radicular cyst is a:
A. Developmental cyst
B. Implantation cyst
C. Inflammatory cyst
D. None

18. Marble bone disease is also known as:

A. Osteopetrosis
B. Albert Schonberg disease
C. Both A and B
D. None

19. Which of the following is used for rapid palatal expansion?

A. Coffin Spring
B. W arch
C. Hyrax
D. Ni Ti expander

20. Which of the following orthodontic wire can be heat treated?

A. Niti
B. Beta titanium
C. Elgiloy
D. Stainless steel

21. Most posterior point of mandible is:

A. Gnathion
B. Pogonion
C. Menton
D. Gonion

22. Drugs to be contraindicated during orthodontic treatment:

A. Antibiotics
B. Corticosteroids
C. NSAIDs
D. Anesthetics

23. Which is not the function of head gear:

A. Distalization of molars
B. Anchorage augmentation
C. For maxillary protrusion
D. Uprighting of tilted molars

24. The easiest tooth movement in orthodontics is:

A. Derotation
B. Intrusion
C. Bodily movement
D. Extrusion

25. Which is the contraindication for serial extraction?

A. Missing deciduous canines on one side
B. Lingual tipping of lateral incisors
C. Missing maxillary canine
D. Proclination of anteriors

26. For uncontrolled tipping the centre of rotation is at:

A. Centre of resistance
B. Infinity
C. Root apex
D. Incisal edge

27. Orthodontic decompensation is done prior to orthognathic surgery to correct inclination of which tooth?

A. Canines
B. Molars
C. Incisors
D. Premolars

28. Movement of tooth with digital pressure with hand is proposed by:

A. Hippocrates B. Bakers
C. Celsius D. Angle

29. The orthodontic wire which exhibits shape memory is:

A. NiTi B. Cobalt Chromium
C. Beta Titanium D. Bakers

30. True about CPITN is:

A. Was observed for the first time by ADA in 1992
B. Measure 6 representative teeth
C. Score of 3 means the treatment involvs oral hygiene instructions, scaling and curettage
D. Scored by a special periodontal probe of length 3 to 5 mm backward for easy visibility

31. Russel periodontal index score ranges from:

A. 0-4 B. 0-2
C. 0-6 D. 0-8

32. Gingival bleeding index is used to assess:

A. Measures periodontal health
B. State of oral hygiene on the day of examination
C. Cumulative effect of the last 15 days of oral hygiene
D. Cumulative effect of last 7 days of oral hygiene

33. Oral Health Status index in 1980 was given by:

A. Rosenban
B. WHO
C. Nazir
D. Marcus, Koch and Gershen

34. Prevention of onset of risk factor is:

A. Primary prevention
B. Secondary prevention
C. Primordial prevention
D. Tertiary prevention

35. In a sample of population maximum observations are concentrated around:

A. Median B. Mean
C. Mode D. Arithmetic mean

36. Least cariogenic among these is:

A. Fructose B. Refined starch
C. Sucrose D. Raw starch

37. **A 4-year-old child living in fluoride deficient area should be given fluoride supplementation as:**
   A. 0.5 mg B. 0.25 mg
   C. 0.75 mg D. 1 mg

38. **Primary consideration in any preventive program is:**
   A. Fluoride application
   B. Diet control
   C. Plaque control
   D. Pit and fissure sealant

39. **Which of the following is commonly missing teeth?**
   A. Mandibular incisors
   B. Mandibular second premolars
   C. Maxillary canine
   D. Maxillary molars

40. **The supplementation of fluoride to get maximum cariostatic effect should start from:**
   A. 3 months after birth
   B. 9 months after birth
   C. 6 months after birth
   D. Birth

41. **Encocranial disturbances affecting eruption timing without causing hypoplasia:**
   A. Hypoparathyroidism
   B. Rickets
   C. Hyperthyroidism
   D. None

42. **Cariogram was given by:**
   A. Aramani B. Brathall
   C. Blatterfein D. Klevin Allen

43. **For stainless steel crown the tooth surface requiring least amount of reduction is:**
   A. Buccal B. Occlusal
   C. Lingual D. Proximal

44. **Partial pulpotomy technique is given by:**
   A. Bowen B. Cvek
   C. Clark D. Willet

45. **On examining of a 9-year-old child, caries prevalence will mostly found in:**
   A. Lingual surface of anteriors

B. Interproximal surface of anteriors
C. Proximal surface of 2nd molar
D. Occlusal surface of 1st molar

46. True about acquired pellicle is:
A. Full of microorganisms
B. Derived from microorganisms
C. Prerequisite for plaque
D. Is inorganic in nature

47. CADIA system is used to check:
A. Furcation involvement
B. Progression of periodontal disease
C. Mobility of teeth
D. Bleeding sites

48. The advantage of natural tooth bristles over nylon bristles is:
A. Easy to clean
B. Flex more than nylon bristles
C. Causes less tooth abrasion
D. Susceptible to fraying

49. Which of the following is osteoinductive material?
A. Freeze dried bone
B. Flex more than nylon bristles
C. Hydroxyapatite
D. Dura

50. Which one of the following condition indicates a periodontal rather than endodontic lesion?
A. Acute pain on percussion with no swelling
B. A deep narrow sulcular pocket to the apex with exudates
C. Pain to lateral percussion with wide sulcular pocket
D. Pain to palpation of the buccal mucosa near the root apex

51. Actinobacillus actinomycetum comitance attachment on tooth surface can be prevented by:
A. Myeloperoxidase B. Collagenase
C. Lactoperoxidase D. None

52. Minimum concentration of chlorhexidine to prevent plaque formation is:
A. 2% B. 0.12%
C. 0.2% D. 0.25%

53. **A splint can be defined as:**
   A. Appliance to prevent movement of mobile teeth
   B. Appliance to be used during flap procedure
   C. A prosthesis to keep graft in place
   D. None

54. **Cells present in stage III gingivitis are:**
   A. Plasma cells
   B. Monocytes
   C. PMNs
   D. Lymphocytes

55. **Degeneration of periodontal tissue without inflammation is called as:**
   A. Chronic periodontitis
   B. Desquamative gingivitis
   C. Periodontosis
   D. Pericoronitis

56. **The most common periodontal fiber which regenerate after injury is:**
   A. Transseptal fibers
   B. Horizontal fibers
   C. Oblique fibers
   D. Apical fibers

57. **McCall's festoon occurs due to:**
   A. Physiological resorption
   B. Inflammatory disease
   C. Poor oral hygiene
   D. Trauma from occlusion

58. **Pathologic migration of tooth occurs:**
   A. Away from bone resorption area
   B. Towards bone resorption area
   C. Incisoocclusal direction
   D. Axioincisal direction

59. **Caries activity test measures:**
   A. Caries susceptibility
   B. Motivational aspect
   C. pH change
   D. None

60. **What is the minimum distance between the nasal vestibule and implant?**
   A. 1 mm
   B. 2.5 mm
   C. 2 mm
   D. 3 mm

61. Non union of fracture is due to:
A. Early mobilization
B. Bone loss due to infection
C. Mobility of fracture site
D. None of the above

62. During inferior alveolar nerve block the needle is inserted in which space?
A. Submandibular space
B. Infratemporal space
C. Masseteric space
D. Pterygomandibular space

63. Floating fracture of maxilla is seen in:
A. Pyramidal fracture of maxilla
B. Fracture of alveolar process
C. Horizontal fracture of maxilla
D. None

64. Drug which can cause the osteonecrosis of the jaw?
A. Calcitonin
B. Alendronate
C. Corticosteroids
D. None

65. The recommended time gap between the radiation and surgery to avoid radio necrosis is:
A. 6-12 months after radiotherapy
B. Immediately after radiotherapy
C. Any time during the course of radiotherapy
D. 4-6 weeks after radiotherapy

66. During exodontia the force applied firstly in which direction?
A. Lingual
B. Apical
C. Buccal
D. Coronal

67. Battle's sign is seen in fracture of:
A. Fracture occipital bone
B. Fracture posterior cranial fossa
C. Fracture zygoma
D. Fracture middle cranial fossa

68. After Cald Wel Luc procedure, intranasal antrostomy is done through:
A. Middle meatus
B. Superior meatus
C. Inferior meatus
D. Floor of the nose

69. **Traumatic injury to nerve causing parasthesia is:**
A. Axonomesis
B. Toxolysis
C. Neurotemesis
D. Neuropraxia

70. **Which of the following is the radiographic feature of TMJ ankylosis?**
A. Mandibular prognathism
B. Deep antigonial notches
C. Increased gonial angle
D. Increased mandibular plane angle

71. **CSF otorrhea is due to fracture of:**
A. Fracture of ethmoid bone
B. Fracture of petrous part of temporal membrane
C. Fracture of cribriform plate
D. Fracture of occipital bone

72. **Which of the following suture material will lead to maximum tissue response?**
A. Silk
B. Nylon
C. Catgut
D. Linen

73. **Infection of the dangerous area of face is commonly leads to:**
A. Osteomyelitis
B. Space infection
C. Ludwig's angina
D. Cavernous sinus thrombosis

74. **All are considered in TNM staging *except*:**
A. Tumor site
B. Tumor size
C. Size of lymph node
D. Metastasis

75. **Ameloblastoma originates from:**
A. Odontogenic ectomesenchyme
B. Odontogenic epithelium
C. Mixed tumor
D. It is not a tumor but is an odontogenic cyst

76. **In adult patient resuscitation follows the order A airway, B breathing, C circulation, D......:**
A. ABCD
B. DACB
C. BACD
D. BCAD

77. **Ormocers are:**
A. Organically modified glass ionomers
B. Organically modified ceramics
C. Glass ionomer modified composites
D. Composite modified glass ionomers

78. **Bevels are given for restoration with cast gold inlay and onlay for:**
A. To remove unsupported enamel rods
B. To enhance edge strength
C. To prevent fracture of teeth
D. Thin margins are easily adaptable

79. **The value of condylar inclination is:**
A. 15-20 degree
B. 20-25 degree
C. 10-15 degree
D. 30-40 degree

80. **The success of removable die system depends upon the:**
A. Length of the dowel pin protruding out of the master cast
B. Precise relocation of die in the working cast
C. Abrasion resistance of the die material
D. Time involved in die construction

81. **When establishing occlusion for partial denture which of the following is an advantage of the functionally generated path technique?**
A. Verification of the recording in the mouth is easy
B. The occlusion of opposing dentures can be developed altogether
C. During the generation of path there is no risk of movement of the distal extension base
D. It eliminates the need for adjusting an articulator with intraoral records

82. **Antibiotic prophylaxis is given to prevent infection endocarditis in case of RHD patient is:**
A. Gingivoplasty
B. Open reduction of fracture by intraoral route
C. Scaling and curettage
D. Extraction of teeth

83. **Acute pancreatitis is due to:**
A. Hepatitis
B. Viral disease
C. Alcoholism
D. None

84. Hypokalemia is blood potassium level below:
A. 4.6 mM B. 3.6 mM
C. 5.6 mM D. 6.6 mM

85. Hyperpyrexia is defined as:
A. Fever > 38 degree C
B. Fever > 40 degree C
C. Fever > 37 degree C
D. Fever > 39 degree C

86. Granulation tissue is replaced by connective tissue by:
A. 7 days B. 14 days
C. 1 month D. 21 days

87. Koplik spots are seen in:
A. Herpes B. Varicella
C. German measles D. Measles

88. Which of the following is radiopaque mass surrounded by radiolucent line?
A. Osteomas B. Osteosarcoma
C. Sialolithiasis D. Compound odontomas

89. The retentive terminals of clasp is normally positioned:
A. At the mesiofacial and distofacial line angles
B. At the mesiolinugal or distolingual line angles
C. Near the labial surface of tooth
D. Near the facial surface

90. The low thermal conductivity of impression compound is overcome by:
A. By heating with ethanol flame and directly placing in patient's mouth
B. Heating in hot water and immediately quenching in water for 20 minutes
C. By melting it in boiling water at 50 degree C for one hour
D. Impression is placed in mouth till it gets cold and sudden removal of the impression

91. Solders in stainless steel differ from that of gold in:
A. KF B. Calcium carbonate
C. Silver nitrate D. Strontium fluoride

92. The radiographic appearance of cherubism is:
A. Unilateral unilocular radiolucency
B. Unilateral multilocular radiolucency

C. Bilateral multilocular radiolucency
D. Bilateral unilocular radiolucency

93. Radiopaque irregularity associated with CEJ of mandibular central incisors most likely represent:
A. Subgingival calculus
B. Hyperplastic cementum
C. Root caries
D. Subgingival pellicle

94. Not a feature of MRI:
A. Bone appear white
B. Brain tissue appear white
C. Tooth appear black
D. Bone marrow appear white

95. Numbers of developmental lobes for primary central incisors are:
A. 1
B. 2
C. 3
D. 4

96. Maximum incidence of developmental defects occurs in:
A. Permanent incisors
B. Permanent mandibular first molar
C. Primary incisors
D. Primary mandibular second molar

97. Root completion occurs after how much time after eruption?
A. 1 year
B. 2-3 years
C. 6 years
D. 6 months

98. Pulp polyp is due to:
A. Reversible pulpitis
B. Acute pulpal infection
C. Chronic pulpal infection
D. None

Answers

1.	B	2.	A	3.	B	4.	D
5.	C	6.	A	7.	A	8.	B
9.	C	10.	C	11.	B	12.	B
13.	B	14.	B	15.	B	16.	A
17.	C	18.	C	19.	C	20.	C
21.	D	22.	C	23.	D	24.	D
25.	B	26.	A	27.	C	28.	C
29.	A	30.	B	31.	D	32.	B
33.	D	34.	C	35.	A	36.	D
37.	A	38.	C	39.	B	40.	D
41.	C	42.	B	43.	C	44.	B
45.	D	46.	C	47.	B	48.	C
49.	A	50.	C	51.	A	52.	B
53.	A	54.	A	55.	C	56.	A
57.	D	58.	B	59.	A	60.	A
61.	B	62.	D	63.	C	64.	B
65.	D	66.	B	67.	D	68.	C
69.	D	70.	B	71.	B	72.	A
73.	D	74.	A	75.	B	76.	A
77.	B	78.	D	79.	B	80.	B
81.	D	82.	B	83.	C	84.	B
85.	B	86.	D	87.	D	88.	D
89.	A	90.	D	91.	A	92.	C
93.	A	94.	A	95.	A	96.	A
97.	B	98.	C				

PGI Paper

June 2014

1. **Cornea is supplied by which fibres?**
   A. A beta
   B. A alpha and C delta fibres both
   C. A delta and C fibres
   D. C delta fibres only

2. **Which of the following is false with respect to systemic hypertension?**
   A. Long standing hypertension causes left ventricular failure
   B. Long standing systemic hypertension cause right ventricular hypertrophy
   C. Pulmonary hypertension causes right ventricular failure
   D. Coarctation of the aorta raises the blood pressure

3. **Forcing in or sucking of air from a tissue is called:**
   A. Emphema B. Abscess
   C. Emphysema D. Asphyxia

4. **Which subunit of troponin binds with tropomyosin to form tropomyosin complex?**
   A. Troposin I B. Troposin M
   C. Troposin C D. Troposin T

5. **Percentage of percutaneous HIV transfer is:**
   A. 13% B. 50%
   C. 2-3% D. 0.2-0.5%

6. **Hyperpyrexia is seen in:**
   A. 31.5 degree Celsius or 96.7 degree F
   B. > 37 degree Celsius or 98 degree F
   C. 38 degree Celsius or 100 degree F
   D. 41.5 degree Celsius or 106.7 degree F

7. **Incision given along which lines for facial skin surgeries?**
   A. Lines of Blaschko B. Lines of Krausi
   C. Lines of Futcher D. Lines of Langer

8. Which of the following option is wrong?

A. Haemophilia B does not occur in females
B. Von Willebrand can occur in woman
C. Half life of factor IX less than factor VIII
D. Half life of factor VIII is less than factor IX

9. All of the following are features of tetanus *except*:

A. Coagulopathy
B. Opisthotonus
C. Trismus
D. Respiratory failure

10. During wound healing the fibroblasts which are found in abundant?

A. Golgi bodies
B. Nucleus increased
C. RER
D. SER

11. Which of the following is least likely to be present in lymphodema?

A. Swelling
B. Chronic eczema
C. Pitting
D. Ulcer

12. What is the major detrimental factor for individual patient's perioperative surgical complication?

A. Duration of anesthesia
B. Anesthesia technique
C. Surgical procedure
D. Surgical procedure length

13. Which of the following is not indication of tracheostomy?

A. Comatose patient
B. Foreign body obstruction in trachea
C. Bronchoscopy in neonates
D. Bronchial toilet in associated ventilation

14. Which of the following is false about silica used in investment material?

A. Beta allotropic form is stable below transition temperature
B. Quarts acts as refractory
C. It regulates setting expansion
D. Quarts and crystoballite are allotropic forms used in denture investments

15. False about non-gypsum die impression material:

A. Metal dies are preferable to high strength gypsum dies for captek restorations
B. All impression materials are compatible with these

C. Polyester produces the best die
D. Epoxy resin are undersized but are used due to high abrasion resistance

16. Which of the following is false regarding setting of plaster procedure?

A. Potassium sulphate 3.4% acts as accelerator and prevent setting expansion
B. Most accurate way of controlling setting expansion is on chairside of patient by adding chemicals
C. Setting expansion which increases with increase in the density
D. Maximum acceleration effect for sodium sulphate is 3.4%

17. For strengthening of the ceramic all of the following are done *except*:

A. Higher thermal coefficient of expansion of ceramic as compared to metal substructure
B. Stiffer supporting material
C. Minimizing number of porcelain firing cycles
D. Three layer laminate technique

18. MTA setting time is:

A. 4 hours 20 minutes B. 2 hours 45 minutes
C. 4 hours D. 2 hours 30 minutes

19. Dark color radiolucency adjacent to the instrument in the main canal of radiograph:

A. Extra canal B. Perforation
C. Extra root D. Lamina dura

20. Aims of access cavity are all *except*:

A. Complete removal of root of the pulp chamber
B. Straight line access to the apex
C. Convergent walls to conserve the tooth structure
D. Removal of all the carious tooth structure

21. Which of the following contraindication for single visit RCT?

A. Draining sinus B. Diabetes mellitus
C. Hypertension D. Acute pulpal inflammation

22. GP sterilization is done by:

A. 2.5 percent glutaraldehyde for 1 minute
B. 5 percent NaOCl for 1 minute

C. 5.25% NaOCl for 5 minutes
D. 2.5 percent glutaraldehyde for 5 minutes

23. The AH sealer is a:
A. Medicated sealer
B. Non resin based sealer
C. Resin based
D. Zinc oxide free sealer

24. Active GP is:
A. Gp + $CaOH_2$
B. Gp + $ZNpO_4$
C. Gp + zoe
D. Gp + glass ionomer

25. Endotec 2 is:
A. BMP preparation
B. Obturation system
C. Access cavity preparation
D. Irrigation device

26. Which of the following is not present in triple antibiotic paste?
A. Minocycline
B. Metronidazole
C. Ciprofloxacin
D. Amoxycillin

27. EDTA C contains:
A. EDTA plus cetavlon
B. EDTA plus Calcium hydroxide
C. EDTA plus Cetrimide
D. EDTA

28. The pain of cracked tooth syndrome is differentiated by:
A. Decrease threshold pain
B. Pain on release of pressure
C. Continuous pain
D. Pain on biting

29. Which of following is not true regarding abrasive used for grinding restoration?
A. Cutting and grinding procedures are purely predominantly unidirectional
B. Carbide bur work by cutting action
C. Tungsten carbide bur is predominantly used for grinding
D. 16 fluted carbide bur causes quick cutting and produces coarse surface

30. The laser used on a crown for debonding orthodontic brackets acts by:
A. Thermal ablation
B. Thermal softening
C. Photoablation
D. Laser debonding

31. Functional matrix theory was forwarded by:

A. Klein
B. Moss
C. Kloff
D. Scott

32. Type 2 forward rotation by Bjork centre of rotation is in:

A. Anterior cranial base
B. Premolars
C. Condyle
D. Mandibular incisors

33. In patient undergoing fixed ortho treatment, fluoride recommended for better oral hygiene is:

A. Sodium fluoride mouthwash 0.05% daily
B. Stannous fluoride mouth rinse
C. 0.2% Naf daily
D. 1.2 ApF weekly

34. The orthopaedic mechanics consist of:

A. Anterior inclined plane
B. Anterior-posterior repositioning device
C. Posterior inclined paste
D. Stabilization appliance

35. In a pre-adjusted edgewise bracket the slot size is 0.022 inches (22 slot bracket). If a 0.0215 inch wire is placed inside it, what will be the play?

A. 0.8°
B. 1.5°
C. 2.8°
D. 3.8°

36. Which appliance is contraindicated in obstructive mouth breathers?

A. Monoblock
B. Twin block
C. Straight wire technique
D. Herbst appliance

37. True about lip pressure and tongue pressure on incisors is:

A. Lip pressure is more on upper incisors but tongue pressure is more on lower incisors
B. Lip pressure is more
C. Tongue pressure is more
D. Tongue pressure is more on upper incisor but lip pressure more on lower incisors

38. **Not a principle of bioprogressive therapy:**
    A. Over correction of malocclusion
    B. Sectional mechanics
    C. Muscular and cortical anchorage
    D. All of the above

39. **Which is false about long face syndrome?**
    A. Increased posterior facial height
    B. High mandibular plane angle
    C. High gonial angle
    D. High occlusal plane angle

40. **The copper NiTi wires Type II are available in the temperature range of:**
    A. 27° B. 15°
    C. 37° D. 40°

41. **Occipital point is used as a landmark on cephalometrics for growth by:**
    A. Frankel B. Tweed
    C. Wilson D. Bjork

42. **According to US FDA, the intraoral X-ray machine is classified as:**
    A. Class 1 B. Class 2
    C. Class 3 D. Class 4

43. **Chin placed anterior to focal spot in OPG is seen as:**
    A. Blurred and constricted
    B. Blurred and magnified vertically
    C. Blurred and magnified horizontally
    D. Neither blurred nor magnified

44. **In X-ray tube focusing cup filament diameter and length respectively:**
    A. 1 cm and 2 mm B. 2 mm and < 1 cm
    C. 2 mm and 3 cm D. 4 mm and 1 cm

45. **How is nicotine stomatitis lesion different from papillary hyperplasia under acrylic denture?**
    A. Peripheral single spot
    B. Peripheral multiple red spot
    C. Multiple central spot
    D. Single red spot centrally

46. Smooth surface lesion arise below epithelium are all *except*:

A. Ranula
B. Intraepithelial bullae in pemphigus
C. Subepithelial bullae in pemphigus
D. Mucocele

47. Which inflammatory mediator has anti-inflammatory properties?

A. Leukotrienes
B. Lipoxins
C. Thromboxanes
D. Prostaglandins

48. Sunburst appearance is seen in:

A. Turner syndrome
B. Osteosarcoma
C. Pemphigus
D. Ewing's sarcoma

49. The Forchheimer spot are seen in:

A. Lichen planus
B. Rubeola
C. Rubella
D. Pemphigus

50. The partially bald tongue is not seen in:

A. Pyogenic stomatitis
B. Reiter disease
C. Psoriasis
D. Atrophic lichen planus

51. Multilocular appearance is seen in:

A. Traumatic bone cyst
B. Dentigerous cyst
C. Ameloblastoma
D. Okc

52. Tennis racket appearance is seen in:

A. Adenomatoid odontogenic tumor
B. Odontogenic myxoma
C. Calcifying epithelial odontogenic tumor
D. Keratocyst

53. About mucous membrane pemphigoid false is:

A. Affect mucous membrane and conjunctiva
B. Antigen are most frequently formed against lamina densa
C. Double frequency in females as compared to males
D. Oral mucosa is most frequently involved

54. A 6-year-old child with the bilateral expansion and involvement of mandible on both sides with floating teeth appearance in the space suggests:

A. Paget's disease B. Cherubism
C. OKC D. None

55. The punched out crater like gingiva is not seen in:

A. ANUG
B. Pyogenic granuloma
C. Gangrenous stomatitis
D. Sickle cell anemia

56. Histological examination of the tissues in desquamative gingivitis would reveal:

A. Loss of basement membrane
B. Hyperkeratosis
C. Elongation of rete pegs
D. No inflammatory response

57. Lactic acid production is because of:

A. Saccharolytic bacteria in supragingival plaque
B. Saccharolytic bacteria in subgingival plaque
C. Non saccharolytic bacteria in subgingival plaque
D. Non saccharolytic bacteria in supragingival plaque

58. Which of the following was false regarding cigarette smoking?

A. Decreased PMN response
B. Increased periodontal breakdown
C. Increased bleeding on probing
D. Decrease response to therapy

59. Which of the following causes initiation of periodontal inflammation?

A. Protease B. Hyaluronidase
C. Endotoxin D. Neuroamidase
E. Deoxyribinuclease

Options

A. A, B and C B. A and B
C. B, C and D D. D

60. Major cause of fracture of implant:

A. Periimplantitis B. Non passive fit
C. Bending overload D. Manufacturing defect

61. Corncob appearance of plaque occurs after how much duration?

A. 1 week
B. 3 weeks
C. 2 weeks
D. 4 weeks

62. Most common side effect of fresh autogenous iliac crest transplant in managing an infrabony periodontal pocket in periodontal surgery:

A. Root resorption
B. Arthus reaction
C. Auto erythro sensitization
D. Infection

63. In root resected in hemisection of maxillary 1st molar which portion of the root is removed?

A. Not root is extracted
B. Mesiobuccal
C. Palatal
D. Distobuccal

64. Full mouth disinfection conducted in how much time:

A. Full mouth scaling in 24 hrs
B. Quadrant wise scaling in 7-10 days
C. Full mouth scaling in 48 hrs
D. Antibiotics for 5 days

65. The occurrence of keratinisation on human gingiva is:

A. Depend on functional stimulation the attached gingiva
B. Lacking in gingival crevice
C. A reflection of inflammation in underlying gingival connective tissue
D. A variable factor directly related with age

66. All of the following regarding eruption cyst are true except:

A. Benign soft tissue associated with permanent or primary unerupted tooth
B. Variant of dentigerous cyst
C. Regress spontaneously
D. Associated with unerupted tooth present in bone

67. Which of the following condition is not characterized by periodontal destruction around primary tooth?

A. Hypophosphotasia
B. Papillon lefevre syndrome

C. Stevens-Johnson syndrome
D. Cystic fibrosis/Sickle cell anemia

68. Most likely cause of syncope in child:
A. Neuro cardiogenic syncope
B. Situational syncope
C. Cerebral syncope
D. Fatigue syndrome

69. The high amount of S. mutans in a child suggest:
A. Risk indicator for caries
B. Low incidence for caries
C. Risk factor for caries
D. Risk predictor for caries

70. A child with deep caries, on radiograph reaching the pulp. The best treatment should be:
A. Direct pulp capping
B. Pulpectomy
C. Pulpotomy
D. Indirect pulp capping

71. The odyophagia is:
A. Difficulty in respiration
B. Pain in the tooth
C. Pain during mastication
D. Pain during swallowing

72. A 40 years patient with endocarditis need extraction for a carious tooth antibiotics should be started:
A. No need of antibiotics
B. 1 hour before extraction
C. 3 days before extraction
D. Six hours before extraction

73. Best treatment of a solid ramus ameloblastoma:
A. En bloc resection of entire mandible
B. Segmental resection
C. Marsupization following excision
D. Enucleation

74. The floor of pterygomandibular space is formed by:
A. Medial pterygoid
B. Pterygomandibular raphe
C. Lateral pterygoid
D. Pterygomasseteric sling

75. **To preserve marginal mandibular branch, best submandibular approach is to save marginal mandibular branch of facial nerve, incision is given:**
   A. Near to submandibular gland
   B. In the platysma
   C. Superficial to platysma
   D. Palpate facial lymph nodes and then give superficial to it

76. **If the tooth fragment is pushed into maxillary sinus during extraction. Which of the following techniques will be used to retrieve it?**
   A. Perform Caldwell procedure to remove the tip
   B. Leave as such till signs of infection appears
   C. Widen the opening and remove the root tip
   D. No treatment required

77. **A 6-year-old child with parasymphyseal fracture with no occlusion disturbance and no mobility, treatment should be:**
   A. Cap splint and fixation
   B. Diet restriction and observe for 2-3 weeks
   C. No active treatment wait and watch
   D. IMF

78. **Infection spread of anterior face triangle include:**
   A. Base of upper lip to lower lip
   B. Upper lip to canine fossa
   C. Medial to the glabella
   D. Lower lip upto canine fossa

79. **A straight elevator is inserted between:**
   A. As deep near cementoenamel junction
   B. Between gingivae and tooth root
   C. Between internal bone and mesiobuccal side of the tooth
   D. Between roots

80. **1 gm of 1000 ppm contains fluoride:**
   A. 1 mg B. 0.25 mg
   C. 0.13 mg D. 0.5 mg

81. **Iceberg concept of disease was first of all given by:**
   A. Pitts and Longbottom
   B. Poulson
   C. Heidmon
   D. Toudd

82. Regarding case control study all of the following are correct, *except*:

A. Risk factors can be identified
B. Used in the study of rare diseases
C. It measures incidence
D. Requires few subjects

83. Colorado stain term given by:

A. Mc Kay
B. Kaithan
C. T Dean
D. Fejerkov

84. The best approach to primary health education:

A. Primary health care
B. Health education approach
C. Service approach
D. Regulatory

85. 21 country, survey is done by:

A. TH Dean
B. Mc Kay
C. Wilson
D. Fejerkov

86. Which is not a part of operating dental auxillary?

A. Dental hygienist
B. School dental nurse
C. Denturist
D. Dental therapist

87. Which is closed dental camp?

A. It is a preselected area like school for camp
B. Open dental camp
C. Serving large number of people
D. The term does not exist

88. Level of public health service are:

A. Initial professional stage
B. Undifferentiated professional stage
C. Differentiated professional stage
D. All of the above

89. The selective fluoride ion-electrode was first given by:

A. Estrond 1970
B. Shyler and Armstrong 1960
C. Frant and Ross 1966
D. Duck and Morgan 1970

90. The usefulness of a screening test depends upon it:

A. Sensitivity
B. Specificity
C. Predictive value
D. Reliability

91. Why regular topical application of concentrated fluoride doesn't cause mottling of teeth?

A. It is not fluoride that cause mottling
B. Teeth are already calcified
C. Mottling occur in bones not in teeth
D. Calcium present in saliva neutralize the fluoride

92. Amount of IgA secreted in colostrum is:

A. 22 mg/ml B. 45 mg/ml
C. 34 mg/ml D. 12 mg/ml

93. Which is false about remounting procedure?

A. It is used to maintain stability
B. It is better over making intraoral correction
C. The semi adjustable articulator is mandatory
D. It is a gold standard for rebasing procedure

94. According to the Cawood and Howell classification, the maxillary ridge with cup shaped alveolar ridge and peripheral horse-shoe shaped appearance of atrophied edentulous maxilla is classified as:

A. Class 3 B. Class 5
C. Class 4 D. Class 6

95. The cusp fossa and cup embrasure relationship is given by:

A. Angle
B. Thomas
C. Huffman and Regenos
D. Charles Stuart

96. Regarding dispersion strengthening:

A. Increasing the strength of ceramic by dispersing their matrix with the crystalline phase of the same material
B. The strengthening is due to polymorphic transformation
C. The crystalline phase works by hindering the crack propagation
D. Cad cam procedures in these materials further decrease their surface flaws

97. Which penicillin is taken orally?

A. Benzpenicillin
B. Penicillin V
C. Aqueous Penicillin G
D. Methicillin

Answers

1.	C	2.	B	3.	C	4.	D
5.	D	6.	D	7.	D	8.	D
9.	A	10.	C	11.	D	12.	C
13.	C	14.	A	15.	C	16.	B
17.	A	18.	B	19.	A	20.	C
21.	A	22.	B	23.	C	24.	D
25.	B	26.	D	27.	C	28.	B
29.	D	30.	D	31.	B	32.	D
33.	C	34.	B	35.	B	36.	A
37.	A	38.	D	39.	D	40.	A
41.	A	42.	B	43.	A	44.	B
45.	D	46.	B	47.	B	48.	B
49.	C	50.	A	51.	D	52.	B
53.	B	54.	B	55.	A	56.	A
57.	A	58.	C	59.	A	60.	C
61.	B	62.	D	63.	D	64.	A
65.	B	66.	D	67.	C	68.	A
69.	C	70.	D	71.	D	72.	B
73.	B	74.	D	75.	C	76.	C
77.	B	78.	B	79.	C	80.	A
81.	A	82.	C	83.	A	84.	B
85.	A	86.	C	87.	A	88.	D
89.	C	90.	A	91.	B	92.	D
93.	D	94.	D	95.	C	96.	C
97.	B						

PGI Paper December 2013

1. **Which of the following is not present in acrosome of spermatozoa?**
   A. Alkaline phosphatase
   B. Acid phosphatase
   C. Acrosomase
   D. Hyaluronidase

2. **Inca bone, Gothe ossicle in skull presents as independent bone in suture is:**
   A. Pterion B. Lambda
   C. Bregma D. Asterion

3. **Maxillary antrum attains its full size with pneumatisation at age of:**
   A. 12 years B. 18-20 years
   C. 2-4 years D. 14-15 years

4. **Most anteriorly placed foramen is:**
   A. Carotid canal
   B. Foramen magnum
   C. Foramen spinosum
   D. Foramen ovale

5. **Which of the following is true about total body water?**
   A. Female and obese person has increase % of body water
   B. Increase muscle mass is associated with decrease body water
   C. Total body water decrease steadily with age
   D. Any person % of TBW is subject to wide physiological variation

6. **Mucin is:**
   A. Glycoprotein B. Nucleoprotein
   C. Phosphoprotein D. Chromo protein

7. Stevens-J ohnson syndrome involves:
A. Type I hypersensitivity reaction
B. Type II hypersensitivity reaction
C. Type III hypersensitivity reaction
D. Type IV hypersensitivity reaction

8. Toll like receptors lipopolysaccharides:
A. TLR-1
B. TLR-2
C. TLR-3
D. TLR-4

9. Red painful mucosa is seen on removal of denture what kind of candidiasis?
A. Atrophic
B. Mucocutaneus
C. Hyperplastic
D. None

10. A 9-year-old child with fever 38°C, vesicles involving hard palate, posterior oropharyngeal wall is suffering from:
A. Herpangina
B. Herpetic gingivostomatitis
C. Diphtheria
D. Aphthous ulcer

11. Which form of osteomyelitis having negative microbiological culture, and doesn't respond to antibiotic treatment is:
A. Acute suppurative osteomyelitis
B. Bidder osteomyelitis
C. SAPHO syndrome
D. Garre's osteomyelitis

12. Which of the following disorder associated with increase in dental caries?
A. Epidermolysis bullosa
B. Down syndrome
C. Turner syndrome
D. Hereditary fructose intolerance

13. Which of these is not related to stress?
A. Syphilis
B. TMJ disorder
C. Pemphigus
D. Lichen planus

14. Mulberry molars is seen in:
A. Primary syphilis
B. Congenital syphilis

C. Secondary syphilis
D. Tertiary syphilis

15. Supernumerary teeth is seen in all *except*:
A. Gardner syndrome
B. Sickel syndrome
C. Apert syndrome
D. Down syndrome

16. Correct sequence:
A. Inoculation, abscess, cellulitis
B. Abscess, inoculation, cellulitis
C. Cellulitis, abscess, inoculation
D. Inoculation, cellulitis, abscess

17. Which of the following is true about lichen planus?
A. Common on extensor surface of skin
B. Most common in females in ratio of Female: Male = 3:2
C. Hepatitis C is most commonly associated
D. Prevalence in general population is 3.7 to 5.8%

18. Gene associated with amelogenesis imperfecta:
A. ENAM
B. DSSP
C. MSX-1/MSH 1
D. PAX-9

19. Hypoplastic hypomaturation type of amelogenesis imperfecta is seen in:
A. Tricho-dento-osseous syndrome
B. Osteogenesis imperfecta
C. Pierre Robin syndrome
D. Cleidocranial dysplasia

20. Main cause of oral submucous fibrosis is:
A. Tobacco
B. Areca nut
C. Alcohol
D. Smoking

21. The best radiographic view of condyle neck is:
A. Towne's view
B. Reverse towne's view
C. Water view
D. Caldwell view

22. Filmbadge in IOPA is a type of:
A. Dosimetry
B. Sonometry
C. Tachometry
D. Identification badge

23. How to reduce magnification in X-ray?
A. Long cone
B. Film placed away from object
C. Short cone
D. Film placed near to object

24. Most common cause of break in canal seen on IOPA radiograph:

A. Calcification of canal
B. Merging of canal
C. Bifurcation of canal
D. Extra canal

25. Proximal caries is best detected by:

A. IOPA B. Bitewing
C. Occlusal D. OPG

26. Brown tumor in hyperparathyroidism resembles:

A. Giant cell tumor B. Benign tumor
C. Malignant tumor D. Vascular malformation

27. Anti mongoloid slant is a feature of which fracture?

A. Lefort 1 B. Lefort 2
C. Lefort 3 D. Naso-orbito-ethmoid fracture

28. What is the color coding of bag in hospitals to dispose human anatomical wastes such as human extracted tooth?

A. Yellow B. Black
C. Blue D. Red

29. Which of the following is sclerosing agent used in TMJ ankylosis?

A. Sodium bicarbonate
B. Sodium tetradecyl sulphate
C. Sodium morrhuate
D. Sodium psylliate

30. Glossopharyngeal neuralgia is also known as:

A. Tic doulourex
B. Frey's syndrome
C. Vago-glossopharyngeal neuralgia
D. Both 1 and 3

31. Which of the following is not associated with increased likelihood of infection after major elective surgery?

A. Age over 70 years
B. Chronic malnutrition
C. Controlled diabetes mellitus
D. Long-term steroid use

32. Most common in syncope:

A. Hypoperfusion B. Hypotension
C. Hypoxia D. All of the above

33. Which of the following is not done in ankylosis treatment?

A. High condylar fracture
B. Ipsilateral coronoidectomy
C. Contralateral coronoidectomy
D. Repositioning of temporal fascia

34. While extracting maxillary 3rd molar which position is not possible?

A. 12'O clock B. 11'O clock
C. 1'O clock D. 9'O clock

35. Pregnant female patient in third trimester is kept in:

A. Left lateral decubitus
B. Right lateral decubitus
C. Supine
D. Sitting

36. When tumor is removed what's done to evaluate the border of residual or resected tumor intraoperatively?

A. Punch biopsy B. Exfoliative cytology
C. Brush biopsy D. Fresh frozen section

37. Which number blade used for incision and drainage and incision is puncture type of incision?

A. No. 11 B. No. 12
C. No. 15 D. No. 20

38. Which of the following is true?

A. Grading of tumor is based upon metastasis
B. Grade I means poorly differentiated tumour
C. Less in numerical value less in tumour differentiation
D. More number of cells, nuclear pleomorphism, and decreased production of keratin shows highly differentiated tumour

39. Patient with an hepatic condition and with full supportive therapy for how much time a patient can survive?

A. 24-48 hours B. 1-2 hours
C. 1 week D. 2-4 weeks

40. The transfusion of fresh frozen plasma (FFP) is indicated for which of the following reasons?

A. Volume replacement
B. As a nutritional supplement
C. Specific coagulation factor deficiency
D. Acute blood loss

41. Amount of fluoride used in amalgam:

A. 1% NaF_2
B. 1% SnF_2
C. 8% SnF_2
D. 10% SnF_2

42. When particle size is used if sandblasting with Al_2O_3/ Aluminium oxide particles sprayed on inner side of porcelain has size:

A. 10 mm
B. 25 mm
C. 50 mm
D. 100 mm

43. Residual monomer content in heat cure resin is:

A. 0.3-0.5%
B. 0.5-1.0%
C. 3-5%
D. 1-2%

44. Chromium when added to steel it doesn't increase:

A. Corrosion resistance
B. Increase hardness
C. Decrease elastic limit
D. Increase tensile strength

45. Coating of bonding agent applied with a brush so that oxygen from air does not pass through/Bonding agent thickness is used to prevent oxygen penetration:

A. 100 micrometer
B. 200 micrometer
C. 150 micrometer
D. 50 micrometer

46. Zinc phosphate cement pH at the time of mixing:

A. 1-2
B. 2.5-4.5
C. 6-7
D. 1.5-3.5

47. Which of the following is not a function of using boric oxide in ceramic restoration?

A. It act as glass modifier
B. It decreases the viscosity of ceramic restoration
C. Remove the unsintered matrix from the ceramic residue
D. Prevent the unreacted particles from being oxidizing in atmosphere

48. Which is not true about ethyl silicate investment material?

A. MgO increase strength
B. Aqueous solution of colloidal silica forms gel after heating
C. Gel silica formed by heating
D. Most user friendly material

49. Which of the following is not a criteria while selecting stainless steel crown for deciduous teeth?

A. Occlusal morphology of crown
B. Greater mesiodistal diameter of crown
C. Greater occlusal height of crown
D. Slight resistance on seating of crown

50. Arch length from deciduous to permanent dentition:

A. Decreases
B. Increases
C. Remains same
D. First increase then decreases

51. All techniques of tooth brushing are done by vibratory method *except*:

A. Fones method
B. Bass method
C. Stillman method
D. Charter method

52. Iodoform 40% + calcium hydroxide 42% use for root canal sealer in primary teeth is in:

A. Vitapex
B. KRI
C. Miasto
D. Walkoff

53. Vitremer is:

A. Metal modified Gic
B. Resin modified Gic
C. Organically modified composite
D. Polyacid modified composite

54. Tetracycline cause tooth discoloration due to:

A. Calcium orthophosphate
B. Tetracalcium phosphate
C. Calcium oxide
D. Dicalcium phosphate dehydrate

55. Self inflicted bites are seen in:

A. Lesch-Nyhan syndrome
B. Friese-Maria syndrome
C. Cockanye syndrome
D. Down syndrome

56. Pacifer sucking is an example of:

A. Bottle sucking
B. Nutritive sucking
C. Non-nutritive sucking
D. Finger sucking

57. Ego centricism and animism is seen in which stage of Piaget's theory?

A. Sensorimotor
B. Concrete operational
C. Pre operational
D. Formal operational

58. Response which is graded by an observer on an agree or disagree continuum is based on:

A. Visual analog scale
B. Guttman scale
C. Likert scale
D. Adjectival scale

59. In epidemiological triad which of the following is not included?

A. Agent
B. Host
C. Disease
D. Environment

60. Most commonly used dye in modified Quigley-Hein index is:

A. Bismark green
B. Two tone dye
C. Basic fuschin
D. Diazoresoricinol

61. Didactic refers to:

A. One way communication
B. Two-way communication
C. Telecommunication
D. Verbal

62. Variability is seen in:

A. Variability constant
B. Square of standard deviation
C. Coefficient of variance
D. Confidence interval

63. 1 ppm fluoride means:

A. 1 mg/liter of H_2O
B. 10 mg/liter of H_2O
C. 1 gm/liter of H_2O
D. 1 gm/ml of H_2O

64. For repetitive study, which group is used?

A. Panel group
B. Case control group
C. Cohort group
D. Control group

65. A community having resistance to particular infection shows:

A. Herd immunity B. Active immunity
C. Passive immunity D. Humoral immunity

66. In Grand Rapid Survey (1945) of water fluoridation, which city was used as control?

A. Evanston B. Oakpark
C. Kingston D. Muskegon

67. Under DMFT index which of the following can't be measured?

A. Number of restored teeth
B. Tooth missing due to decay
C. Extent of caries
D. Tooth require restoration

68. Minimum angulation of implant to bone to prevent shear stresses is i.e. To decrease the shear force transmitted to bone, implant angulation should be less than:

A. 15 degree B. 20 degree
C. 25 degree D. 30 degree

69. In FPD patient, while cementing a crown:

A. It is easy to remove because compressive strength of cement is more, shear strength is more
B. It is easy to remove because compressive strength of cement is more, tensile strength is less
C. Cement is the weakest part in prosthesis
D. Increased thickness of cement will cause less flow compared to small thickness

70. Nesbit prosthesis is:

A. Unilateral removable prosthesis
B. Silicone based nasal prosthesis
C. Guidance device for hemi-mandibulectomy patient
D. Ear prosthesis

71. In complete denture patient V sound is used for:

A. Anteroposterior relation of maxillary mandibular teeth
B. Freeway space
C. Closest speaking space
D. Maxillary-mandibular relation of teeth

72. Impression is commonly repeated if:

A. Improper positioning of tray
B. Too less or excess material
C. Voids that is irreparable
D. Improper mixing

73. Enamel is permeable to:

A. Bacteria B. Bacterial products
C. Peroxides D. Retrovirus

74. Enamel loss over molars and incisors is described as:

A. Qualitative
B. Quantitative
C. Post eruptive deformity
D. Quantitative and qualitative

75. 5 outer wires rotated around single axial core is called:

A. Coaxial wire B. Braided wire
C. Twisted wire D. Axial wire

76. Angle's line of occlusion tells malocclusion is in which planes?

A. Sagittal B. Vertical
C. Transverse D. Transverse and vertical

77. For bodily movement, the centre of resistance is:

A. Infinity B. Apical 1/3
C. Mid point of root D. Cervical third

78. Mushroom arch wire is used in:

A. Edge wise B. Begg's
C. Straight wire D. Lingual

79. Difference between total rotation and matrix rotation representing remodelling at the lower border of mandible:

A. Intramatrix rotation
B. Apparent rotation
C. Angular remodelling of lower border
D. Internal rotation

80. The wire which is more ductile and resilient and on heating whose deformation resistance increases:

A. Red elgiloy B. Blue elgiloy
C. Green elgiloy D. Yellow elgiloy

81. Secondary displacement of maxilla is due to:
A. Cortical drift B. Growth at synchondrosis
C. Suture D. Functional matrix

82. Wire used in pendulum appliance:
A. 0.032" TMA B. 0.032" SS
C. 0.036" SS D. 0.036" TMA

83. Which of the following drugs affect orthodontic treatment?
A. Tetracycline B. Aspirin
C. Metronidazole D. Amoxicillin

84. 150 forward rotation of core of mandible, mandibular plane angle will be:
A. Increases 6-8° B. Increases 2-4°
C. Decreases 6-8° D. Decreases 2-4°

85. Which of the following contains primer and bonding agent in a single bottle and is known as "Single Component System"?
A. 3 B. 4
C. 5 D. 6

86. Sinus tract exit on buccal or lingual side depends upon:
A. Approximation of root apex to cortical bone
B. Bone density
C. Thickness of soft tissue
D. Thickness of cortical bone

87. How much G.P. should be left to provide leakage for post placement?
A. 4 mm B. 1 mm
C. 2 mm D. 1.5 mm

88. Filler size in microfilled composite:
A. 0.1-1 mm B. 2-5 mm
C. 0.01-0.04 mm D. 1-0.4 mm

89. In inlay preparation the cavosurface angle is:
A. Right angle B. Beveled
C. Chamfer D. Feather edge

90. Which of the following bacteria do not invade connective tissue?
A. P. Gingivalis B. T. Denticola
C. P. Intermedia D. F. Nucleatum

91. Piezo-electric scaler has wavelength of:
A. 6000-9000 Hz B. 9000-12000 Hz
C. 20000-30000 Hz D. 20000-45000 Hz

92. Glycated Hb test before any periodontal treatment is done for:

A. Anemia B. Controlled diabetes
C. Untreated diabetes D. Haemoglobinopathy

93. Which drug has higher levels in periodontal tissue and has good effect as compared to plasma?

A. Tetracycline B. Augmentin
C. Metronidazole D. Penicillin

94. Bleeding on probing without color change is seen in:

A. Stage I gingivitis B. Stage II gingivitis
C. Stage III gingivitis D. Stage IV gingivitis

95. Flossing method most commonly used is:

A. Winding B. Spiral
C. Spool D. Knutson

96. To reinforce the thin bony trabeculae by occlusal forces, bone formed is:

A. Buttressing bone formation
B. Condensing osteitis
C. Reinforced bone formation
D. Ledge

97. A young patient having bone loss in incisor and molar region with pus discharge and calculus which doesn't respond to antibiotic therapy is suffering from:

A. Local juvenile periodontitis
B. Aggressive periodontitis
C. Refractory periodontitis
D. None

98. In periodontal supportive therapy which is not included?

A. No of teeth < 28
B. Bleeding on probing
C. Furcation involvement
D. Pocket depth > 4 mm

99. Which inflammatory mediator has anti-inflammatory properties?

A. Prostaglandins B. Thromboxanes
C. Leukotrienes D. Lipoxins

100. Which is autoimmune gastritis?

A. Type a B. Type b
C. Type c D. Reflux

Answers

1.	A	2.	B	3.	B	4.	D
5.	C	6.	A	7.	C	8.	D
9.	A	10.	A	11.	C	12.	A
13.	A	14.	B	15.	B	16.	D
17.	B	18.	A	19.	A	20.	B
21.	B	22.	A	23.	A	24.	C
25.	B	26.	A	27.	C	28.	A
29.	A	30.	C	31.	C	32.	A
33.	A	34.	A	35.	A	36.	D
37.	A	38.	A	39.	A	40.	C
41.	B	42.	B	43.	A	44.	C
45.	D	46.	A	47.	C	48.	D
49.	A	50.	A	51.	A	52.	A
53.	B	54.	A	55.	A	56.	C
57.	C	58.	C	59.	C	60.	C
61.	A	62.	B	63.	A	64.	C
65.	A	66.	D	67.	C	68.	C
69.	A	70.	A	71.	A	72.	A
73.	C	74.	B	75.	A	76.	A
77.	C	78.	D	79.	A	80.	B
81.	B	82.	A	83.	B	84.	D
85.	C	86.	A	87.	A	88.	C
89.	B	90.	C	91.	D	92.	B
93.	A	94.	B	95.	C	96.	A
97.	C	98.	C	99.	D	100.	A

PGI Paper
June 2013

1. **Which of the following is a pneumatic bone?**
   A. Maxilla B. Mandible
   C. Nasal D. Occipital

2. **Multipennete order is not seen in which of the following muscle?**
   A. Masseter B. Deltoid
   C. Medial pterygoid D. Temporalis

3. **Which of the following has least regenerative capacity?**
   A. Collagen B. Bone
   C. Liver D. Striated muscle

4. **Not true about osteoporosis is:**
   A. Hypervitaminosis B. Chronic malnutrition
   C. Adult age D. Corticosteroids

5. **For pulmonary maturation which is required during gestation?**
   A. Surfactant B. Acetylcholine
   C. Cortisol D. Meconium

6. **Hair on end appearance is seen in all *except*:**
   A. Sickle cell anaemia
   B. Thalassemia
   C. Cooley anemia
   D. Paget's disease

7. **Inverted 'Y' shape of Ennis seen in which area of radiograph?**
   A. Maxillary central incisor
   B. Maxillary canine region
   C. Maxillary posterior
   D. Mandibular posterior

8. Well developed and properly stored X-ray film look like:

A. Cloudy
B. Total dark
C. Foggy and blue tint
D. Clear and slight blue tint

9. Contrast is effected by:

A. Kvp B. mA
C. Exposure time D. Developing time

10. Number of radiographs film for 6-9 years required for full mouth examination is:

A. 4 B. 12
C. 14 D. 20

11. Film size 0 for bitewing radiograph is:

A. 22 × 35 B. 24 × 32
C. 32 × 36 D. 30 × 40

12. Curettage in furcation area is done by:

A. Nabers probe B. Hu-friedy small 5 curette
C. Universal curette D. Hu-friedy mini 5 curette

13. The metabolite of one of the following is lethal to AA comitans is:

A. S. Sanguis B. S. Mitis
C. S. Mutans D. S. Salivarius

14. Maximum stability while scaling and root treatment is provided by:

A. Scaler B. Hoe scaler
C. Chiael D. Files

15. Calculus present in anterior region of mandible is:

A. Brushite
B. Magnesium whitlockite
C. Calcium phosphate
D. Hydroxyapatite

16. Cul-de-sac is seen in following graduation of furcation:

A. 2 B. 1
C. 3 D. 4

17. All of the following are true *except*:

A. 2/3 mandibular defect-osseous craters
B. 1/3 of all defect are osseous craters

C. 80%- Facial and lingual height of crest have been found to be identical
D. Occurs twice as often in anterior segment as in posterior segment

18. Experimental gingivitis is given by:
A. Loe and Sillness
B. Loe and Thielke
C. Green and Vermellion
D. Ainamo and Bay

19. Actinobacillus actinomycetem commitans attachment of tooth surface can be prevented by:
A. Myeloperoxidase
B. Lactoperoxidase
C. Collagenase
D. Leukotoxin

20. In hemi-mandibulectomy vertical dimension is best determined by:
A. Lips closure and unstrained facial expression
B. Facial silhouette
C. Facial photography
D. All of the above

21. In patient with palatal obturator occlusion plan of complete denture should be:
A. Balanced on affected side
B. Monoplane
C. Lingualized
D. Cusp in fossa

22. Custom tray all true *except*:
A. More accurate than stock trays
B. Do not require much impression material
C. It should be easy to remove
D. It should have similar colour to adjacent tissues

23. The amount of occlusal surface reduction required for gold crown is:
A. 1.5 mm
B. 2 mm
C. 1 mm
D. 0.5 mm

24. All of the following statements are all true *except*:
A. A pterygomaxillary seal extends from hamular notch to mucogingival junction
B. Pterygomaxillary seals covers hamular notch width

C. Pterygomaxillary seal extends distal to maxillary tuberosity
D. Pterygomaxillary seal extend distal to the hamular notch

25. CAD-CAM, time taken in processing of crown:
A. 5 mins B. 20 mins
C. 30 mins D. 60 mins

26. Marginal fit of cast crown is:
A. 100 micron B. 200 micron
C. 300 micron D. 400 micron

27. Most sensitive fluorosis index is among the following:
A. TFI index
B. Community Fluorosis index
C. Deans index
D. Public Health Fluorosis index

28. Which is not a school dental nurse duty?
A. Oral examination B. Prophylaxis
C. Take X-ray D. Fluoride application

29. Most common used in dentifrices:
A. Sodium mono fluorophosphate
B. Sodium difluorophosphate
C. Sodium trifluorophosphate
D. Sodium tetrafluorophosphate

30. Periodic screening and referrals comes under:
A. Primordial prevention
B. Primary prevention
C. Secondary prevention
D. Tertiary prevention

31. Which of the following is a factor common in all component of epidemiology?
A. Agent B. Host
C. Disease D. Environment

32. Gingival bleeding occurs in AINAMO and BAY INDEX is considered positive within:
A. 10 sec B. 20 sec
C. 30 sec D. None

33. Number of teeth examined CPITN of age group under 16-19 years is:
A. 10 B. 6
C. 12 D. 14

34. A test for proportion:
A. Chi square test
B. Student 't' test
C. Anova
D. 'F' test

35. Range of OHI is:
A. 0-6
B. 1-3
C. 0-12
D. 0-6

36. The rectus abdominal graft has a blood supply of:
A. Inferior epigastric artery
B. Iliolumbar artery
C. Superior thoracic artery
D. Thoracoacromian artery

37. All of the following regarding the Ludwig angina are true *except*:
A. Includes sublingual and submaxillary spaces
B. It is mostly bilateral involvement in the nature
C. Mostly dental in origin
D. Spread by lymphatics

38. Interstitial arthroplasty material for TMJ ANKYLOSIS includes all *except*:
A. Osseous graft
B. Buccal fat
C. Temporalis
D. Abdominal pad

39. The location for reduction click of zygomatic fracture is:
A. Infraorbital margin
B. Zygomatico-frontal suture
C. Zygomatico maxillary
D. Zygomatico temporal

40. Radicular cyst is:
A. Developmental
B. Inflammatory
C. Non epithelial
D. Non odontogenic

41. Sagittal split fracture of condyle, treatment is:
A. No treatment
B. Open reduction
C. Closed reduction for 4 weeks
D. Closed reduction of 2 weeks with guided physiotherapy

42. Distraction osteogenesis. True is:
A. Applied when bone growth is not yet completed
B. Synonym is distraction histogenesis
C. No effect on soft tissue
D. Rate of distraction osteogenesis is 4 mm per day

43. In a condylar fracture and bone plate synthesis to counteract the dynamic tension and compression zone. The most acceptable place for plating is:

A. A plate fixed laterally in the neck of condyle
B. One plate on posterior border of condyle only
C. One plate on anterior border and one on posterior pole of condyle

44. Treatment for brown tumour is:

A. Curettage
B. Intralesional steroid
C. Parathyroidectomy
D. Surgical excision

45. All are true about superior orbital syndrome *except*:

A. Blindness
B. Parasthesia
C. Ophthalmoplegia
D. Ptosis

46. Torquing is resisted by denture via:

A. Adhesion
B. Cohesion
C. Adequate border seal
D. Interfacial surface tension

47. Synthetic absorbable suture is:

A. Silk
B. Vicryl
C. Chronic catgut
D. Polypropelene

48. Raccoon eyes are seen in all *except*:

A. Le Fort 1
B. Le Fort 2
C. Le Fort 3
D. Nasoethmoidal fracture

49. Hecks disease is known as:

A. Focal epithelial hyperplasia
B. Dematophyses
C. Lingual Nigrosa
D. Lingua Villosa

50. In hairy tongue which papilla is mostly involved hypertrophied?

A. Fungiform
B. Filiform
C. Circumvallate
D. All

51. Osteopetrosis is also known as:

A. Albers-Schönberg disease
B. Marble bone

C. Gorham disease
D. Both A and B

52. **Most common benign tumor of connective tissue:**
A. Fibroma
B. Papilloma
C. Lipoma
D. Acanthoma

53. **Precancerous potential is not seen in:**
A. Lichen planus
B. Leukoplakia
C. Pemphigus
D. Erythroplakia

54. **Which of the following is true about intraosseous hemangioma?**
A. True neoplasm
B. It is a vascular malformation
C. Surgical treatment should be avoided
D. Most common cause is trauma

55. **Increased salivary secretion seen in:**
A. Acrodynia
B. Bells palsy
C. Gastroesophageal reflex disease
D. All of the above

56. **Radiographic feature of pindborg's tumor is:**
A. Soap bubble appearance
B. Snow driven appearance
C. Sun burst appearance
D. Onion peel appearance

57. **True about cystic fibrosis is:**
A. Increase incidence of caries
B. Increased tendency for staining with systemic fluorides
C. Habit of mouth breathing
D. Higher incidence of children

58. **In preparing a primary molar for a stainless steel crown, the surface requiring the least amount of reduction is:**
A. Occlusal
B. Lingual
C. Mesial
D. Facial

59. **Fear of closed spaces like "dental clinics" is called as:**
A. Nyclophobia
B. Zoophobia
C. Xenophobia
D. Claustrophobia

60. **Riga-Fede's disease seen in:**
A. Infant
B. Children
C. None
D. Adolescent

61. Which of the following is most anticariogenic?

A. Milk B. Cheese
C. Butter D. Tomato

62. According to the Sigmund Freud, mixed dentition and character development occurs in which stage?

A. Oral B. Phallic
C. Latency D. Concrete operational

63. Cvek pulpotomy refers to:

A. Partial pulpotomy
B. Non vital pulpotomy
C. Glutaraldehyde pulpotomy
D. Formocresol pulpotomy

64. Child with IQ of 20-50 called as:

A. Moron B. Imbelicile
C. Genius D. Idiot

65. Stainless steel crown introduced in dentistry by:

A. Humphrey in 1950-1953
B. Davison in 1967, 1988
C. Macmillan in 1987
D. Thomson in 1953

66. Role of peer group is maximum at which age?

A. Pre-adolescence B. Adolescence
C. Teenage D. Juvenile

67. Most common material used for obturation in primary teeth:

A. ZOE B. ZOE and Gutta-percha
C. Gutta-percha D. ZOE plus Calcium hydroxide

68. Low calorigenic sweetner is:

A. Asparatame, lactulose
B. Sucralose, mannitol
C. Asparatame, sucralose
D. Sucralose, mannitol

69. All of the following are features of tetanus *except*:

A. Trismus B. Respiratory failure
C. Coagulopathy D. Opisthotonus

70. Which of the following stage shows negative nitrogen phase?

A. Catabolism B. Anabolism
C. Ebb phase D. None

71. The characteristic changes that follow a major surgical procedure or trauma do not include the following:

A. Hypermetabolism B. Tachypnea
C. Hyperphagia D. Negative nitrogen balance

72. The best diagnostic feature of acute pylonephritis:

A. Bacteremia
B. Focal scar in kidney
C. Fever flecking pain
D. Altered renal function

73. Which will not be used in patient suffering from anaphylactic reaction?

A. Adrenaline injection
B. Antihistaminic
C. Beta adrenergic agonist
D. Blood transfusion

74. The component of irreversible hydrocolloid component which cause allergic reaction is?

A. Phenolpthalein B. Sodium fluorotitanate
C. $CaSO_4$ D. MgO

75. The amount of luting agent to be filled in the crown:

A. ½ of inner cavity of crown
B. 2/3 of inner cavity of the crown
C. Complete filling to eliminate air
D. It should be applied just as liner to inner surface of the crown

76. Alloys used in PCM all are true *except*:

A. Characterized by high sag resistance
B. Have high solidus temperature
C. Coefficient of thermal contraction metal alloys is less than that of porcelain
D. Chemical bond

77. True statement regarding using 50% H_2PO_4 in acid etching for 45 sec is:

A. Type 1 pattern occur
B. Type 2 pattern occur
C. Type 3 pattern occur
D. Adherent monocalcium PO_4 layer

78. Dental lamina arise from which part of gum pad?

A. Transverse groove B. Dental groove
C. Labial groove D. Lingual groove

79. Most common missing permanent teeth:

A. Mandibular second premolar
B. Maxillary 1st molar
C. Mandibular 1st molar
D. Maxillary central incisors

80. In which year child has 6 permanent and 6 deciduous teeth?

A. 4.5 B. 6.5
C. 8.5 D. 11.5

81. False of wound fibroblast is:

A. Derived from blood precursor cell
B. With fibrin form scaffold
C. Thick blood clot prevents fibrin or fibroblast penetration and delay healing
D. Fibroblast forms collagen

82. Which of the following are pure opoid antagonists?

A. Naloxone B. Pentazocine
C. Nalorphine D. Bupenorphine

83. Gates glidden drill used in mid canal region is:

A. 5 B. 2
C. 3 D. 7

84. Agent used to kill Enterococcus fecalis is:

A. Irrigate with normal saline water
B. Irrigate with chlorhexidine 2%
C. Irrigate with CHX + ca (oh)2
D. Irrigate with 5.25% NaOCl

85. Which of the following is true of spreader extension during biochemical preparation?

A. Extends 0.5 mm short of working length
B. Extends 1 short of working length
C. Extends 2 mm short of working length
D. Extends to fullest working length

86. Pain by thermal application on traumatic teeth indicates:

A. Pulpal inflammation
B. Pulpal necrosis

C. Pal inflammation
D. Pal necrosis

87. Least related to pathogenicity of endodontic flora is:
A. Microbial interaction action
B. Endotoxin released by dead bacteria
C. Endotoxin released by living bacteria
D. Enzymes released by bacteria

88. In pin retained restorations, amount of pin in dentine and restoration:
A. 1 mm B. 1.5 mm
C. 2 mm D. 3 mm

89. "C" shaped configuration is seen in:
A. Maxillary 1st molar
B. Mandibular 1st premolar
C. Maxillary 1st premolar
D. Mandibular 1st molar

90. Form and function concept of craniofacial structure was given by:
A. Petrovic B. Scott's
C. Enlow and Bang D. Moss

91. Anderson gave which wire?
A. Nitinol B. Chinese niti
C. TMA D. Beta titanium

92. Primary bone grafting done in:
A. 6 months-1 year B. < 2 years
C. 2-4 years D. 4-15 years

93. The terminology forward and backward rotators is given by:
A. Shudy B. Profitt
C. Bjork and Skeiller D. Solow and Houston

94. Corpus rotation w.r.t cranium is used:
A. Matrix B. Internal rotation
C. Intramatrix D. Apparent rotation

95. Rotation centered within the body of the mandible is called as:
A. Apparent rotation B. True rotation
C. Total rotation D. Intramatrix

96. Root shape before and after ortho treatment with radiographic evidence is first given by:

A. Ketcham AH
B. Malmgren and Levander
C. Kaley and Philips
D. Newman and Profitt

97. Orthodontic treatment done in mixed dentition for class II dental malocclusion so that it itself correct skeletal II:

A. RME device
B. Serial extraction
C. Hawley appliance with anterior bite plane
D. None of the above

98. Average enamel lost by acid etching:

A. 3-10 micron
B. 10-15 micron
C. 1-5 micron
D. 20-30 micron

99. Tooth positioned is used as a retainer in posterior teeth. Most beneficial effect is:

A. Esthetics due to its clearness
B. Gingival massage inflamed during orthodontic treatment
C. Final settling of occlusion
D. Used in uncooperative patient

100. Permanent canines are palatally deflected if:

A. A mild space discrepancy
B. Moderate space discrepancy
C. Severe discrepancy of space
D. Lateral incisor anomalous

Answers

1.	A	2.	D	3.	D	4.	A
5.	A	6.	D	7.	B	8.	D
9.	A	10.	C	11.	A	12.	D
13.	A	14.	B	15.	D	16.	A
17.	D	18.	B	19.	A	20.	A
21.	B	22.	D	23.	C	24.	D
25.	B	26.	A	27.	A	28.	C
29.	A	30.	C	31.	C	32.	A
33.	B	34.	A	35.	C	36.	A
37.	D	38.	A	39.	A	40.	B
41.	D	42.	A	43.	C	44.	D
45.	A	46.	C	47.	B	48.	A
49.	A	50.	B	51.	D	52.	A
53.	C	54.	D	55.	D	56.	B
57.	B	58.	B	59.	D	60.	A
61.	B	62.	C	63.	A	64.	B
65.	A	66.	C	67.	A	68.	C
69.	C	70.	A	71.	C	72.	C
73.	D	74.	A	75.	A	76.	C
77.	D	78.	B	79.	A	80.	C
81.	A	82.	A	83.	C	84.	B
85.	C	86.	A	87.	C	88.	C
89.	D	90.	D	91.	A	92.	B
93.	C	94.	B	95.	D	96.	A
97.	C	98.	A	99.	B	100.	D

PGI Paper
December 2012

1. **Regarding periosteum which of the following is false?**
   - A. Inner layer is called cambium layer
   - B. Outer layer is fibrous
   - C. Inner layer consists of osteo-progenitor cells
   - D. Single layered

2. **Keisselbach's plexus is present:**
   - A. Anteroinferior surface of nasal septum
   - B. Anterosuperior surface of nasal septum
   - C. Anteroinferior surface of lateral nasal septum
   - D. Anterosuperior surface of lateral nasal septum

3. **Muller's muscle is:**
   - A. Muscles of nasal tip
   - B. Muscles of upper eyelid
   - C. Muscles of lower eyelid
   - D. Muscles of medial canthus

4. **Medial pterygoid palpation is done:**
   - A. At rest position
   - B. Close mouth
   - C. Mouth open as wide as possible
   - D. Half open with mandible movement to opposite side

5. **Which of the following contributes to the buccinator mechanism?**
   - A. Superior constrictor
   - B. Inferior constrictor
   - C. Middle constrictor
   - D. Palatopharyngeus

6. **Classification of malocclusion according to etiology was given by:**
   - A. Angle
   - B. Lischer
   - C. Bennett
   - D. Dewey

7. **Remodeling theory of Craniofacial Growth was given by:**
   A. Vander CLAUF B. Sicher
   C. Brash D. John Hunter

8. **In Moyer's classification, type D class II indicates:**
   A. Orthognathic Mandible and Maxilla
   B. Prognathic Maxilla, Orthognathic Mandible
   C. Orthognathic Maxilla, Retrognathic Mandible
   D. Retrognathic Maxilla, Retrognathic Mandible

9. **Maximum familial tendency is seen in:**
   A. Protruded max. incisors
   B. Deep bite
   C. Open bite
   D. Cross bite

10. **Lip thickness of males is maximum at which age?**
    A. 21 years B. 18 years
    C. 16 years D. 25 years

11. **Ratio of width of nose to height of nose is:**
    A. 62% B. 65%
    C. 66% D. 70%

12. **Attritional theory of malocclusion was given by:**
    A. P.R. Begg B. Tweed
    C. Story and Smith D. Angle

13. **Resorption of which will not occur during high intermittent force application?**
    A. Enamel resorption
    B. Dentin resorption
    C. Cementum resorption
    D. Bone resorption

14. **Collum angle increased in:**
    A. Bimaxillary protrusion
    B. Class II div 1
    C. Class II div 2
    D. Mandibular retrusion

15. **In pendulum appliance, at 90 degree activation how much force is generated?**
    A. 75 gm B. 125 gm
    C. 250 gm D. 350 gm

16. According to Fishman skeletal maturity indicator how many sites are involved?

A. 4 B. 6
C. 10 D. 8

17. %age of cranial cavity formed in a 5 years child:

A. 78% B. 82%
C. 90% D. 98%

18. Earnest Klein has classified habits into:

A. Compulsive and non-compulsive
B. Intentional and non-intentional habits
C. Primary and secondary
D. Pressure and non-pressure

19. Archial analysis facial type III include:

A. Anterior cranial base plane doesn't pass through O
B. Palatal plane doesn't pass through O
C. Mandibular plane doesn't pass through O
D. Occlusal plane doesn't pass through O

20. During orthodontic treatment tooth movement is inhibited by using:

A. RANK B. RANKL
C. OPG-FC D. Vitamin K

21. Epigenetic factors controlling the growth of skeleton are:

A. Genetic factors present within the skeleton
B. Genetic factors present outside the skeleton
C. Local non-genetic factors
D. General non-genetic factors

22. Development of face occurs in the following planes:

A. Transverse Sagittal Vertical
B. Sagittal Vertical, Transverse
C. Sagittal Transverse, Vertical
D. Vertical Transverse Sagittal

23. At what age, maxillary intercanine dimension is essentially complete in boys and girls during growth?

A. 15 years in boys and 10 years in girls
B. 10 years in boys and 12 years in girls
C. 18 years in boys and 12 years in girls
D. 15 years in boys and 15 years in girls

24. In periodontally compromised tooth, which of the following movements is done very carefully?

A. Tipping
B. Intrusion
C. Uprighting
D. Proclination

25. Sure Smile Commercial Orthodontic service is related to:

A. Cleft palate and lip care
B. Smile designing
C. Clear retainer
D. Customized band prescription arch wire

26. Which of the following is not present on the mandible?

A. Porion
B. Pogonion
C. Menton
D. Gonion

27. Behavior shaping includes all *except*:

A. Desensitization
B. Contingency management
C. Modelling
D. Voice control

28. Operant conditioning theory was given by:

A. Pavlov
B. Skinner
C. Freund
D. Massler

29. The term Pedodontic triangle was given by:

A. Finn
B. Wright
C. McDonald
D. Jordan

30. Atraumatic restorative treatment (ART) was first given by:

A. McLean
B. McDonald
C. McLevan
D. McKay

31. Newborn infant is:

A. Obligatory nasal breather
B. Obligatory mouth breather
C. Obstructive nasal breather
D. Obligatory mouth breather

32. Permanent and deciduous teeth can be differentiated by:

A. Size of the teeth
B. Thickness of enamel and dentin
C. Direction of enamel rods cervically
D. Direction of roots below CEJ

33. Role of peer group is maximum at which age?
A. Pre-adolescence B. Adolescence
C. Teenage D. Juvenile

34. In a 9 years old child, an hour old Ellis Class III fracture with a small pulp exposure. Treatment is:
A. Direct pulp capping
B. Pulpotomy
C. Pulpectomy
D. Apexification

35. Most common material used for obturation in primary teeth:
A. ZOE B. ZOE and Gutta-percha
C. Gutta-percha D. ZOE plus Calcium hydroxide

36. Bond between tooth surface and pit and fissure sealants is:
A. Mechanical
B. Chemical
C. Chemical and Mechanical
D. None

37. Retention of stainless steel crown is mainly by:
A. Chamfer
B. Shoulder
C. Parallel mesial and distal walls
D. Crimping

38. Non-invasive method to measure blood flow is:
A. Electric pulp test
B. Percussion
C. Radiograph
D. Laser Doppler Flowmetry

39. Size of rubber dam sheet used for pedo patient:
A. 5 × 5" B. 6 × 6"
C. 3 × 3" D. 8 × 8"

40. Fear from strangers that fear of dentist on first visit:
A. Xenophobia B. Acrophobia
C. Arthrophobia D. Claustrophobia

41. According to the Sigmund Freud, mixed dentition and character development occurs in which stage?
A. Oral B. Phallic
C. Latency D. Concrete operational

42. Fear of child patient related to dentistry is primarily:
A. Subjective
B. Objective
C. Subjective and objective
D. Psychological

43. Lap to Lap position is used at the age of:
A. 0-1 years
B. 1-3 years
C. 4-5 years
D. 6-7 years

44. Odontogenic keratocyst now called as:
A. Odontogenic ghost cell cyst
B. Dentigerous cyst
C. Keratocystic odontogenic tumor
D. Both A and B

45. Which of the following is true about intraosseous-hemangioma?
A. Dental extraction can cause exsanguinations
B. It is a vascular malformation
C. Surgical treatment should be avoided
D. Most common cause is trauma

46. Radiographic feature of pindborg's tumor is:
A. Soap bubble appearance
B. Snow driven appearance
C. Sun burst appearance
D. Onion peel appearance

47. Stress can be one of the cause of following conditions *except*:
A. OSMF
B. Lichen planus
C. Syphilis
D. Pemphigus

48. Submucosal cleft is best seen by:
A. Clinical laminography
B. Cephalographic laminography
C. Palpation
D. Lateral cephalogram

49. In Dentinogenesis imperfecta Type II which is not true:
A. Early exposure of pulp due to high pulp horn
B. Decreased diameter of dentinal tubule
C. DEJ shape changes/defective DEJ shape
D. Attrition of teeth occur/wear of teeth occurs at early ages

50. Critical temperature above which necrosis of bone occurs?

A. 60°C B. 47°C
C. 30°C D. 55°C

51. Ocular dystopia is:

A. Unequal size of pupil
B. Unequal level of pupil
C. Increased distance between medial canthus
D. Double vision

52. Anisocoria is:

A. Unequal size of pupil
B. Unequal level of pupil
C. Increased distance between medial canthus
D. Double vision

53. Raccoon eyes are seen in all *except*:

A. Le Fort 1 B. Le Fort 2
C. Le Fort 3 D. Nasoethmoidal fracture

54. All are used after condylectomy as inter-positional graft material *except*:

A. Abdominal fat pad B. Osseous graft
C. Buccal pad of fat D. Temporal fascia

55. Jacob's disease:

A. Syngnathia
B. Hemifacial microsomia
C. Unilateral enlargement of tongue
D. Osteochondroma

56. Distance between implant shoulder and facial curvature of arch at the level of gingival margin should be:

A. 1 mm B. 1.5 mm
C. 2 mm D. 3 mm

57. In a fracture champy line extended upto condyle; line of treatment will be:

A. One miniplate B. Two miniplate
C. Lag screw D. No fixation of condyle

58. After inferior alveolar nerve block [IANB] the success of block is checked at:

A. Attached gingiva unilaterally from midline to premolar
B. Attached gingiva unilaterally from midline to molar

C. Attached gingiva unilaterally posterior to premolar
D. Gingiva of tooth to be extracted

59. Which of the following method is not used in the treatment of TMJ ankylosis?
A. Ipsilateral condylectomy
B. Inter-positional gap arthoplasty
C. High condylar shave
D. Contralateral condylectomy

60. The roof of pterygomandibular space is formed by:
A. Temporalis muscle
B. Medial pterygoid
C. Cranial base
D. Lateral pterygoid

61. Which of the following is not used in the treatment of OSMF?
A. Chondroitin sulphate
B. Hyaluronidase
C. Corticosteroids intra-lesional
D. Pentoxyphyline

62. Keen's technique used in zygomatic complex fracture is:
A. Gillies extraoral temporal approach
B. Intraoral approach through an incision in buccal sulcus
C. Extraoral approach through stab incision in cheek
D. Disimpaction of maxilla

63. Initial clicking in TMJ while opening is due to:
A. Condyle in anterior position ahead of disc
B. Disc in anterior position ahead of condyle
C. Perforated disc
D. Rough surface of eminence

64. For a 9 years old child with TMJ ankylosis the treatment of choice is:
A. Gap Arthroplasty
B. Condylectomy
C. Gap Arthroplasty with costochondral graft
D. Treatment not required in such cases

65. Supraperiosteal plating is done in:
A. Condylar fracture
B. Geriatrics patient
C. Pedo patient
D. Communited fracture

66. Which of the following is not considered in TNM staging?

A. Tumor size B. Tumor size
C. Lymph node size D. Metastasis

67. Distance between occlusal level and residual alveolar ridge for implant supported overdenture is:

A. 12 mm B. 10 mm
C. 15 mm D. 18 mm

68. Which is not considered as 3rd point in face bow?

A. Orbitale B. Menton
C. Alar of nose D. Nasion

69. In case of implant placement which metal should not be used for screwing of abutment analogue?

A. Stainless steel B. Co-Cr
C. Brass D. Cp-Titanium

70. Which of the following procedures done first after transferring face how records to articulator?

A. Articulate maxillary case first
B. Articulate mandibular case first
C. Both simultaneously at CR position
D. Both simultaneously at protrusive position

71. Fastest and most appropriate method of recording condylar axis is:

A. Kinematic B. Earpiece
C. Fascia type D. None

72. In microwave curing of resin denture residual monomer content is:

A. Less than 1% B. Greater than 1%
C. Less than 10% D. Greater than 10%

73. Head position of patient during recording the centric relation is:

A. Upright
B. Supine
C. Neutral head position (NHP)
D. None

74. For rest position of mandible which is not true?

A. It is constant
B. It is highly variable
C. Varies with stress
D. Not reliable for the measurement of vertical dimension of occlusion

75. For denture stability all of the following are done *except*:

A. Harmonious occlusion
B. Improved fit
C. Proper extension
D. Increase weight of mandibular denture

76. Which of the following is an objective for guided prosthesis?

A. Restoration of speech
B. Restoration of esthetics
C. Establishment of occlusion and proprioception
D. Help in swallowing

77. Neutral zone phenomenon is seen in:

A. Multiple CD patients
B. Multiple, unstable, less retentive CD patients
C. Combination syndrome
D. Multiple failed cast partial denture cases

78. Calcification of permanent molar starts:

A. At 1st week of uterine life
B. At birth
C. 6 months after birth
D. 10 months after birth

79. Odontoblasts show inward movement of the tubules when:

A. Mechanical irritation
B. Overheating
C. Dehydration of dentine
D. None

80. Pulp horn exposure in deciduous teeth:

A. MB horn of maxillary first molar
B. MB horn of maxillary second molar
C. DB horn of maxillary first molar
D. DB horn of maxillary second molar

81. If the adult dose is 30 mg. Age of child is 3 years, then child dose is:

A. 5 mg B. 6 mg
C. 10 mg D. 12 mg

82. Long-term intake of corticosteroids lead to:

A. Congestive heart failure
B. Osteoporosis

C. Hypertension
D. Renal failure

83. All of the following are false about fluoride fluxes *except*:
A. They are protective fluxes
B. They remove only stable oxides
C. They dissolve gold alloys
D. They are type III fluxes

84. Which of the following has coefficient of thermal expansion closest to dentin?
A. Amalgam
B. Alumina porcelain
C. Silicane
D. Bio-commercial titanium

85. In dilatants material; how viscosity is related to shear strain rate:
A. Increases with decrease in shear strain rate
B. Increases with increase in shear strain rate
C. Viscosity remains same
D. Increases at some rate and then becomes constant

86. Durometer is used to:
A. Measure hardness of O ring
B. Initial hardness of POP
C. Thickness of dura mater
D. None

87. Which of the following is most accurate method for rinsing gypsum cast?
A. Water bath saturated with disinfectant
B. Water bath saturated with calcium sulphate
C. Under running water till 20 minutes
D. Water at the room temperature

88. In comparison with admixed and low copper silver amalgam alloy one hour compressive strength of single composition alloy is:
A. Four times
B. Double
C. Half
D. One fourth

89. Pin-hole porosity is:
A. Due to inclusion of hydrogen ion
B. Due to inclusion of oxygen ion
C. Prevented by flaring the sprue
D. Lower casting temperature or mould temperature

90. Increased humidity in environment manifested the first effect in POP as:

A. Color changes
B. Increased setting time
C. Decreased setting time
D. None

91. Adhesive used in special tray for elastomeric impression material is for the purpose of:

A. Interchange between elastomers
B. Influence the uniform polymerization of impression
C. Minimize the distortion on removal
D. None

92. Which one of the following is least accurate method of Inlay wax pattern?

A. Directly in the mouth
B. Indirect over the die/tooth
C. Direct/Indirect
D. Type of wax

93. Coronoid fracture best seen on which radiograph?

A. Postero-anterior view of skull
B. Water's view
C. Lateral skull view
D. Reverse town view

94. Most common cause seen in all shocks is:

A. Tachycardia
B. Bradycardia
C. Fluid loss
D. Hypoperfusion

95. Matted lymph nodes are seen in:

A. Sarcoidosis
B. Hodgkin lymphoma
C. Tuberculosis
D. Non-Hodgkin lymphoma

96. Critical factor for pulp integrity during cavity preparation is:

A. Heat generation
B. Vibrations
C. Pressure/load
D. Speed of bur

97. Which of the following fracture has best prognosis?

A. Cervical root fracture
B. Apical root fracture
C. Middle root fracture
D. None

98. Sutton's disease is:

A. Major apthous ulcers
B. Minor apthous ulcers
C. Recurrent herpetiform ulcers
D. All of these

99. Palatal perforation is seen in case of:

A. Tertiary syphilis
B. Major apthous
C. Scrofula
D. Sialadenitis

100. Which of the following is not significant doing immediately after trauma?

A. Radiographic examination
B. Clinical examination
C. Pulp vitality testing
D. History taking

Answers

1.	D	2.	A	3.	B	4.	C
5.	A	6.	C	7.	C	8.	C
9.	B	10.	B	11.	D	12.	A
13.	A	14.	C	15.	C	16.	B
17.	C	18.	B	19.	D	20.	C
21.	B	22.	A	23.	C	24.	B
25.	D	26.	A	27.	D	28.	B
29.	B	30.	A	31.	A	32.	B
33.	C	34.	A	35.	A	36.	A
37.	C	38.	D	39.	A	40.	A
41.	C	42.	A	43.	B	44.	C
45.	A	46.	B	47.	C	48.	C
49.	B	50.	B	51.	B	52.	A
53.	A	54.	B	55.	D	56.	B
57.	B	58.	A	59.	C	60.	D
61.	A	62.	B	63.	B	64.	C
65.	B	66.	A	67.	A,B	68.	B
69.	D	70.	A	71.	B	72.	A
73.	A	74.	A	75.	D	76.	C
77.	B	78.	B	79.	C	80.	A
81.	B	82.	B	83.	D	84.	D
85.	B	86.	A	87.	B	88.	B
89.	B	90.	C	91.	C	92.	B
93.	A	94.	D	95.	C	96.	A
97.	B	98.	A	99.	A	100.	C

PGI Paper

June 2012

1. **Hyaline cartilage is developed from:**
   A. Ectoderm B. Endoderm
   C. Mesoderm D. Ectomesoderm

2. **Platysma is supplied by:**
   A. Cervical branch of facial nerve
   B. Cervical branch of accessory nerve
   C. Ansacervicalis
   D. Mandibular nerve

3. **Submandibular ganglion is anatomically related to:**
   A. Hypoglossal nerve
   B. Chorda tympani nerve
   C. Facial nerve
   D. Lingual nerve

4. **Period of embryo is:**
   A. Fertilization to 2 weeks
   B. 2-8 weeks
   C. 8 weeks to birth
   D. 4-16 weeks

5. **Hemifacial microsomia occurs during:**
   A. Formation of germ layer
   B. Migration of neural crest cells
   C. Formation of organ system
   D. Final differentiation of tissue

6. **Whole blood is stored at:**
   A. 0 °C B. 4-8 °C
   C. 18-22 °C D. At room temperature

7. **Tremors on movement (intention tremors) is seen in:**
   A. Spinal cord injury B. Internal capsule injury
   C. Thalamus injury D. Cerebellum injury

8. **Methemoglobinemia is caused by which of the following drugs?**
   A. Phenacetin
   B. Paraphenitidin
   C. Desferrioxamine
   D. Paracetamol

9. **Fetal alcohol syndrome occurs during:**
   A. Formation of germ layers and initial organization of structure
   B. At the time of organ formation
   C. Neural tube formation
   D. Final differentiation of tissue

10. **Glycated Hb test before initiating periodontal treatment is done for:**
   A. Anemia
   B. Hemoglobinopathy
   C. Untreated diabetes
   D. Controlled diabetes

11. **Prolonged carbohydrate deficiency leads to:**
   A. Ketoacidosis
   B. Metabolic alkalosis
   C. Vitamin C deficiency
   D. Respiratory acidosis

12. **Mucin is a:**
   A. Nucleoprotein
   B. Glycoprotein
   C. Phosphoprotein
   D. Chromoprotein

13. **Which of the following is associated with prolonged drug use or which of the following is drug induced anemia?**
   A. Nutritional anemia
   B. Aplastic anemia
   C. Pernicious anemia
   D. Hemolytic anemia

14. **In hypertension, end organ involvement depends upon:**
   A. Systolic blood pressure
   B. Diastolic blood pressure
   C. Mean capillary blood pressure
   D. Decreased elasticity of blood vessel

15. **Pansystolic Murmur is a feature of all of the following *except*:**
   A. Mitral stenosis
   B. Mitral regurgitation
   C. Ventricular septal defect
   D. Atrial septal defect

16. **In epidemiological triad which of the following is not included?**
A. Agent B. Host
C. Disease D. Environment

17. **DMFT score by 2025 will be:**
A. 2 B. 1.5
C. 1 D. 0

18. **Toxoid is given in:**
A. Oral polio vaccine B. Hepatitis A
C. Rabies D. Diphtheria

19. **A community having resistance to particular infection shows:**
A. HERD immunity B. Passive immunity
C. Active immunity D. Humoral immunity

20. **Didactic refers to:**
A. One way communication
B. Two way communication
C. Verbal
D. Telecommunication

21. **Screening is a better indicator of:**
A. Sensitivity B. Specificity
C. Reliability D. Validity

22. **Knutson technique uses:**
A. NaF B. SnF2
C. Duraphat D. APF

23. **2% NaF is:**
A. Slightly acidic in nature
B. Acidic in nature
C. Basic in nature
D. Neutral

24. **In Grand Rapid Survey (1945) of water fluoridation, which city was used as control?**
A. Evanston B. Oakpark
C. Kingston D. Muskegon

25. **Salt fluoridation uses:**
A. 250 mg/kg of salt
B. 100 mg/kg of salt
C. 700 mg/kg of salt
D. 50 mg/kg of salt

26. **1 ppm fluoride means/amount of fluoride in 1 ppm:**
A. 1mg/liter of H_2O B. 1 gram/liter of H_2O
C. 1 gram/ml of H_2O D. 1 mg/ml of H_2O

27. **Measure to prevent the emergence or development or risk factors of a distance in a community:**
A. Primary prevention
B. Secondary prevention
C. Tertiary prevention
D. Primordial prevention

28. **For repetitive study, which group is used?**
A. Panel group
B. Cohort group
C. Case control group
D. Control group

29. **Which of the following country have 100% artificially fluoridated water?**
A. Spain and France B. Thailand and Polland
C. Thailand and Spain D. Hong Kong and Singapore

30. **Preterm baby is referred to:**
A. Babies born before the end of 37 weeks
B. Babies born before the end of 30 weeks
C. Babies born at completion of 42 weeks
D. Babies born before the end of 38 weeks

31. **Discoloration of tooth in tetracycline therapy is due to formation of:**
A. Calcium orthophosphate
B. Dicalcium phosphate dehydrate
C. Calcium oxide
D. Tetracalcium phosphate

32. **Pulse oximetry is used:**
A. Laser wavelength for estimation of blood flow
B. Probe with diode is used to measure oxygen saturation
C. Blood volume
D. Blood coefficient

33. **Most common injury in child:**
A. Complicated crown fracture
B. Crown root fracture
C. Root fracture
D. Luxation

34. Self inflicted bites are seen in:

A. Lesch-Nyhan syndrome
B. Friese Maria syndrome
C. Beckwith-Wiedemann syndrome
D. Cockanye syndrome

35. From mixed dentition to permanent dentition arch length:

A. Increases
B. Decreases
C. Increases the decreases
D. Remains same

36. Initiation of calcification of 2nd maxillary lateral incisor begins in:

A. 4th month in utero
B. 3-4 months after birth
C. 10-12 months after birth
D. 4-5 years after birth

37. Most mature enamel is found at:

A. Incisal edge and cusp tip
B. Cervical region
C. Middle region
D. Apical region

38. Incidence of 3rd root in upper 1st premolar:

A. Less than 1% B. 6%
C. 10% D. 12%

39. In IOPA image magnification can be reduced by:

A. Long cone
B. Short cone
C. Film place away from object
D. Film placed near to tooth

40. Proximal caries is best detected by:

A. IOPA B. Bitewing
C. Occlusal D. Panoramic

41. Hair or end appearance is seen in all *except*:

A. Cooley's anemia B. Thalassemia
C. Paget's disease D. Sickle cell anemia

42. Crowe's sign is seen in:

A. Von Recklinghausen's disease of bone
B. Von Recklinghausen's disease of skin
C. Fracture of mandible
D. Cholecystitis

43. Brown tumour in hyperparathyroidism resembles:

A. Vascular malformation
B. Giant cell granuloma
C. Benign tumour
D. Malignant tumour

44. Which of the following is true?

A. Grading of tumour based upon metastasis
B. Grade I means poorly differentiated tumour
C. Less in numerical value less in the tumour differentiation
D. More number of cells, nuclear pleomorphism, decreased production of keratin shows highly differentiated tumour

45. For myositis ossificans, main cause is:

A. Infection
B. Trauma
C. Benign pathology
D. Hereditary

46. Grinspan syndrome includes:

A. Leukoplakia
B. Lichen planus
C. Pemphigus
D. Pemphigoid

47. True about lichen planus:

A. More common in females in ratio of female : male = 3 : 2
B. Prevalence in general population is 3.7 to 5.8%
C. Skin lesions occur commonly on extensor surfaces of limbs
D. Hepatitis C is commonly seen in it

48. Sutton's disease is:

A. Major aphthous ulcer
B. Minor aphthous ulcer
C. Herpetiform ulcer
D. All options

49. Which of the following occurs in OSMF?

A. Vesicles, melanosis and xerostomia
B. Stomatopyrosis
C. Blanched, pallor, hard, subepithelial stiffness
D. All of these

50. OSMF occurs due to:

A. Tobacco
B. Alcohol
C. Areca nut
D. None of these

51. Percentage of cleft lip and palate in total cases of cleft:

A. 10
B. 30
C. 80
D. 50

52. A 9-year-old child with fever 38 °C, vesicles involving palate, posterior oropharyngeal wall is suffering from:

A. Herpangina
B. Herpetic gingivostomatitis
C. Diphtheria
D. None

53. Ameloblastoma originates from:

A. Odontogenic epithelium
B. Odontogenic ectomesenchyme
C. Mixed tumour
D. It is not a tumor but is an odontogenic cyst

54. Not a feature of cavernous sinus thrombosis:

A. Evidence of septicemia
B. Known site of infection
C. Signs of venous obstruction in the retina, conjunctiva or eye lid
D. Evidence of meningeal irriation

55. Which of the following is correct about facial nerve?

A. UMN lesion affects ipsilateral lower half
B. UMN lesion affects contralateral lower half
C. LMN affects contralateral complete half of face
D. LMN affects ipsilateral lower half

56. Best radiographic view for condyle and ramus fracture:

A. Water's view
B. Towne's view
C. Reverse Towne's view
D. Caldwell view

57. Antimongoloid slant is a feature of which fracture?

A. Lefort 1
B. Lefort 2
C. Lefort 3
D. Naso-orbito-ethmoid fracture

58. Which of the following is not done in treatment of ankylosis?

A. High condylar shave
B. Ipsilateral coronoidectomy
C. Contralateral coronoidectomy
D. Repositioning of temporal fascia

59. While extracting maxillary 3rd molar which position is not possible?

A. 12'O clock
B. 9'O clock
C. 11'O clock
D. 1'O clock

60. Pregnant female patient in third trimester is kept in:

A. Left lateral decubitus
B. Right lateral decubitus
C. Supine
D. Sitting

61. Cidex contains:

A. Formaldehyde
B. Gluteraldehyde
C. Hypochlorite
D. Phenol

62. Pulp polyp is:

A. Chronic hyperplastic pulpitis
B. Irreversible pulpitis
C. Reversible pulpitis
D. All

63. G.P. is best sterilized by:

A. Full concentration of sodium hypochlorite
B. Ethyl alcohol
C. Dry heat
D. Hot salt sterilizer

64. Hot tooth is:

A. Tooth in line of fracture
B. Vertical line fracture
C. Difficult to anaesthetize
D. Very sensitive to heat test

65. How much G.P. should be left to prevent leakage for post placement?

A. 1 mm
B. 4 mm
C. 2 mm
D. 1.5 mm

66. After a major oral surgery, the phase of acute injury catabolic phase lasts for:

A. 1-2 days B. 2-5 days
C. 4-7 days D. 5-10 days

67. Vitremer is:

A. Polyacid modified composites
B. Organically modified composites
C. Metal modified GIC
D. Resin modified GIC

68. Filler size in microfilled composite is:

A. 0.1-1 m B. 2-4 m
C. 0.01-0.04 m D. 1-5 m

69. Amount of fluoride in amalgam:

A. 10% $SanF_2$ B. 1% SnF_2
C. 8% SnF_2 D. 1% NaF

70. In inlay preparation the cavosurface angle is

A. Right angle B. Beveled
C. Feather edge D. Chamfer

71. A-Suffix for Rubber Dam denotes

A. Deciduous teeth B. Partially erupting teeth
C. Winged clamp D. Wingless clamp

72. Advantage of NiTi over K-files:

A. Increased flexibility
B. Resistance to breakage
C. Low resiliency
D. Not recalled

73. Which of the following drugs affect orthodontic treatment?

A. Tetracycline B. Metronidazole
C. Aspirin D. Amoxycillin

74. APDI is:

A. 81.4 + 3.79 B. 89.3 + 4.79
C. 78.4 + 3.79 D. 91.2 + 3.27

75. For bodily movement centre of resistance is:

A. Infinity B. Mid-point of root
C. Cervical third D. Apical third

76. In pendulum appliance which wire is used:

A. 0.032" TMA
B. 0.032" SS (Stainless steel)
C. 0.036" SS
D. 0.036" TMA

77. Angle's line of occlusion tells malocclusion in which direction?

A. Sagittal
B. Vertical
C. Transverse
D. Transverse and vertical

78. Secondary displacement of maxilla is due to:

A. Suture
B. Functional matrix
C. Drift
D. Growth at synchondrosis

79. Centre of Resistance of 6 Maxillary anterior teeth is:

A. Midline between two central incisor
B. Between central and lateral incisor
C. Between 1st and 2nd premolar
D. Between canine and premolar

80. Velar sound like k.g.ng useful to check:

A. Interference in palatal thickness
B. Vertical dimension of occlusion
C. Freeway space
D. Have no effect on denture

81. In complete denture patient V sound is used for determining:

A. Anteroposterior relation of maxillary mandibular teeth
B. Freeway space
C. Closest speaking space
D. Vertical relationship

82. Altered cast technique is used in:

A. Class II
B. Class III
C. Class II Modification 2
D. Class IV

83. Widest PPS is seen in:

A. Class I
B. Class II
C. Class III
D. Varies according to operator's experience

84. Precision attachment are given in:

A. For extra retention

B. Distal extension denture base
C. Edentulous area with periodontally stable teeth anterior and posteriorly
D. Where abutment teeth with large pulp chamber

85. Frequency curve or probability curve resembles:
A. Curve of Monson B. Anti Monson
C. Curve of Spee D. Curve of Wilson

86. Impression is repeated most commonly when:
A. Improper positioning of tray
B. Too less or excess material
C. Voids that are irrepairable
D. Improper mixing

87. Nesbit prosthesis is:
A. Removable prosthesis
B. Silicon based nasal prosthesis
C. Guidance device or hemimandibulectomy patient
D. Ear prosthesis

88. Minimum protrusion required for condylar guidance adjustment:
A. 3 mm B. 4 mm
C. 6 mm D. 8 mm

89. Bleeding on probing without color change is seen in:
A. Stage I gingivitis B. Stage II gingivitis
C. Stage III gingivitis D. Stage IV gingivitis

90. First implant system developed:
A. Noble Biocare-Branemark
B. ITI-Strauman
C. Nobel Biocare-Sterrioss
D. Astra

91. A child is having bone loss around molars and incisor region with pus discharge and calculus which can't be treated by medication is suffering from:
A. Aggressive Periodontitis
B. Juvenile Periodontitis
C. Refractory Periodontitis
D. None

92. Stillman and Bass method is:
A. Vibratory B. Roll
C. Vertical D. Scrub

93. **Which drug has higher levels in periodontal tissue and has good effect as compared to plasma?**
A. Metronidazole B. Penicillin
C. Amoxycillin D. Tetracycline

94. **Chromium when added to steel does not:**
A. Increase corrosion resistance
B. Increases hardness
C. Decrease elastic limit
D. Increase tensile strength

95. **Which of the following wires does not obey Hook's law?**
A. TMA B. Nitimol
C. A-NiTi D. M-NiTi

96. **Supernumerary teeth is seen in all *except*:**
A. Apert's syndrome B. Down syndrome
C. Sickel syndrome D. Gardner syndrome

97. **In treatment of ANUG which of the following is not indicated on first days?**
A. Subgingival scaling
B. Ultrasonic scaling
C. Topical anaesthetic
D. Removal of pseudomembrane

98. **Piezo electric scaler has a wavelength of:**
A. 6000-9000 Hz B. 9000-12000 Hz
C. 20000-30000 Hz D. 20000-45000 Hz

99. **Modified gingival index with moderate inflammation glazing, redness, edema/or hypertrophy of marginal or papillary gingiva. Score will be:**
A. 1 B. 2
C. 3 D. 4

100. **Probe enters buccally and reaches palatally or distally and is covered by soft tissue denoted by:**
A. Grade I furcation B. Grade II furcation
C. Grade III furcation D. Grade IV furcation

Answers

1.	C	2.	A	3.	D	4.	B
5.	B	6.	B	7.	D	8.	B
9.	A	10.	D	11.	A	12.	B
13.	B	14.	B	15.	A	16.	C
17.	C	18.	D	19.	A	20.	A
21.	A	22.	A	23.	D	24.	D
25.	A	26.	A	27.	D	28.	B
29.	D	30.	A	31.	A	32.	B
33.	D	34.	A	35.	B	36.	C
37.	A	38.	B	39.	A	40.	B
41.	C	42.	B	43.	B	44.	A
45.	B	46.	B	47.	A	48.	A
49.	D	50.	C	51.	D	52.	A
53.	A	54.	A	55.	B	56.	C
57.	C	58.	A	59.	A	60.	A
61.	B	62.	A	63.	A	64.	B
65.	B	66.	B	67.	D	68.	C
69.	B	70.	B	71.	B	72.	A
73.	C	74.	A	75.	B	76.	A
77.	A	78.	D	79.	C	80.	D
81.	A	82.	A	83.	A	84.	C
85.	B	86.	A	87.	A	88.	C
89.	B	90.	A	91.	C	92.	A
93.	D	94.	C	95.	C	96.	C
97.	A	98.	D	99.	C	100.	C

PGI Paper December 2011

1. **Anterior ethmoidal sinus drains into:**
   A. Superior meatus
   B. Middle meatus
   C. Inferior meatus
   D. None

2. **An area having multipotent cell can give rise to cells of:**
   A. Any 2 of germ layers which become permanent
   B. 1 germ layer only
   C. Any of 3 germ layers
   D. Gives rise to embryo and placenta

3. **Modiolus at the cortex of mouth is formed by all *except*:**
   A. Triangularis
   B. Buccinator
   C. Orbicularis oris
   D. Alaque Nasi

4. **Which is incorrect?**
   A. U-V rays help in formation of Vit. D in skin
   B. Renal failure leads to increase in parathormone release
   C. 25-hydroxycholecalciferol undergoes hydroxylation in kidney
   D. 25-hydroxycholecalciferol is used in treatment of renal failure

5. **Which bacteria will not cause food borne infection?**
   A. E.Coli
   B. Salmonella
   C. Campylobacter
   D. Pseudomonas

6. **Which is most antigenic?**
   A. Hapten
   B. Nucleic acid
   C. Lipids
   D. Proteins

7. **All of the following is added as an accelerator in ZOE cement *except*:**
   A. Acetic acid
   B. Zinc acetate dehydrate
   C. $CaCl_2$
   D. Bromoglycerine

8. Which of the following decreases with strain hardening?
A. Surface hardness B. Strength
C. Proportional limit D. Corrosive resistance

9. Tampering of steel causes:
A. Increases its toughness
B. Increases hardness
C. Increases ductility
D. Decreases toughness

10. For a porcelain fused to metal crown, porcelain and metal should have:
A. Equal hardness
B. Equal coefficient of linear thermal expansion
C. Equal fusion expansion
D. Equal fusion temperature

11. In quartz tungsten light cure device, minimum output of energy should not be less than:
A. 300 mw/cm^2 B. 350 mw/cm^2
C. 400 mw/cm^2 D. 450 mw/cm^2

12. Wavelength at which camphorquinone activity is maximum, in visible light cure system is:
A. 402 nm B. 474 nm
C. 484 nm D. 464 nm

13. Which of the following is added in composites to provide opacity?
A. BIS-GMA B. TEG-DMA
C. TiO_2 (Titanium oxide) D. None

14. In measuring Vickers hardness number, which of the following is used?
A. Spherical indenter
B. Steel ball indenter
C. Rhomboid shaped indenter
D. 136 degree diamond pyramid

15. ZOE is not used for permanent cementation because of:
A. Less strength B. High solubility
C. Poor marginal seal D. Poor pulpal protection

16. Which of the following orthodontic wire can be heat treated?
A. Stainless steel B. B-titanium
C. Elgiloy D. NiTi

17. Self etching adhesives:

A. Incorporates the smear layer into the surface
B. Removes the smear layer
C. Fixes the smear layer
D. Makes impregnation in the smear layer by acidic molecules but does not remove it

18. Which of the following laser has wavelength in visible light spectrum?

A. Er : YAG
B. Nd : YAG
C. Argon
D. CO_2

19. Normal flow rate of saliva is:

A. 1.1 ml/5 min.
B. 5.6 ml/5 min.
C. 3.7 ml/5 min.
D. 2.5 ml/5 min.

20. Maximum incidence of developmental defects is seen in:

A. Primary incisor
B. Permanent incisors
C. Permanent mandibular first molar
D. Primary mandibular second molar

21. Tooth erupting by the time of first birthday of infant:

A. Early infancy tooth
B. Dentitia precox
D. Natal teeth
D. Neonatal teeth

22. Molar-incisor hypoplasia in primary teeth at the occlusal level is due to developmental defect occurring during:

A. Birth to 12 months
B. 4th month intrauterine to birth
C. 22 months to 26 months
D. 24 months to 48 months

23. Most accepted sequence of serial extraction is:

A. C4D
B. D4C
C. CD4
D. DC4

24. Cariogram was given by:

A. Armani
B. Blatterfein
C. Barthall
D. Kelvin allen

25. In Class II cavity preparation for primary teeth, gingival seat is:

A. Bevelled as in permanent teeth
B. Bevelled at an angle more acute than permanent teeth
C. Not bevelled
D. None

26. **Which of the following is most likely to occur after trauma in primary dentition?**
   A. Intrusion
   B. Extrusion
   C. Complicated crown fracture
   D. Subluxation

27. **Iron requirement in children is:**
   A. 2-5 mg/kg of body weight
   B. 8-10 mg/kg of body weight
   C. 20-25 mg/kg of body weight
   D. 50-70 mg/kg of body weight

28. **Atropine is used in preanesthetic medication to:**
   A. Reduce pain
   B. Reduce salivary secretion and depress vagal reflexes
   C. Relieve anxiety
   D. Reduce bronchial secretion

29. **Which of the following is not a ureidopenicillin?**
   A. Piperacillin B. Mezlocillin
   C. Azlocillin D. Flucloxacillin

30. **Which of the following permanent tooth is first to calcify?**
   A. Maxillary permanent 1 molar
   B. Mandibular permanent 1 molar
   C. Maxillary C.I.
   D. Mandibular C.I.

31. **Resorption of dental tissues is caused by:**
   A. Osteoblast B. Odontoblasts
   C. Osteoclasts D. Odontoclasts

32. **Most common cells of connective tissues are:**
   A. Fibroblast B. Plasma cells
   C. Basal cells D. Histiocytes

33. **IL-1 and TNF-α during inflammation are secreted by:**
   A. Plasma cells
   B. Lymphocytes
   C. Activated macrophages
   D. Platelets

34. **White radiating line on buccal mucosa seen in:**
   A. Leukoplakia B. Lichen planus
   C. Erythroplakia D. Erythema multiforme

35. **Most common benign tumour occurring in oral cavity:**
A. Papilloma B. Fibroma
C. Adenoma D. Epulis

36. **A patient aged 50 years presented with a history of jaw expansion and enlargement of maxilla:**
A. Paget's disease B. Acromegaly
C. Fibrous dysplasia D. Hyper parathyroidism

37. **Most common soft tissue benign tumour of oral cavity is:**
A. Lipoma B. Fibroma
C. Adenoma D. Epulis

38. **Koplik spots are seen in:**
A. Measles B. Mumps
C. Herpes D. Varicella

39. **True about syphilis is:**
A. Oral lesions are seen at any age
B. Clinical manifestations occur after few months of exposure
C. VDRL test is positive in early days of primary syphilis
D. Penicillins are ineffective

40. **Hydropic degeneration of the basal cell layer of stratum germinatum is a feature of:**
A. Lichen planus B. Pemphigus
C. Syphilis D. Leukoplakia

41. **Giant cell lesions of periodontium are best considered as:**
A. Benign neoplasm
B. Non-neoplasm reactive lesion
C. Malignant neoplasm
D. None

42. **Bence Jones proteins are found in which condition?**
A. Malignant melanoma B. Multiple myeloma
C. Hodgkin's lymphoma D. None

43. **Granulation tissue is replaced by connective tissue in:**
A. 7 days B. 14 days
C. 21 days D. 1 month

44. **Which type of carcinoma develops in marjolin ulcer?**
A. BCC B. Fibrosarcoma
C. Adenocarcinoma D. None

45. Antibiotic prophylaxis is not used for:

A. Child under 15 years B. In renal failure patient
C. In liver failure patient D. HIV patient

46. In which of the following fractures of mandible, tongue falls back and causes respiratory obstruction?

A. Symphysis
B. Bilateral mandibular body
C. Bilateral parasymphysis
D. Bilateral angle

47. First sensation to be lost following administration of L.A. is:

A. Pain B. Touch
C. Temperature D. Proprioception

48. A patient who faints during extraction should be kept in:

A. Lateral position
B. Horizontal position
C. Trendlenberg position
D. None

49. Partial thromboplastin time is prolonged in:

A. Warfarin therapy B. Hemophilia
C. Heparin therapy D. Hypofibrinogenemia

50. After Caldwel Luc procedure, intranasal antrostomy is done through:

A. Superior meatus B. Floor of nose
C. Middle meatus D. Inferior meatus

51. In treatment of syncope, ammonia function as:

A. Vagal stimulation
B. Cardiac stimulation
C. Respiratory stimulation
D. Bronchodilatation

52. Maxillary antrum dips in the region of:

A. Between 2nd premolar and 1 molar
B. Between buccal roots of furcation of 1st molar
C. Between 1 and 2 premolar
D. Between 1 and 2 molars

53. What is untrue about Ludwig angina?

A. It spreads bilaterally
B. Most common cause is dental infection

C. It involves submandibular and sublingual spaces
D. Involvement of submandibular gland and lymph nodes is common

54. During inferior alveolar nerve block needle is inserted into which space?
A. Infratemporal space
B. Submandibular space
C. Pterygomandibular space
D. Masseteric space

55. Hematoma formation during or immediately following a posterior superior nerve block is most likely a result of damage to the:
A. Facial artery
B. Maxillary artery
C. Pterygoid venous plexus
D. Small capillaries and arterioles

56. Most common cause of TMJ ankylosis is:
A. Trauma
B. Chronic pain
C. Arthritis
D. Infection

57. Hematoma is more frequently seen with:
A. IANB
B. PSA
C. Greater palatine nerve block
D. Infra-orbital nerve block

58. In a 10 years old body in TMJ ankylosis, which material has given the best results: Or in a child with TMJ ankylosis, treated with interpositional arthroplasty which is best?
A. Silicone
B. Titanium mesh
C. Costochondral graft
D. None

59. Which nerve is near to mandibular third molar (Medial aspect) and is likely to be damaged while removing 3rd molar?
A. Inferior alveolar nerve
B. Buccal nerve
C. Masseteric nerve
D. Lingual nerve

60. Radiographic sign which appears in acute case of osteomyelitis?
A. Radiolucency in relation to bone
B. No appreciable change

C. Sunray appearance
D. None

61. Apthous like ulcers are seen in:
A. Behcet syndrome
B. Sweet syndrome
C. PFAPA
D. All of the above

62. Gnawing radiating pain is a feature of:
A. Herpetic gingivostomatitis
B. ANUG
C. Chronic periodontitis
D. None

63. Botulinum toxin causes:
A. Tachycardia
B. Bilateral cranial nerve involvement
C. Fever
D. Hypertension

64. In systemic inflammatory response syndrome (SIRS) which is not seen?
A. Temperature < 36°C or > 38°C
B. Blood pressure < 110/70 mm Hg.
C. Respiratory rate > 20 min.
D. $PaCO_2$ > 32 mPl.

65. What is true about acute rheumatic fever?
A. Mitral valve is invariably associated
B. Earliest symptom is migratory arthritis
C. Sydenham's chorea is always present
D. It follows streptococcal skin infection

66. Radiographically sequestrum formed in osteomyelitis is:
A. More radiopaque than healthy bone
B. Less radiopaque than healthy bone
C. Same radiopaque than healthy bone
D. None

67. Radiation induced caries occurs in:
A. 1 month
B. 3 months
C. 6 months
D. 9 months

68. Best technique to locate an impacted maxillary canine:
A. Occlusal radiograph
B. Periapical radiograph with tube shift technique
C. CBCT
D. OPG

69. **Structure that resembles PDL of maxillary second molar on radiographs is:**
   A. Zygomatic arch and zygomatic process
   B. Nasal fossa
   C. Greater palatine foramen
   D. None

70. **Which microorganisms is increased in pregnancy gingivitis?**
   A. Porphyromonas gingivalis
   B. Provetella intermedia
   C. Capnocytophage
   D. Actinomyces

71. **Minimum concentration of chlorhexidine for plaque control:**
   A. 0.2% B. 0.12%
   C. 0.4% D. 0.25%

72. **McCall's festoon result from:**
   A. Normal physiological process
   B. Tooth brush trauma
   C. Trauma from occlusion
   D. Food impaction

73. **Which of the following condition indicate periodontal rather an endodontic lesion?**
   A. Acute pain on vertical percussion with no swelling
   B. Pain to lateral percussion with wide sulcular pocket
   C. A deep narrow sulcular pocket to the apex with exudates
   D. Pain to palpation of the buccal mucosa near the tooth apex

74. **Actinobacillus actinomycetemcomitans attachment to tooth surface can be prevented by:**
   A. Myelo peroxidase B. Lacto peroxidise
   C. Collagenase D. None

75. **Total arch length reduced due to mesial migration of teeth:**
   A. 1 cm B. 3 cm
   C. 0.5 cm D. 0.15 cm

76. **Which of the following is an intra matrix procedure?**
   A. Rotation of Mandibular base in relation to cranium
   B. Rotation of Mandibular plane in relation to cranium

C. Rotation of Mandibular plane in relation to core of Mandible
D. Rotation of Mandibular base in relation to Maxilla

77. Period of adolescent growth in boys is:

A. 3 years B. 3.5 years
C. 4 years D. 5 years

78. Andrew's 5th key of occlusion is:

A. Curve of spee
B. Tight contacts
C. Incisor inclination
D. Molar-Interarch relationship

79. Type A growth pattern is:

A. Maxillary excess or midface grows more than the lower face
B. Mandibular excess or lower face grows more than the midface
C. Growth of maxilla and mandible is equal
D. Prognosis is poor

80. Most posterior point on mandible is:

A. Gonion B. Menton
C. Pogonion D. Gnathion

81. Time period of growth spurt in girls occur at:

A. 3, 6-7, 11-14 years B. 3, 6-7, 11-13 years
C. 3, 7-9, 11-13 years D. 3, 7-8, 11-14 years

82. According to Veau's classification of cleft lip and palate, isolated cleft palate falls under:

A. Group I B. Group II
C. Group III D. Group IV

83. A sound which is most affected in patient of class III malocclusion:

A. Linguoalveolar consonants
B. Sibilant sounds
C. Linguoalveolar fricatives
D. Labio dental fricatives

84. Most commonly used slot size in orthodontic brackets is:

A. 0.018 × 0.022 B. 0.017 × 0.021
C. 0.014 × 0.024 D. 0.010 × 0.020

85. Spontaneous space closure is expected upto how many millimetres of midline diastema?

A. 1 mm B. 2 mm
C. 1.5 mm D. 3 mm

86. For uncontrolled tipping centre of rotation is at:

A. Infinity B. Root apex
C. Centre of resistance D. Incisal edge

87. AO and BO in wits appraisal signify:

A. Relationship of maxilla to cranial base
B. Relationship of mandible to cranial base
C. Relationship of maxilla to mandible
D. Relationship of maxilla and mandible to face

88. The patient experiencing pain at the appointment of jaw relation, which may be used as treatment option for such condition?

A. Using a jig to train jaw movements
B. Manual manipulation of jaw
C. Using bite plane to correct relationship of jaws
D. Either A or C

89. Pulp cavity tests are used to check:

A. Pulp blood supply B. Afferent nerve fibres
C. Efferent nerve fibres D. None

90. A disease which involves large group of population within short time is known as:

A. Epizoonotic B. Endemic
C. Epidemic D. Sporadic

91. Best method to checking on effectiveness of diet counselling is:

A. Lactobacillus count
B. Synder's test
C. Latest dietary history
D. Salivary reductase test

92. The name of the sample group of individuals when followed for successive examination to evaluate the effect of oral prevention programme is:

A. Panel group B. Cohort group
C. High risk group D. Prospective group

93. Prevention of onset of risk factor is:

A. Primary prevention
B. Secondary prevention
C. Tertiary prevention
D. Primordial prevention

94. 0.05% NaF has F^{++} in concentration of:

A. 900 ppm
B. 9000 ppm
C. 225 ppm
D. 250 ppm

95. 0.2% NaF mouth rinse is recommended:

A. Once daily
B. Weekly
C. Fortnightly
D. Twice daily

96. Effectiveness of systemic fluoridation in prevention of caries is:

A. 20%
B. 30%
C. 80%
D. 60%

97. In a sample of population maximum observation is concentrated around:

A. Mean
B. Median
C. Mode
D. Arithmatic mean

98. Prevalence is defined as:

A. All new cases of a specific disease occurring during a specified period
B. Rate of disease transmission
C. Cumulative effect of a disease in an area
D. Proportion of population affected by the disease

99. Primary consideration in any oral health preventive programme:

A. Fluoride application
B. Diet control
C. Plaque control
D. Pit and fissure sealant

Answers

1.	B	2.	C	3.	D	4.	D
5.	D	6.	D	7.	D	8.	D
9.	A	10.	B	11.	A	12.	B
13.	C	14.	D	15.	A	16.	C
17.	D	18.	C	19.	B	20.	B
21.	D	22.	A	23.	C	24.	C
25.	C	26.	D	27.	C	28.	B
29.	D	30.	A	31.	D	32.	A
33.	C	34.	B	35.	B	36.	A
37.	B	38.	A	39.	A	40.	A
41.	B	42.	B	43.	C	44.	A
45.	A	46.	C	47.	A	48.	C
49.	B	50.	D	51.	C	52.	A
53.	D	54.	C	55.	C	56.	A
57.	B	58.	C	59.	D	60.	B
61.	D	62.	B	63.	B	64.	D
65.	B	66.	A	67.	B	68.	C
69.	C	70.	B	71.	B	72.	C
73.	B	74.	C	75.	C	76.	C
77.	D	78.	B	79.	C	80.	A
81.	C	82.	B	83.	D	84.	A
85.	B	86.	C	87.	C	88.	D
89.	B	90.	C	91.	C	92.	B
93.	D	94.	A	95.	C	96.	D
97.	B	98.	D	99.	C		

PGI Paper

June 2011

1. **Kiesselbach's plexus is present in:**
   A. Superior part of lateral nasal wall
   B. Antero-inferior part of lateral nasal wall
   C. Superior part of nasal septum
   D. Antero-inferior part of nasal septum

2. **Which of the following structure is not located medial to submandibular gland?**
   A. Facial vein B. Hypoglossus
   C. Styloglossus D. Mylohyoid

3. **Which of the following passes through the foramen rotundum?**
   A. Maxillary nerve
   B. Maxillary artery
   C. Mandibular nerve
   D. Middle meningeal artery

4. **Which muscle helps in protrusion of tongue?**
   A. Hyoglossus B. Genioglossus
   C. Hyoglossus D. Styloglossus

5. **Type of collagen present in circummaxillary suture:**
   A. Type I B. Type II
   C. Type III D. Type IV

6. **In acute hepatitis infection, the first marker of infectivity:**
   A. HbsAg B. Anti HbcIgM
   C. HbcAg D. Anti HbeAg

7. **Nosocomial infections are:**
   A. Hospital acquired infection
   B. Supra infections
   C. Maternally acquired infections
   D. Acquired from home

8. According to OSHA maximum permissible amount of nickel in dental clinic environment is:

A. 1 mg B. 2 mg
C. 3 mg D. 4 mg

9. Change in hue with change in light intensity:

A. Metamerism B. Bezold-Brucke effect
C. Light scatter D. Fluorescence

10. Maximum tear strength is seen in:

A. Polyether
B. Polysulfide
C. Condensation silicon
D. Addition silicon

11. Amount of tin in low copper amalgam is:

A. 5% B. 25-28%
C. 63-70% D. 13-25%

12. Which among the following is the only impression material that can be electroplated?

A. Addition silicone B. Hydrocolloid
C. Polyether D. Polysulfide

13. Glossy smooth margins of casting are due to:

A. Shrinkage of alloy on cooling
B. Investment breakdown
C. Incomplete gas elimination
D. Incomplete wax elimination

14. Most biocompatible material:

A. Commercially pure titanium
B. Silver
C. Tin
D. Chromium

15. Prolonged corticosteroid therapy leads to:

A. Adrenal insufficiency
B. Cardiac failure
C. Myocardial infarction
D. Pneumonia

16. Drug which is safe in pregnancy is:

A. Fluoroquinone B. Sulfadiazine
C. Tetracycline D. Penicillin

17. Goldenhar syndrome is:

A. Facial deformity, auricular abnormalities and vertebral deformity
B. Facial deformity, auricular abnormalities, vertebral deformity and genital lesion
C. Facial and auricular abnormalities only
D. Auricular abnormalities only

18. Fordyce's granules/spots are:

A. Ectopic mucous gland
B. Ectopic sweat gland
C. Ectopic dermoid cyst
D. Ectopic sebaceous gland

19. Atropine and red tongue is geographic tongue is due to:

A. Eosinophilic infiltration
B. Neutrophilic infiltration
C. Both
D. None of these

20. All are considered in TNM staging *except*:

A. Tumor size
B. Tumor site
C. Lymph nodes
D. Metastasis

21. Granularity of oncocyte is due to:

A. Over abundance of mitochondria
B. Over abundance of golgi bodies
C. Deficiency of mitochondria
D. Deficiency of golgi bodies

22. Icterus occurs in sclera because of:

A. Increased collagen
B. Increased elastin
C. White in color
D. Exposed to sunlight

23. In a patient with full blown AIDS, the CD_4 count is:

A. Less than 800
B. Less than 200
C. Less than 600
D. Less than 400

24. Diamond Blackfan anemia is:

A. Inherited thrombocytopenia
B. Inherited leucopenia
C. Inherited erythrocytopenia
D. All of these

25. **Reed Sternberg cells are seen in:**
A. Hodgkin lymphoma
B. Non Hodgkin lymphoma
C. Multiple myeloma
D. Burkitt's lymphoma

26. **Matted lymph nodes are seen in:**
A. T.B. (Tuberculosis)
B. Non Hodgkin lymphoma
C. Sarcoidosis
D. Hodgkin lymphoma

27. **Lupus vulgaris is:**
A. Tuberculosis lesion (skin) on the face
B. Syphilitic lesion on the face
C. Generalized collagen disease
D. Localized collagen disease

28. **The new name of odontogenic keratocyst is:**
A. Odontogenic ghost cell
B. Keratocyte ghost cell
C. Keratocysticodontogenic tumour
D. None

29. **Vazirani Akinosi technique is used to anaesthetize:**
A. Inferior Alveolar Nerve
B. Maxillary Nerve
C. Posterior Superior alveolar Nerve
D. Mandibular Nerve

30. **Infraorbital nerve block will anaesthetize:**
A. Anterior Superior Alveolar and Middle Superior Alveolar Nerve
B. Middle Superior Alveolar, Posterior Superior Alveolar Nerve
C. Anterior Superior Alveolar, Posterior Superior Alveolar
D. Posterior Superior Alveolar Nerve

31. **Most stable wiring in close reduction is:**
A. Arch bar
B. Eyelid
C. Direct
D. IMF screws

32. **Which of the following is not a part of Glassgow Coma Scale?**
A. Eye opening
B. Motor disturbance
C. Verbal response
D. Sensory level

33. Keen's approach is used for:

A. Extra-oral reduction of zygomatic arch
B. Intra-oral reduction of zygomatic arch
C. Disimpaction of maxilla
D. Disimpaction of nasal bone

34. Which of the following is not anesthetized with mental nerve block?

A. First molar B. Permanent molars
C. Canines D. Incisors

35. Blow out fracture with enopthalmos is seen with:

A. Medial wall
B. Floor of orbit
C. Orbital floor or medial wall
D. Roof or orbit

36. Which of the following condition is not associated with exophthalmosis?

A. Blow out fracture B. Blow in fracture
C. Hyperthyroidism D. Thyrotoxicosis

37. An 8-year-old child having unilateral condyle fracture with chronic pain and normal occlusion; what will be the treatment modality?

A. IMF for 2 weeks
B. IMF for 4 weeks
C. Active jaw movements
D. Open reduction

38. Which of the following is not a parameter for basic life support/or not involve vital statistics?

A. B.P. B. Airway
C. Breathing D. Circulation

39. Remaining bone associated which implant papillary level of single tooth implant is denoted by:

A. Bone level surrounding adjacent natural bone height
B. 5 mm of implant abutment junction
C. 5 mm of implant bone level
D. According to bone height of implant

40. After inferior alveolar nerve block the success of block is checked at:

A. Site of injection
B. Gingiva of tooth to be extracted

C. Attached gingival over premolar
D. Not recalled

41. Which of the following is used cut the bone in lingual split bone technique?

A. Osteotome B. Bur
C. Chisel D. Straight elevator

42. Necrotizing fasciitis involves which of the following?

A. Fascia B. Skin
C. Muscle D. All of the above

43. Which of the following needle is used for irrigation?

A. 23 B. 25
C. 26 D. 29

44. What is the rotation of speed of Ni-Ti rotary system?

A. 250-300 rpm B. 150-300 rpm
C. 200-250 rpm D. 800-1000 rpm

45. Which of the following denotes No. 20 GT taper size?

A. 0.06, 0.07, 0.08, 0.09
B. 0.006, 0.008, 0.010, 0.012
C. 0.06, 0.08, 0.10, 0.12
D. 0.2, 0.8, 1.0, 1.2

46. Filling motion of K-file is:

A. Watch winding B. Rotational
C. Linear D. Linear and Rotational

47. In case of retreatment which is ideal for removal of G.P.?

A. H-file B. K-file
C. GT-file D. Lentulospiral

48. AH plus and AH 26 are used as:

A. Root canal fillers
B. Root canal cements
C. Root canal medicaments
D. Root canal irrigants

49. Which file is used along with irrigation of ultrasonic system?

A. 8 B. 10
C. 15 D. 20

50. Before replanting an avulsed tooth, it is treated with Sodium Hypochlorite followed by:

A. 2% NaF for 5 minutes
B. 10% NaF for 2 minutes
C. 2% SnF_2 for 5 minutes
D. 10% SnF_2 for 10 minutes

51. Avulsed tooth is not kept in water because:

A. Water is hypotonic and causes rapid cell lysis
B. Water is isotonic and cause rapid cell lysis
C. Water is hypertonic
D. Water is infectious to periodontal ligament

52. Maximum demineralization of enamel occurs at a depth of:

A. 20-30 mm B. 30-50 mm
C. 10-20 mm D. 100-200 mm

53. In which of the following patient there is 10-20 fold increased risk of leukemia during infancy?

A. Down syndrome
B. Pierre Robin syndrome
C. Fragile X syndrome
D. None

54. High viscosity GIC was discovered in:

A. 1990 B. 1980
C. 1970 D. 2000

55. Window of infectivity period for caries is:

A. 24-30 months B. 19-33 months
C. 12-30 months D. 6-21 months

56. 2½ years old child with severe horizontal bone resorption and normal cementum is suffering from:

A. Hypophosphatasia
B. Precocious periodontosis
C. Down syndrome
D. Generalized periodontitis

57. First active metabolite of chloral hydrate is:

A. Monochloroethanol
B. Dichloroethanol
C. Ethanol
D. Trichloroethanol

58. In X-ray tube cathode is:

A. Copper B. Molybdenum
C. Tin D. Aluminium

59. What is the S.I. unit of effective dose?

A. Sievert B. Gray
C. Becquerel D. Roentgen

60. Intensity of radiation at a distance of 4 cm is R. At the distance of 2 cm, the intensity will be:

A. 1/2 R B. R
C. 2 R D. 4 R

61. Digital OPG as compared to conventional OPG reduces radiation exposure by:

A. 80% B. 70%
C. 60% D. 50%

62. Experimental gingivitis was given by:

A. Herald Loe B. Carranza
C. Newman D. None of these

63. Causative organism is localized aggressive periodontitis is:

A. Porphyromonas gingivalis
B. B forsythus
C. Capnocytophaga
D. Actinomycetem comitans

64. In susceptible females, pregnancy gingivitis occurs in which month?

A. 1st B. 4th
C. 8th D. 9th

65. Paper points, micropipette and....... are used to collect:

A. GCF B. Saliva
C. Bacteria D. Serum

66. As compared to a non smoker, in a smoker the increased incidence of gingivitis is:

A. 2-6% B. 6-10%
C. 15-20% D. 25-30%

67. Which of the following is related to gingivitis?

A. Plaque
B. Calculus
C. Tooth brush trauma
D. Abrasive powder

68. Type of cells which predominate in the Stage-III lesion of gingivitis are:

A. PMN B. Macrophages
C. Plasma cells D. Lymphocytes

69. CHF and periodontitis shows:

A. Positive relation
B. Negative relation
C. Weakly positive relation
D. No relation

70. Dentist : Population ratio in India is:

A. 1:55000 B. 1:25000
C. 1:17000 D. 1:13000

71. If odds ratio = 1, then which of the following is true?

A. Positive co-relation
B. Negative co-relation
C. No association
D. High association

72. Type 1 error is:

A. Null Hypothesis is false but rejected
B. Null Hypothesis is true but rejected
C. Null Hypothesis is false but accepted
D. Null Hypothesis is true but accepted

73. All are true of about case control studies *except*:

A. Requires regular follow up of patient
B. Cost-effectiveness
C. Retrospective
D. Rapid

74. Severity of disease is measured by:

A. Case fatality rate B. Proportional mortality rate
C. Relative risk D. Attributable risk

75. All are in close proximation to median *except*:

A. 2nd quartile B. 2nd Tertile
C. 50th Percentile D. 5th decile

76. A scatter diagram uses the following:

A. Pie chart
B. Line diagrams
C. Distribution of various variable/co-relation between two variable
D. t-variable

77. First fluoride dentifrices contains:

A. NaF
B. SnF2
C. Amine fluoride
D. Sodium mono fluorophosphates

78. The confirmation of disease in a positive test is described as:

A. Specificity
B. Sensitivity
C. Positive predictivity
D. Negative predictivity

79. Which of the following does not show existing data?

A. Medical records of hospital
B. Survey of people living in an area
C. World health report
D. Health information of India

80. Concentration of fluoride in first fluoride varnish:

A. 2%
B. 8%
C. 10%
D. 2.26%

81. The type of periodontitis which persist even after repeated treatments?

A. Aggressive Periodontitis
B. Refractive Periodontitis
C. Juvenile Periodontitis
D. G. Periodontitis

82. Least interference is encountered in which position?

A. Centric relation
B. Centric occlusion
C. Maximum protruded position
D. None

83. Finish line in all ceramic veneer is:

A. Shoulder on both sides
B. Chamfer on both sides
C. Buccal chamfer and Palatal shoulder
D. Palatal chamfer and Buccal shoulder

84. In pier abutment, male part of non-rigid connector is in:

A. Mesial surface of distal pontic
B. Distal surface of mesial pontic

C. Mesial surface of distal abutment
D. Distal surface of mesial abutment

85. Distance travelled in bone by erupting premolars in 4-5 months:

A. 1 mm B. 2 mm
C. 3 mm D. 4 mm

86. Endodontically treated tooth is difficult to move because:

A. Activity of osteoclast is hampered secondary to non vital pulp
B. Atrophy of periodontal ligament
C. Dentin is hardened and brittle
D. Fluoride level is more at apex

87. Pendulum appliance is used for:

A. Distalisation of molars
B. Derotation
C. Uprighting
D. Correcting open bite

88. Amount of Pressure/Force exerted by lip on maxillary incisors:

A. 10-15 gm/cm^2 B. 20-25 gm/cm^2
C. 25-30 gm/cm^2 D. 30-35 gm/cm^2

89. In a perfect smile, the ratio of which to height of maxillary incisor is:

A. 8 : 10 B. 6 : 8
C. 10 : 14 D. 20 : 25

90. The pharyngeal structure established in early age and remain constant throughout life is:

A. Depth of oropharynx
B. Depth of nasopharynx
C. Width of nasopharynx
D. Width of oropharynx

91. In Tweed's Analysis if FMA is 35 degrees, what will be FMIA?

A. 65° B. 63°
C. 60° D. 68°

92. Three quarter profile photograph is used to detect:

A. Lip in competence B. Mandibular asymmetry
C. Midline D. Mid face deformity

93. Angle formed between F.H. plane and occlusal line:

A. 25° B. 100°
C. 10° D. Both are parallel

94. Which of the following is used to measure the mineral bone density of mandible?

A. Microradiography
B. Auto radiography
C. Finite element modelling
D. Nuclear volume morphometry

95. Shape memory in A-NiTi is because of change:

A. From austenitic to martensitic as a result of stress
B. From martensitic to austenitic as a result of stress
C. From austenitic to martensitic as a result of temperature
D. From martensitic to austenitic as a result of temperature

96. Hand, foot and mouth disease is caused by:

A. Coxsackie A 16 B. Coxsackie A 10
C. Coxsackie A 4 D. Coxsackie B 4

97. Staghorn appearance is seen in:

A. Hemangiopericytoma
B. Histiocytoma
C. Both
D. Histoplasmosis

98. Osteitis fibrosa cystica is:

A. Hypoparathyroidism
B. Hyperparathyroidism
C. Hyperthyroidism
D. Hypothyroidism

99. Osteoclast in bone remodelling has receptor for:

A. Parathyroid hormone
B. Calcitonin
C. Growth hormone
D. None of these

100. Which of the following is not a type of leukoplakia?

A. Bullous B. Ulcerative
C. Speckled D. Homogenous

101. In a five-year-old child which of the following foramen is located in posterior cranial fossa?

A. Foramen Rotundum
B. Foramen Spinosum
C. Foramen Lacerum
D. Jugular Foramen

102. NRHM was formed in:

A. 2002
B. 2005
C. 2011
D. 2008

Answers

1.	D	2.	A	3.	A	4.	B
5.	C	6.	A	7.	A	8.	A
9.	B	10.	B	11.	B	12.	D
13.	D	14.	A	15.	A	16.	D
17.	A	18.	D	19.	B	20.	B
21.	A	22.	B	23.	B	24.	C
25.	A	26.	A	27.	A	28.	C
29.	D	30.	A	31.	A	32.	D
33.	B	34.	B	35.	C	36.	A
37.	C	38.	A	39.	A	40.	C
41.	C	42.	D	43.	C	44.	B
45.	C	46.	A	47.	A	48.	B
49.	C	50.	C	51.	A	52.	C
53.	A	54.	A	55.	B	56.	B
57.	D	58.	B	59.	A	60.	C
61.	B	62.	A	63.	D	64.	C
65.	A	66.	A	67.	A	68.	C
69.	A	70.	D	71.	C	72.	B
73.	A	74.	A	75.	B	76.	C
77.	B	78.	C	79.	B	80.	D
81.	B	82.	A	83.	A	84.	A
85.	A	86.	C	87.	A	88.	B
89.	A	90.	B	91.	A	92.	D
93.	C	94.	A	95.	A	96.	A
97.	A	98.	B	99.	B	100.	A
101.	D	102.	B				

PGI Paper December 2010

1. **An area having multipotent cells can give rise to cells of:**
   A. Any 2 of germ layers which become permanent
   B. 1 germ layer only
   C. Any of 3 germ layers
   D. Gives rise to embryo and placenta

2. **The anterior displacement of articular disc is by which muscle?**
   A. Masseter
   B. Temporalis
   C. Medial pterygoid
   D. Lateral pterygoid

3. **Type of epithelium in nasopharynx, trachea and respiratory mucosa is:**
   A. Pseudostratified ciliated columnar
   B. Stratified squamous
   C. Stratified columnar
   D. Pseudostratified columnar

4. **Anterior ethmoidal sinus drains into:**
   A. Superior meatus
   B. Middle meatus
   C. Inferior meatus
   D. None

5. **Which of the following is true about hemoglobin?**
   A. Consist of 4 polypeptide chains
   B. It has 4 heme molecules, 2 alpha and 2 beta chains
   C. It has 2 heme molecules, 4 polypeptide chains
   D. It has 1 heme and 1 globin molecule

6. **Activator of receptors for ANP increases in target cell:**
   A. Cyclic AMP
   B. IP_3
   C. Protein kinase A activity
   D. Guanyl cyclase activity

7. **Which of the following is most antigenic?**
   A. Proteins
   B. Lipids
   C. Nucleic acids
   D. Hapten

8. **Which bacteria will not cause food borne infection?**
   A. E. coli
   B. Salmonella
   C. Campylobacter
   D. Pseudomonas

9. **Koplik spots are seen in:**
   A. Measles
   B. German Measles
   C. Herpes
   D. Varicella

10. **Cells responsible for resorption of dental hard tissue are:**
   A. Osteoclasts
   B. Odontoclasts
   C. Giant cells
   D. Fibroblasts

11. **Maximum incidence of developmental defects are seen in:**
   A. Primary incisor
   B. Permanent incisors
   C. Permanent mandibular first molar
   D. Primary mandibular second molar

12. **What is normal average eruption time period of permanent mandibular 1st molar?**
   A. 0-6 months
   B. 6-10 months
   C. 10-14 months
   D. 14-18 months

13. **Von Ebner's gland are:**
   A. Pure mucous gland
   B. Mixed glands with predominant mucous acini
   C. Pure serous gland
   D. Mixed glands with predominant serous acini

14. **Number of developmental lobes for primary central incisor are:**
   A. 1
   B. 2
   C. 3
   D. 4

15. **The last primary tooth to be replaced by a permanent tooth is:**
   A. Maxillary canine
   B. First premolar
   C. Maxillary incisor
   D. Mandibular 1st molar

16. **Which of the following is an example of child maltreatment?**

A. Munchausen syndrome by proxy
B. Blue baby syndrome
C. Kanner syndrome
D. Stockholm syndrome

17. Tooth start erupting corresponding to which Nolla's stage?

A. 4
B. 5
C. 6
D. 7

18. Teeth present in the oral cavity on the date of first birthday of a child are:

A. Ghost teeth
B. Natal teeth
C. Neonatal teeth
D. Enamel teeth

19. Cariogram was given by:

A. Armani
B. Blatterfein
C. Barthall
D. Kelvin allen

20. Pulp cavity tests are used to check:

A. Pulp blood supply
B. Afferent nerve fibres
C. Efferent nerve fibres
D. None

21. McCall's festoons occur due to:

A. Trauma from occlusion
B. Inflammation
C. Poor oral hygiene
D. Physiological resorption

22. Sulcular epithelium is:

A. Always keratinized
B. Always not keratinized
C. Is non keratinized but become keratinized or removal of inflammation or exposure into oral cavity
D. Is keratinized but become non-keratinized or removal of inflammation or exposure to oral cavity

23. Specific plaque hypothesis for etiology of periodontal disease was given by:

A. Glickman
B. Socransky
C. Listgarten
D. Loesche

24. Which of the following microorganism increases in pregnancy gingivitis?

A. Porphyromonas gingivalis
B. Prevotella intermedia
C. Capnocytophage
D. Actinobacillus

25. Which of the following salivary factor is not bactericidal?

A. Ca^{2+} and PO_4^{2-}
B. Lactoperoxidase
C. Lysozyme
D. IgA

26. Giant cell lesions of the periodontium are best considered:

A. Benign neoplasm
B. Non-neoplastic reactive lesion
C. Malignant neoplasm
D. Herpangina

27. Most common benign neoplasm of oral cavity:

A. Myxoma
B. Lipoma
C. Fibroma
D. Papilloma

28. True about syphilis is:

A. Oral lesions are seen in any stage
B. Clinical manifestations occur after few months of exposure
C. VDRL test is positive in early stages of primary syphilis
D. Penicillins are effective

29. A patient aged 50 years presented with history of jaw expansion and increased size of maxilla. The diagnosis is:

A. Paget's disease
B. Fibrous dysplasia
C. Acromegaly
D. Hyperthyroidism

30. Giant cell lesions of the periodontium are best considered as:

A. Benign neoplasm
B. Malignant neoplasm
C. Non-neoplastic reactive lesion
D. Herpangina

31. Oral lesions similar to apthous ulcers are seen in:

A. Behcet syndrome
B. PFAPA syndrome
C. Sweet syndrome
D. All of the above

32. Disuse atrophy of periodontium occurs in all *except*:

A. Erythema Multiforme
B. Lupus Erythematosus

C. Herpangina
D. Chicken pox

33. The tooth preparation for laminates extends:

A. Labial to contact
B. Lingual to contact
C. Upto contact
D. None

34. In tooth preparation procedure the foremost principle is:

A. Retention form
B. Resistance form
C. Convenience form
D. Conservation of what is remaining

35. Self etching adhesives:

A. Incorporates the smear layer into the surface
B. Removes the smear layer
C. Fixes the smear layer
D. Makes impregnation in the smear layer by acidic molecules but does not remove it

36. Acid used for micro-abrasions technique recommended by croll is:

A. H_2SO_4 10%
B. HCl 18%
C. Citric acid 10%
D. HNO_3 8%

37. During jaw relation, protrusion records are used for:

A. Condylar inclination measurement of one side
B. Condylar inclination measurement of both sides
C. Records centric relation
D. Records retruded contact position

38. Immediate Bennett side shift is used to define the shift when it occurs:

A. Immediately after the forward movement is completed
B. In the first 5-6 mm of the forward movement
C. Before any forward movement of the orbiting condyle
D. Throughout the range of motion

39. Centre of rotation for bodily movement is at:

A. Root apex
B. Infinity
C. Centre of resistance
D. Incisal edge

40. Andrews 5th key of occlusion is:

A. Absence of incisor rotation
B. Labio-lingual inclination
C. Tight contacts
D. Curve of spee

41. In Farkas anthropometric analysis, which of the following is true?

A. Interpupillary distance is equal to width of mouth
B. Intercanthal distance is equal to width of mouth
C. Nasolabial angle is more in boys than in girls
D. Distance between pupil and midface is equal to width of mouth

42. Which of the following is a tissue borne appliance?

A. Activator
B. Bionator
C. Frenkel regulator
D. Herbst appliance

43. AO and BO in wits appraisal is relationship of:

A. Maxilla to cranium
B. Mandible to cranium
C. Maxilla to mandible
D. Maxilla and mandible to face

44. Most posterior points on the mandible is:

A. Gonion
B. Menton
C. Pogonion
D. Gnathion

45. Intra matrix rotation is:

A. Rotation of Mandibular base in relation to cranium
B. Rotation of Mandibular plane in relation to cranium
C. Rotation of Mandibular plane in relation to core of Mandible
D. Rotation of Mandibular base in relation to Maxilla

46. Force applied in maxillary protrusion is:

A. 0-100 gm
B. 300-600 gm
C. 600-900 gm
D. None

47. Tooth movement requiring maximum force value?

A. Intrusion
B. Extrusion
C. Root uprighting
D. Rotation

48. In gnathological diagnosis, what is the normal gap between maxillary and mandibular incisors when the mandible is in centric occlusion?

A. 0.005”
B. 0.0005”
C. 0.005”
D. 0.5”

49. Which of the following is an example of fixed functional appliance?

A. Activator
B. Bionator
C. Frenkel regulator
D. Herbst appliance

50. The time period of growth spurts in girls occur during?

A. 3, 7, 11-13 years of age
B. 3, 7-9, 11-13 years of age
C. 3, 6-7, 11-12 years of age
D. 3, 7-9, 13-14 years of age

51. For uncontrolled tipping the centre of rotation is at:

A. Infinity
B. Root apex
C. Centre of resistance
D. Incisal edge

52. Teeth that are extracted last in full mouth extraction:

A. Incisors
B. Canines
C. Premolars
D. Molars

53. The type of anchorage used in maxillary expansion by Quad Helix is:

A. Simple
B. Reinforced
C. Reciprocal
D. Complex

54. All of the following are used as an accelerator in zinc oxide, eugenol cement *except*:

A. Acetic acid
B. Zinc acetate dehydrate
C. Calcium chloride
D. Bromoglycerine

55. Tempering heat treatment produces following change in wire:

A. Increases its toughness
B. Increases hardness
C. Increases ductility
D. Decreases toughness

56. In measuring Vicker hardness number, which of the following is used?

A. Spherical indenter
B. Steel ball indentation
C. Rhomboid shaped indenter
D. 136 degree diamond pyramid

57. Which of the following decreases with strain hardening?

A. Hardness B. Strength
C. Proportional limit D. Ductility

58. Which of the following decreases with strain hardening?
(Question was repeated twice in the exam)

A. Hardness B. Strength
C. Proportional limit D. Ductility

59. To prevent tensile forces in porcelain, which of the following in a metal ceramic crown should nearly be equal?

A. Coefficient of thermal expansion of metal and porcelain
B. Compressive strength of metal and porcelain
C. Amount of fillers
D. None

60. Which impression material have poor surface representation?

A. Reversible hydrocolloid
B. Polyether
C. Irreversible hydrocolloid
D. Zinc oxide eugenol

61. ZoE is not used for permanent cementation because of:

A. Less strength
B. High solubility
C. Poor marginal seal
D. Poor pulpal protection

62. Amount of filler in flowable composite is:

A. 36 B. 46
C. 56 D. 66

63. Botulinum toxin causes:

A. Tachycardia
B. Bilateral cranial nerve involvement
C. Fever
D. Hypertension

64. Hypokalemia is not present in which condition?

A. Vomiting
B. Diarrhoea
C. Patient on diuretics
D. Chronic renal failure

65. IL-1 and TNF-α are secreted by:
A. Lymphocytes
B. PMN's
C. Fibroblasts
D. Activated macrophages

66. In β-thalassemia major, the blood picture shows:
A. Normocytic-Normochromic anemia
B. Microcytic-Hypochromic anemia
C. Normocytic-Hypochromic anemia
D. Microcytic-Normochromic anemia

67. Atropine is drug used for preanaesthetic medication because:
A. It decreases bronchial secretions
B. To reduce pain
C. To relieve anxiety
D. Decrease salivary secretions and depress vagal reflex

68. Normal prothrombin time is:
A. 6-10 sec.
B. 14-16 sec.
D. 15-20 sec.
D. 20-30 sec.

69. Fall back of tongue after an accident occurs due to:
A. Bilateral parasymphyseal fracture
B. Bilateral angle fracture
C. Bilateral condylar fracture
D. Symphysis fracture

70. The recommended position to keep a person who faints during extraction:
A. Horizontal position
B. Lateral position
C. Trendelenberg position
D. Dorso sacral

71. Most of the cases of hematoma occurs during which nerve block?
A. Inferior alveolar nerve block
B. Postero-superior block
C. Infra-orbital nerve block
D. Long buccal nerve block

72. Complications of osteomyelitis include:
A. Ludwig's angina
B. Cavernous sinus thrombosis

C. Parotid gland involvement
D. All of the above

73. **TMJ ankylosis in an 8-year-old child is treated by:**
A. Gap arthroplasty and costochondral graft
B. Gap arthroplasty
C. Interpositional gap arthroplasty
D. None

74. **Inverted L-shaped osteotomy is used for:**
A. In case of mandibular prognathism
B. Deformities of mandible not involving the occlusion
C. Correction of maxillary deformities
D. Chin correction

75. **Trismus results from infection of which space?**
A. Submandibular space
B. Sublingual space
C. Submasseteric space
D. Buccal space

76. **Which cardiac conditions associated with highest risk for infective endocarditis?**
A. Mitral valve prolapsed without regurgitation
B. Ventricular septal defect
C. Previous history of extraction
D. Coronary artery disease

77. **Feature of fracture of infraorbital margin is characterized by:**
A. Anaesthesia of upper lip
B. Paralysis of muscles of cheek
C. Paralysis of muscles of lower eyelid
D. None

78. **Topical anesthesia used are effective upto the depth of:**
A. 0.5-1 mm B. 1-2 mm
C. 2-3 mm D. 1.5 mm-2.5 mm

79. **Hematoma formation during or immediately following a posterior superior alveolar nerve block anesthesia is most likely a result of damage to the:**
A. Facial artery
B. Pterygoid venous plexus
C. Internal maxillary artery
D. Small capillaries and arterioles

80. After Caldwel Luc procedure, intranasal antrostomy is done through:

A. Superior meatus
B. Middle meatus
C. Inferior meatus
D. Floor of nose

81. Which of the following is most important for bone degeneration?

A. Periosteum
B. Cementum
C. Bone
D. PDL

82. Iron requirement of a child is:

A. 0.5-0.1 mg/kg body weight
B. 25 mg/kg body weight
C. 100-200 mg/kg body weight
D. 500 mg/kg body weight

83. Which of the following is not a ureidopenicillin?

A. Piperacillin
B. Mezlocillin
C. Azlocillin
D. Meficloxacillin

84. Radiopaque mass is seen attached to the tooth near cervical region continuous with cementum. It is most likely:

A. Hyperplastic cementum
B. Calculus
C. Root caries
D. Subgingival pellicle

85. Radiographically sequestrum appear as:

A. Less radiopaque than normal bone
B. More radiopaque than normal bone
C. Same radiopaque than normal bone
D. None

86. The type of study involving repetitive examination of a sample is:

A. Cohort study
B. Retrospective study
C. Prospective study
D. Panel study

87. Proportion of population once affected by a disease at point of time is called:

A. Incidence
B. Prevalence
C. Point prevalence
D. Period prevalence

88. 0.2% concentration of NaF is used:

A. Once daily
B. Twice daily
C. Once weekly
D. Once fortnightly

89. Sever dental fluorosis not associated with skeletal fluorosis:

A. 1 ppm
B. 3 ppm
C. 8 ppm
D. 10 ppm

90. Concentration of labile fluoride in dentifrices is:

A. 700 ppm
B. 1000 ppm
C. 1200 ppm
D. 1400 ppm

91. In diet counselling to reduce caries in a subject of rampant caries:

A. Sugar restricted to one time a day
B. Restricted to only liquid sugar
C. No sugar content for 21 days
D. Sugar restricted to meal time only

92. The concentration of fluoride in 0.05% NaF mouthwash is:

A. 225 ppm
B. 250 ppm
C. 500 ppm
D. 1000 ppm

93. When disease spreads rapidly from one person to another in a region in a given period of time, it is termed as:

A. Pandemic
B. Endemic
C. Epidemic
D. Sporadic

94. Prevalence is defined as:

A. New cases of a particular disease occurring during a specified period
B. Proportion of population affected by disease
C. Rate of disease transmission
D. Cumulative number of cases in an area

95. What is true about case control study?

A. Retrospective study
B. Prospective study
C. Measures incidence
D. None

96. Prevention of onset of risk factor is:

A. Primary Prevention
B. Secondary Prevention
C. Tertiary Prevention
D. Primordial Prevention

97. Most common complication after use of general anesthesia is:

A. Hypertension
B. Atelectasis
C. Renal failure
D. Cardiac failure

98. Untrue among the following for class I occlusion is:

A. Mesiobuccal cusp tip if the maxillary permanent first molar falls within the groove between the mesial and middle cusps of the mandibular permanent first molar
B. Mesiolingual cusp of the maxillary permanent first molar seats in the central fossa of the mandibular permanent first molar
C. In Angle's class I molar relation, maxillary molar is slightly distal the mandibular counterparts.
D. Not recalled

99. Which of the following nerve passes through 2 heads of lateral pterygoid muscles?

A. Buccal branch of mandibular nerve
B. Masseteric nerve
C. Nerve to pterygoid muscle
D. Inferior alveolar nerve

Answers

1.	C	2.	D	3.	A	4.	B
5.	B	6.	D	7.	A	8.	D
9.	A	10.	B	11.	B	12.	D
13.	C	14.	A	15.	A	16.	A
17.	C	18.	C	19.	C	20.	B
21.	A,B	22.	C	23.	D	24.	B
25.	A	26.	B	27.	C	28.	A
29.	A	30.	C	31.	D	32.	C
33.	A	34.	D	35.	D	36.	B
37.	B	38.	C	39.	B	40.	C
41.	A	42.	C	43.	C	44.	A
45.	C	46.	C	47.	C	48.	B
49.	D	50.	B	51.	C	52.	B
53.	C	54.	D	55.	A	56.	D
57.	D	58.	D	59.	A	60.	C
61.	A	62.	B	63.	B	64.	D
65.	D	66.	B	67.	D	68.	B
69.	A	70.	C	71.	B	72.	D
73.	A	74.	A	75.	C	76.	C
77.	A	78.	C	79.	B	80.	C
81.	A	82.	B	83.	D	84.	B
85.	B	86.	D	87.	C	88.	D
89.	B	90.	A	91.	C	92.	A
93.	C	94.	B	95.	A	96.	D
97.	B	98.	D	99.	A		

PGI Paper

June 2010

1. **Maxillary antrum dips in the region of:**
   A. Between 2nd premolar and 1 molar
   B. Between buccal roots of furcation of 1st molar
   C. Between 1 and 2 premolar
   D. Between 1 and 2 molars

2. **Anterior ethmoidal sinus drains into:**
   A. Superior meatus
   B. Middle meatus
   C. Inferior meatus
   D. None

3. **Injury to which of the following will cause tongue to deviate to left when protruded?**
   A. Left hypoglossal nerve
   B. Right hypoglossal nerve
   C. Left glossopharyngeal nerve
   D. Right glossopharygeal nerve

4. **Type of epithelium in nasopharynx, trachea and respiratory mucosa is:**
   A. Pseudostratified ciliated columnar
   B. Stratified squamous
   C. Stratified columnar
   D. Pseudostratified columnar

5. **Anterior displacement of the articular disc is due to:**
   A. Masseter muscle
   B. External pterygoid
   C. Internal pterygoid
   D. Temporalis

6. **Feature of iron deficieny anemia is:**
   A. Increased Mean corpuscular volume
   B. Increased Hemoglobin levels
   C. Decreased Mean corpuscular volume
   D. Increased Mean corpuscular haemoglobin concentration

7. **Which of the following is incorrect?**
   A. U-V rays help in formation of Vitamin D in skin
   B. Renal failure leads to increase in parathormone release
   C. 25-hydroxycholecalciferol undergoes hydroxylation in kidney
   D. 25-hydroxycholecalciferol is used in treatment of renal failure

8. **PTT is prolonged in case of:**
   A. Hemophilia-A
   B. Warfarin therapy
   C. Hyper fibrinogenemia
   D. None

9. **Which of the following is true about hemoglobin?**
   A. Consist of 4 polypeptide chains
   B. It has 4 heme molecules, 2 alpha and 2 beta chains
   C. It has 2 heme molecules, 4 polypeptide chains
   D. Has 1 heme and 1 globin molecule

10. **Neutral zone concept for the arrangement of posterior teeth was given by:**
    A. Bell B. Fish
    C. Smith D. Boucher

11. **In a complete denture patient, graphic method of recording centric relation is preferred over interocclusal check record method when:**
    A. Ridges are excessively flabby
    B. Patient has uncontrollable mandibular movements
    C. Ridges are well built and related normally to each other
    D. Jaws are not related normally

12. **In RPD, functionally generated path technique has the advantage that:**
    A. The occlusion of opposing dentures can be developed together
    B. It eliminates the need for adjusting an articulator with intra-oral records
    C. Verification of the records in the mouth is easy
    D. During the generation of the path there is no risk of movement of a distal extension base

13. **All other factors remaining same, an F.P.D. with a span of 2 pontics compared to FPD with span of one pontic would flex:**

A. 2 times
B. 4 times
C. 6 times
D. 8 times

14. Retentive terminal of a clasp is placed at:

A. Either at the mesiolingual or mesiofacial line angle
B. Either at the mesiolingual or distolingual line angle
C. Either at the mesiofacial or distofacial line angle
D. Near the facial surface

15. Floating fracture of the maxilla is seen in:

A. Horizontal fracture of Maxilla
B. Pyramidal fracture of Maxilla
C. Alveolar process fracture
D. None

16. Battle's sign is seen in:

A. Fracture of anterior cranial fossa
B. Fracture of middle cranial fossa
C. Fracture of posterior cranial fossa
D. None

17. Hematoma formation during or immediately following a posterior superior alveolar nerve block is due to involvement of:

A. Pterygoid venous plexus
B. Internal maxillary artery
C. Ophthalmic vein
D. None

18. Atropine in premedication is used for:

A. To increase heart rate
B. To reduce pain
C. To reduce anxiety
D. To decrease salivation

19. During parotid gland surgery, injury to auriculotemporal nerve leads to:

A. Horner syndrome
B. Frey's syndrome
C. Facial palsy
D. Trigeminal neuralgia

20. All are true about Ludwig's angina *except*:

A. It spreads bilaterally
B. Most common cause is dental infection
C. It involves sub mandibular and sublingual spaces
D. Involvement of sub mandibular gland and lymph nodes is common

21. **Best incision to expose TMJ is:**
A. Preauricular incision
B. Risdon incision
C. Alkayat Bramley incision
D. Blair incision

22. **Infection in danger area of face most commonly leads to:**
A. Ludwig's angina
B. Cavernous sinus thrombosis
C. Space infection
D. Osteomyelitis

23. **Which of the following does not require antibiotic prophylaxis?**
A. Child under age of 15 years
B. Patient requiring liver transplantation
C. Patient having chronic renal disease
D. HIV posterior patient

24. **In TMJ ankylosis, in a child patient, what should be done?**
A. Gap arthroplasty
B. Condylectomy
C. Gap arthroplasty with costochondral grafting
D. None

25. **First sensation to be lost after administration of local anesthesia is:**
A. Pain
B. Temperature
C. Touch
D. Proprioception

26. **During 3rd trimester of pregnancy, if antibiotics are required, it should be:**
A. Reduced to half
B. Same dose is given
C. Doubled
D. Not to be given

27. **According to Veau's classification on a cleft lip and palate, isolated cleft palate falls under:**
A. Group I
B. Group II
C. Group III
D. Group IV

28. **Osteomyelitis begin in:**
A. Medullary bone
B. Periosteum

C. Cortical bone
D. All of the above spontaneously

29. After Caldwell-Luc procedure, intranasal antrostomy is done through:

A. Superior meatus B. Middle meatus
C. Inferior meatus D. Floor of nose

30. Which of the following is a tissue borne appliance?

A. Activator B. Bionator
C. Frankel regulator D. Herbst appliance

31. First step in orthodontic triage is:

A. To assess facial asymmetry
B. To assess profile of the patient
C. To separate outpatient with facial syndromes
D. Evaluation of dental development

32. Wits appraisal is relationship of:

A. Maxilla to cranium
B. Mandible to cranium
C. Maxilla to mandible
D. Maxilla and mandible to face

33. Active retainer is indicated for:

A. Maintenance of midline diastema
B. Realignment of irregular lower incisors
C. Initial lower incisor crowding during growth phase
D. Crossbite case

34. Total duration of adolescent growth in boys is:

A. 3½ years B. 5 years
C. 4 years D. 2 years

35. In a case of anterior-open bite, which sounds get distorted?

A. F B. V
C. Ch D. T

36. A single tipping force is applied to tooth, the centre of rotation is:

A. 1/3rd distance between apex and cervical line of tooth
B. 1/3rd distance between apex and incisal edge
C. 2/3rd distance between apex and cervical line of tooth
D. At apex

37. **Most commonly used slot size in orthodontic bracket is:**
A. 0.018 × 0.022 B. 0.017 × 0.021
C. 0.014 × 0.024 D. 0.010 × 0.020

38. **In a patient with normal maxilla, moderately prognathic mandible, what is the indicated treatment?**
A. Face mask B. Chin cup
C. Surgery D. Head gear

39. **In boys, fat spurt indicates:**
A. Beginning of adolescent growth
B. Height spurt beginning
C. Peak velocity in height
D. End of growth spurt

40. **In a pre-adjusted edgewise bracket the slot size is 0.022 inches (22-slot bracket). If a 0.0215 inch wire is placed inside it, what will be the play?**
A. 0.8° B. 1.8°
C. 2.8° D. 3.8°

41. **Spontaneous space closure to expected upto how many millimetres of midline diastema:**
A. 1 mm B. 2 mm
C. 1.5 mm D. 3 mm

42. **What is Roll?**
A. Transverse cant of occlusal plane
B. Up-ward deviations around anteroposterior axis
C. Left-right deviation around the vertical axis
D. Play obliquely

43. **Point representing the mid-point of symphysis (of mandible):**
A. Point-Xi B. Point-D
C. Gonion D. Gnathion

44. **Posterior most point at angle of mandible:**
A. Gonion B. Gnathion
C. Xi-point D. Point-A

45. **Which of the following orthodontic wire can be heat treated?**
A. β-titanium B. Stainless steel
C. Elgiloy D. Ni-Ti

46. What is a feature of Type-A growth pattern?

A. Maxillary Excess or Midface grows more than the lower face
B. Mandibular Excess or lower face grows more than the midface
C. Angle ANB remains same
D. Prognosis is poor

47. Hyperthyroidism in children is not associated with which of the following dental finding?

A. Periodontal destruction
B. Precocious eruption of teeth
C. Mandibular retrognathism
D. Osteoporosis

48. Development defects in enamel is usually seen with which teeth?

A. Permanent anteriors/incisors
B. Primary anteriors/incisors
C. Permanent molars
D. All

49. Molar-incisor hypoplasia in primary teeth at the occlusal level is due to developmental defect occurring during:

A. Birth to 12 months
B. 4th month intrauterine to birth
C. 22 months to 26 months
D. 24 months to 48 months

50. Which permanent tooth is first to calcify?

A. Maxillary 1st molar
B. Mandibular 1st molar
C. Canine
D. 1st premolar

51. Which of the following is least likely to occur after trauma in primary dentition?

A. Intrusion
B. Extrusion
C. Complicated crown fracture
D. Subluxation

52. Maximum part of leeway space is provided by which tooth?

A. Primary canine
B. Primary 1 molar

C. Primary 2 molar
D. Primary 1 and 2 molar contribute equally

53. **Most commonly affected by caries in a 9 years old child is:**
A. Occlusal surface of 1 molar
B. Occlusal surface of 2 molar
C. Lingual surface of anteriors
D. Interproximal surface of anteriors

54. **Destruction resorption of dental hard tissue is caused by:**
A. Odontoclasts B. Osteoclasts
C. Odontoblasts D. Osteoblasts

55. **When a primary hue is mixed with its complementary hue, the result is:**
A. Grey B. Intensification
C. Hue sensitivity D. Third hue

56. **Coefficient of thermal expansion of dental amalgam relative to tooth enamel is:**
A. 2 times than enamel
B. 2.5 times than enamel
C. 3.5 times than enamel
D. 3.0 times than enamel

57. **Which of the following is most hydrophobic?**
A. Polysulfide B. Hydrocolloid
C. Addition silicone D. Polyether

58. **Most hydrophilic material is:**
A. Hydrocolloids B. Addition silicone
C. Polyether D. Polysulfide

59. **In measuring Vicker hardness number which is used?**
A. Spiral indenter
B. Rhomboid indenter
C. 136 degree diamond pyramid
D. Stainless steel ball indenter

60. **Which of the following reduces with strain hardening?**
A. Resistance to corrosion
B. Strength
C. Surface hardness
D. Proportional limit

61. Which of the following is added in composites to provide opacity?

A. BIS-GMA
B. TEG-DMA
C. TiO_2 (Titanium dioxide)
D. None

62. In Quartz tungsten light cure device, minimum output of energy should not be less than:

A. 300 mw/cm^2 B. 350 mw/cm^2
C. 400 mw/cm^2 D. 450 mw/cm^2

63. Wavelength at which camphorquinone activity is maximum, in visible light cure system is?

A. 402 nm B. 474 nm
C. 484 nm D. 464 nm

64. Which of the following acts as an agent that removed oxides from noble metals in molten state?

A. Zinc B. Barium
C. Chromium D. Cobalt

65. Free gingival graft is placed on:

A. Bone B. Cementum
C. PDL D. Periosteum

66. Which of the following indicates a periodontal rather than endodontic lesion?

A. Acute pain on percussion with no swelling
B. Pain to lateral percussion with wide sulcular pocket
C. Deep narrow sulcular pocket to apex with exudates
D. Pain to palpation of buccal mucosa

67. The best way to prevent dehiscence during gingival graft procedure is:

A. Elevate partial thickness flap
B. Elevate full thickness flap
C. Elevate coronally positioned flap
D. Elevate double flap

68. Which micro-organism is most abundant in patients of pregnancy gingivitis?

A. P. Gingivalis B. P. Intermedia
C. Actinobacillus D. Streptococci

69. Most common implant related complication, which is mild, reversible, suprabony and present in soft tissue is:

A. Peri-implantitis
B. Peri-implant mucositis
C. Peri-implant hyperplasia
D. Fistula

70. Sulcular epithelium is:

A. Keratinized
B. Non-keratinized
C. Non-keratinized but becomes keratinized in presence of inflammation
D. Keratinized but becomes non-keratinized when exposed to oral cavity

71. Gnawing radiating pain is feature of:

A. Herpetic gingivostomatitis
B. ANUG
C. Chronic periodontitis
D. None

72. Normal salivary flow rate is:

A. 1 ml per 5 minutes
B. 3.7 ml per 5 minutes
C. 5.7 ml per 5 minutes
D. 6.5 ml per 5 minutes

73. Cells predominantly present in Stage-III gingivitis:

A. Polymorphonuclear leukocytes
B. Lymphocytes
C. Plasma cells
D. Neutrophils

74. Which of the following causes least decrease in pH?

A. Sucrose
B. Glucose
C. Fructose
D. Lactose

75. In a study, if a sample is examined on successive occasions, such a study design is called as:

A. Cohort
B. Panel
C. Prospective
D. Case control

76. 0.2% concentration of fluoride mouth rinse is used:

A. Weekly
B. Once fortnightly
C. Daily
D. Only monthly

77. In controlled trials, for how long the patient is advised to keep layer of fluoride varnish over tooth surface:

A. 1 hour after placement
B. 2 hours after placement
C. 8 hours after placement
D. 12 hours after placement

78. Prevention of onset of risk factor is:

A. Primordial Prevention
B. Primary Prevention
C. Secondary Prevention
D. Tertiary Prevention

79. Primary consideration in any oral health prevention programme:

A. Fluoride application
B. Diet contol
C. Plaque control
D. Pit and fissure sealant

80. Prevalence is defined as:

A. All new cases of a specific disease occurring during a specified period
B. Rate of disease transmission
C. Cumulative effect of a disease in an area
D. Proportion of population affected by the disease

81. Best method of checking on effectiveness of diet counselling of:

A. Lactobacillus count
B. Synder'test
C. Latest dietary history
D. Salivary reductase test

82. Dental fluorosis not associated with skeletal fluorosis:

A. 1 PPM
B. 3 PPM
C. 8 PPM
D. 10 PPM

83. Effectiveness of systemic fluoridation is:

A. 20%
B. 30%
C. 40%
D. 60%

84. Concentration of free fluoride in dentifrices is:

A. 700 ppm
B. 1000 ppm
C. 2000 ppm
D. 3000 ppm

85. After how much time, pH of root canal drops, after $Ca(OH)_2$ is placed?

A. 1 week
B. 2 weeks
C. 6 weeks
D. 4 weeks

86. Acid used for microabrasion technique recommended by croll is:

A. H_2SO_4 10%
B. HCl 18%
C. Citric acid 10%
D. HNO_3 8%

87. Type of carcinoma that develops in Marjolin ulcer:

A. BCC
B. Fibrogenic sarcoma
C. Adenocarcinoma
D. None

88. Best technique to locate an impacted canine:

A. Occlusal radiograph
B. Periapical radiograph with tube shift technique
C. CBCT
D. OPG

89. Radiographically, sequestrum appears:

A. More radiolucent than normal bone
B. Less radiopaque than normal bone
C. More radiopaque than normal bone
D. Same radiopacity as that of normal bone

90. Which structure resembles radiographically with PDL of maxillary 2nd molar?

A. Median palatine foramen
B. Anterior palatine foramen
C. Zygomatic process
D. Angle of maxilla

91. Which papillae are absent in familial dysautonomia?

A. Filiform and fungiform
B. Circumvallate
C. Fungiform and Circumvallate
D. Fungiform only

92. All are true about hypophosphatasia *except*:

A. Autosomal recessive disorder
B. Increased chances of infection
C. Increased alkaline phosphatase in serum
D. Premature exfoliation of primary teeth

93. **True about compound odontoma:**
A. Tooth like denticles
B. Tooth with in tooth appearance
C. Crown is enlarged at expense of root
D. Irregular diffuse radiopaque lesion, surrounded by radiolucent lines

94. **Which of the following is not true regarding Papillon Lefevre syndrome?**
A. Autosomal recessive disorder
B. Quantitative defect of neutrophils
C. Elisa can be used as diagnostic method
D. There is early exfoliation of primary teeth much before the eruption of permanent teeth

95. **Which of the following has polygenic inheritance?**
A. Cleft palate
B. Cleft tongue
C. Bifid rib
D. Not recalled

96. **Patient with cotton-wool appearance, hypercementosis of teeth loss of visual acuity, is suffering from:**
A. Paget's disease
B. Osteogenesis Imperfecta
C. Dentinogenesis Imperfecta
D. Cleidocranial dysplasia

97. **Acrodynia occurs due to:**
A. Exposure to minute amount of lead
B. Exposure to minute amount of mercury
C. Zinc toxicity
D. Excessive accumulation of copper

98. **Herpes zoster is characterized by:**
A. Unilateral occurrence
B. Severe burning pain
C. Crusting vesicles
D. Subepithelial bullae formation

99. **Hydropic degeneration of the basal cell layer of stratum germinativum is seen in:**
A. Lichen planus
B. Pemphigus
C. Syphilis
D. Leukoplakia

100. **Enlargement of maxilla, in a middle aged male patient indicates:**
A. Marfan syndrome
B. Paget's disease
C. Cleidocranial dysplasia
D. Ehlers-Danlos syndrome

Answers

1.	A	2.	B	3.	A	4.	A
5.	B	6.	C	7.	D	8.	A
9.	B	10.	B	11.	C	12.	B
13.	D	14.	C	15.	A	16.	B
17.	A	18.	D	19.	B	20.	D
21.	C	22.	B	23.	A	24.	C
25.	A	26.	B	27.	B	28.	A
29.	C	30.	C	31.	C	32.	C
33.	B	34.	B	35.	C	36.	A
37.	A	38.	B,C	39.	A	40.	B
41.	B	42.	A	43.	B	44.	A
45.	C	46.	C	47.	C	48.	A
49.	A	50.	A	51.	C	52.	C
53.	A	54.	A	55.	A	56.	B
57.	C	58.	A	59.	C	60.	A
61.	C	62.	A	63.	B	64.	A
65.	D	66.	B	67.	A	68.	B
69.	B	70.	B	71.	B	72.	C
73.	C	74.	D	75.	B	76.	B
77.	D	78.	A	79.	C	80.	D
81.	B	82.	B	83.	D	84.	A
85.	A	86.	B	87.	A	88.	C
89.	C	90.	B	91.	C	92.	C
93.	A	94.	B	95.	A	96.	A
97.	B	98.	A	99.	A	100.	B

PGI Paper December 2009

1. **Which of the following muscles leads to protrusion of tongue?**
   A. Genioglossus
   B. Styloglossus
   C. Palatoglossus
   D. Geniohyoid

2. **Anterior ethmoidal sinus drains into:**
   A. Superior meatus
   B. Middle meatus
   C. Inferior meatus
   D. None

3. **Which type of cells are present in trigeminal ganglion?**
   A. Pseudounipolar
   B. Bi-polar
   C. Uni-polar
   D. Multi polar

4. **Which of the following is most antigenic?**
   A. Proteins
   B. Lipids
   C. Hapten
   D. Nucleic acids

5. **Endotoxins are:**
   A. Lipopolysaccharides
   B. Proteins
   C. Antigenic
   D. Both A and B

6. **Rickettsial disease of the following is:**
   A. Relapsing fever
   B. Scrub typhus
   C. Q fever
   D. Weil's fever

7. **Which of the following is true about haemoglobin?**
   A. Consists of 4-polypeptide chains
   B. Has 2 heme molecules and 4 polypeptide chains
   C. Has 4 heme molecules and 2 alpha and 2 beta chains
   D. Has 1 heme and 1 globin molecule

8. **Purine that is found in relatively high concentration in saliva is:**
   A. Uric acid
   B. Amino acid
   C. Thymine
   D. Adenosine

9. **All of the following are used as accelerator in zinc oxide eugenol cement *except*:**
   A. Acetic acid
   B. Zinc acetate dehydrate
   C. $CaCl_2$
   D. Bromoglycerine

10. **The low thermal conductivity of impression compound can be overcome by:**
    A. By melting in boiling water at 50°C for 1 hour
    B. Impression is placed in mouth till it gets cold and sudden removal of impression
    C. By heating with ethanol flame and directly placing in patients mouth
    D. Heating in hot water and immediately quenching in water for 20 min

11. **Inhibitor is added in the monomer of self cure acrylic resin to:**
    A. Prolong the shelf life
    B. Decrease the shrinkage of acrylic
    C. Increase the time of tough stage
    D. Prevent porosity in acrylic

12. **Flux not used in stainless steel solder:**
    A. Potassium fluoride
    B. Sodium fluoride
    C. Borax
    D. Boric acid

13. **Vicker's hardness number is determined by:**
    A. Spherical indenter
    B. Steel ball indenter
    C. Rhomboid shaped indenter
    D. 136 diamond pyramid

14. **Which of the following is true about the salivary peroxidase enzyme present in the saliva?**
    A. Secreted by acinar cells of sublingual salivary gland
    B. Secreted by acinar cells of minor salivary gland

C. Secreted by acinar cells of parotid and submandibular gland
D. None of these

15. Cells responsible for resorption of dental hard tissues are:

A. Osteoclasts B. Odontoclasts
C. Giant cells D. Fibroblasts

16. Most common cells present in connective tissue are:

A. Fibroblasts B. Basket cells
C. Plasma cells D. Histocytes

17. Which of the following leads to gnawing radiating pain?

A. ANUG
B. Herpengina
C. Diptheria
D. Acute herpetic gingivostomatitis

18. The type of incision for periodontal surgery depends upon:

A. Probing depth
B. Frenal attachments
C. Width of attached gingiva
D. Presence of bony defects

19. Concentration of chlorhexidine commonly used as mouth wash:

A. 0.2% B. 2%
C. 0.12% D. 0.02%

20. Attachment of actinomycetemcomitans to the tooth surface can be prevented by:

A. Myeloperoxidase B. Lactoperoxidase
C. Collagenase D. None

21. Probing force used during periodontal examination:

A. 25 gm B. 75 gm
C. 50 gm D. 35 gm

22. Specific plaque hypothesis for etiology of periodontal disease was given by:

A. Glickman B. Jenco
C. Listgarten D. Loesche

23. Which of the following salivary factor is most bactericidal?

A. Ca^{2+} and PO_4^{2-} B. Lactoperoxidase
C. Lysozyme D. IgA

24. Attached gingiva is:

A. From depth of pocket to gingival margin
B. From free gingival margin to the mucogingival junction
C. From base of sulcus to mucogingival junction
D. None

25. IL-1 and TNF-α are secreted by:

A. Lymphocytes
B. PMN's
C. Fibroblasts
D. Activated macrophages

26. Bence Jones proteins are seen in:

A. Multiple myeloma
B. Malignant melanoma
C. Hodgkin's lymphoma
D. None

27. Teratoma is:

A. Originate from mesodermal tissue
B. Hamartous development manifestation consisting of 3 different layers
C. Occurs most commonly in stomach and lungs
D. Associated with very painful condition

28. Giant cell lesions of the periodontium are dental update best considered as:

A. Benign neoplasm
B. Malignant neoplasm
C. Non-neoplastic reactive lesions
D. None

29. Most common cleft defect in lip is:

A. Midline defect
B. Unilateral left cleft
C. Unilateral right cleft
D. Bilateral cleft

30. True about syphilis is:

A. Oral lesions are seen at any stage
B. Clinical manifestation occur after few months of exposure

C. VDRL test is positive in early stages of primary syphilis
D. Penicillins are ineffective

31. Rhabdomyosarcoma is the tumour of:
A. Benign tumour of skeletal muscles
B. Benign tumour of smooth muscles
C. Malignant tumour of smooth muscles
D. Maligant tumour of skeletal muscles

32. Wound healing is impaired by:
A. Steroids
B. Vitamin C
C. Diet high in minerals
D. Analgesics

33. Most commonly used fixative agent for biopsy sample is:
A. 10% formaline
B. 10% alcohol
C. 20% formaline
D. 20% alcohol

34. Ventilation perfusion ratio test would be most required in case of which of following disease?
A. Eosinophilic pneumonia
B. Pulmonary embolism
C. Chronic bronchitis
D. Pneumonia

35. Treatment of hemophilia includes:
A. Factor 8 and 9 replacement
B. Factor 8 replacement
C. Thrombin replacement
D. Fresh frozen plasma

36. Disuse atrophy of periodontium occur in all *except*:
A. Erythema multiforme
B. Lupus erythematous
C. Herpangina
D. Chicken pox

37. In SIRS (Systemic inflammatory response syndrome) there is all *except*:
A. Temperature < 36 or > 38 degree
B. Blood pressure > 110/70
C. Respiratory rate > 20/minute
D. Abnormal white blood cell count > 12000/mm^3 or < 4000/mm^3

38. **Most accepted sequence of extraction to serial extraction is:**
A. CD4 B. 4CD
C. C4D D. D4C

39. **Which of the following is bactericidal substitute for sugars?**
A. Xylitol B. Sorbitol
C. Mannitol D. Glycerol

40. **In a patient of rampant caries, diet modification should be:**
A. Sugar exposure only to meal times
B. Sugar exposure only to meal times for 21 days
C. No sugar for 21 days
D. Restrict only sticky sugars

41. **Tooth start erupting corresponding to which Nolla's stage?**
A. 4 B. 5
C. 6 D. 7

42. **How much variation in eruption of molars is considered normal?**
A. 0-6 months B. 6-12 months
C. 12-18 months D. 18-24 months

43. **Partial pulpotomy technique was given by:**
A. Bowen B. Glark
C. CVEK D. Willet

44. **Which of the following is an example of child maltreatment?**
A. Munchausen syndrome by proxy
B. Blue baby syndrome
C. Kenner syndrome
D. Sending the child to school

45. **Most reliable histologic criteria for the diagnosis of squamous cell carcinomas:**
A. Invasion B. Pleomorphism
C. Encapsulation D. Degeneration

46. **Tracheostomy is done through:**
A. 1st tracheal ring
B. 2nd to 4th tracheal ring

C. Cricothyroid membrane
D. Thyrohyoid ligament

47. Trauma to nerve resulting in parasthesia is termed as:
A. Neuropraxia B. Neurotenesis
C. Axonotmesis D. None

48. Type of carcinoma that develop in marjolin ulcer is:
A. Basal cell carcinoma
B. Adenosarcoma
C. Ameloblastoma
D. Fibrosarcoma

49. Iron requirement in children is:
A. 2-5 mg/kg of body weight
B. 8-10 mg/kg of body weight
C. 20-25 mg/kg of body weight
D. 50-70 mg/kg of body weight

50. Atropine is used in preanesthetic medication for:
A. It decreases bronchial secretion
B. To reduce pain
C. To relieve anxiety
D. Decrease salivary secretions and depress vagal reflex

51. In a normal distribution curve the SD = 2 excludes how much value?
A. 93.4% B. 95.7%
C. 4.6% D. 99.3%

52. How much million people of world are using fluoridated tooth paste?
A. 100 B. 500
C. 700 D. 900

53. Type of study involving repeated examination of group is:
A. Cohort study
B. Panel study
C. Cross-sectional study
D. Retrospective study

54. 0.2% NaF is used:
A. Once daily B. Once weekly
C. Once fortnightly D. Once monthly

55. **When a disease spreads rapidly from one person to another person in a region in a given period of time is termed as:**
A. Pandemic
B. Endemic
C. Epidemic
D. Sporadic

56. **Index age groups according to WHO national path finder survey is:**
A. 5, 15, 25, 35, 65-75 years
B. 5, 10, 15, 30, 60-70 years
C. 5, 12, 15, 35-44, 65-74 years
D. 5-10, 15-35, 40-45 years

57. **Effectiveness of systemic fluoridation in caries is:**
A. 60%
B. 40%
C. 30%
D. 10%

58. **The critical pH of caries ranges from:**
A. 3.5-5.5
B. 4.5-5.5
C. 5.0-5.5
D. 4.0-5.0

59. **ART was invented in Tanzania by:**
A. Je Franken
B. Mclean
C. McDonald
D. Eversole

60. **Which of the following indicate caries incidence?**
A. Caries activity
B. Caries attack rate
C. Caries increment
D. All of the above

61. **Caries activity test measures:**
A. Caries activity
B. pH
C. Motivational aspects
D. Penetration

62. **Carisolv is used for:**
A. Staining of carious lesion
B. Enamel caries detection
C. To study histologic sections of teeth
D. Softening of dentin for removal of carious lesion

63. **Type I acid etching of enamel refers to:**
A. Removal of enamel prism cores with prism peripheries relatively intact
B. Periphery is removed leaving the core intact
C. Prism less enamel
D. Complete removal of enamel

64. In Class II cavity for amalgam in pediatric patients, gingival line angle is:

A. Left unbevelled
B. Beveled as in permanent teeth
C. Beveled to increase retention
D. None

65. Pore volume of the dark zone of enamel caries is:

A. 1% B. 4%
C. 5-24% D. More than 25%

66. Minimum depth of the lesion to be visible on radiograph is:

A. 40 m B. 50 m
C. 100 m D. 500 m

67. What could be the reason for a semicircular radio-opacity present in an IOPA?

A. Artifact B. Contamination
C. Cone cutting D. Eburnation

68. Which of the following will give best view of articular disc?

A. Plane CT B. Cone beam CT
C. Spiral CT D. MRI

69. Most penetrating rays are:

A. Hard rays B. Soft rays
C. Grenz rays D. None

70. Zygomatic arch fracture are best visualized by:

A. Submentovertex view
B. Occipitomental view
C. Reverse Towne's view
D. PA view

71. Which of the following is not a contrast radiography?

A. Sialography
B. Single photon emission computed technology
C. Tomogram
D. Arthrogram

72. Cardiac condition requiring antibiotic prophylaxis for infective endocarditis:

A. Coronary heart disease
B. Cardiac pace makers

C. Rheumatic heart disease
D. Hypertensive heart disease

73. Latency period in distraction osteogenesis is:
A. 4-7 days B. 7-10 days
C. 1-2 days D. 14-20 days

74. Inverted L-shaped osteotomy is done to treat:
A. In case of mandibular prognathism
B. Deformities of mandible not involving the occlusion
C. Correction of maxillary deformities
D. Chin deformity

75. During inferior alveolus nerve block needle is inserted in:
A. Submandibular space
B. Pterygomandibular space
C. Masseteric space
D. Infratemporal space

76. Recommended time gap between the radiation exposure and surgery to avoid osteoradionecrosis is:
A. 4-6 weeks
B. 4-12 months
C. Immediately after exposure
D. Any time

77. What is the minimum distance between the nasal vestibule and implant?
A. 1 mm B. 2 mm
C. 2.5 mm D. 3.0 mm

78. Fall back of tongue after an accident occurs due to:
A. Bilateral parasymphyseal fracture
B. Bilateral single fracture
C. Bilateral condylar fracture
D. Symphysis fracture midline

79. Most common complications of open fracture is:
A. Bleeding
B. Thrombophlebitis
C. Muscular contracture
D. Infection

80. A patient is on warfarin therapy, which factor should be evaluated before taking up oral surgical procedures?

A. Bleeding time
B. Clotting time
C. Partial thromboplastin time
D. Prothrombin time

81. Hematoma formation during or immediately following a posterior superior alveolar nerve block is most likely a result of damage to the:
A. Facial artery
B. Pterygoid venous plexus
C. Internal maxillary artery
D. Capillaries and arterioles

82. Which of the following suture material will lead to maximum tissue response?
A. Liner
B. Catgut
C. Silk
D. Nylon

83. Fracture of floor of the orbit is characterized by:
A. Anesthesia of upper lip
B. Paralysis of muscles of neck
C. Paralysis of muscles of lower eyelid
D. None

84. In 8-year-old child of TMJ ankylosis, should be treated by:
A. Gap arthroplasty and costochondral graft
B. Gap arthroplasty
C. Interpositional gap arthroplasty
D. None

85. Which of the following can be used for controlling the bleeding from an extraction socket?
A. Bone wax
B. Vitamin K
C. Suturing of wound margins
D. None

86. Syndrome associated with Gustatory sweating:
A. Eagle syndrome
B. Trotter syndrome
C. Frey's syndrome
D. Reiter's syndrome

87. **Antibiotic prophylaxis is mandatory in case of:**
A. Open reduction of fracture mandible
B. Scaling and root planning
C. RCT
D. Extraction

88. **In the treatment plan of a conventional immediate complete denture the anterior teeth are extracted:**
A. At the first appointment
B. Before making immediate denture
C. Before extracting the posterior teeth
D. After making the immediate denture

89. **Compared to cast cirumferential clasp the main disadvantage of combination clasp is that:**
A. It can flex in all spatial planes
B. More prone to breakage and damage
C. It is less acceptable esthetically
D. Has greater contact with tooth surface

90. **Tooth preparation for laminates extends upto:**
A. Labial to contact
B. Lingual to contact
C. At the contact
D. None

91. **Neutral zone concept for the arrangement of posterior teeth was given by:**
A. Bell
B. Fish
C. Smith
D. Boucher

92. **In the clasp of an RPD support is provided by:**
A. Rest
B. Reciprocal arm
C. Auxillary arm
D. None

93. **Modiolus at the corner of mouth is formed by all of the following muscles *except*:**
A. Triangularis
B. Buccinator
C. Orbicularis oris
D. Alaque Nasi

94. **Success of removable die system is based upon:**
A. Abrasion resistance of the die material
B. Length of dowel protruding out of master cast
C. Time involved in construction
D. Precise relocation of the die in working cast

95. Tooth movement requiring maximum force value:

A. Intrusion
B. Extrusion
C. Root up righting
D. Rotation

96. Chemical mediators that play role in orthodontic tooth movement:

A. Interleukins
B. Prostaglandins
C. Histamines
D. Serotonin

97. Ossification centers present at birth are:

A. Humerus
B. Proximal end of tibia
C. Distal end of femur
D. All

98. Maximum part of leeway space is provided by which tooth?

A. Primary canine
B. Primary 1 molar
C. Primary 2 molar
D. Primary 1 and 2 molar contribute equally

99. The AO and BO in wit's appraisal is relationship of:

A. Maxilla to cranium
B. Mandible to cranium
C. Maxilla to mandible
D. Maxilla and mandible to face

100. Cartilage differs from bone in that:

A. Apposition growth pattern
B. Interstitial growth pattern
C. Growth of cells in lacunae
D. None

Answers

1.	A	2.	B	3.	A	4.	A
5.	A	6.	B,C	7.	C	8.	A
9.	D	10.	B	11.	A	12.	B
13.	D	14.	C	15.	B	16.	A
17.	A	18.	C	19.	A	20.	A
21.	A	22.	D	23.	A	24.	A
25.	D	26.	A	27.	B	28.	C
29.	B	30.	A	31.	D	32.	A
33.	A	34.	B	35.	A	36.	C
37.	B	38.	A	39.	A	40.	C
41.	C	42.	D	43.	C	44.	A
45.	A	46.	B	47.	A	48.	A
49.	C	50.	D	51.	C	52.	B
53.	B	54.	B	55.	C	56.	C
57.	A	58.	C	59.	A	60.	D
61.	A,C	62.	D	63.	A	64.	A
65.	B	66.	D	67.	C	68.	D
69.	A	70.	A	71.	C	72.	C
73.	A	74.	A	75.	B	76.	A
77.	A	78.	A	79.	D	80.	D
81.	B	82.	B	83.	A	84.	A
85.	A,C	86.	C	87.	A	88.	D
89.	B	90.	A	91.	B	92.	A
93.	D	94.	D	95.	C	96.	B
97.	D	98.	C	99.	A	100.	B

PGI Paper
June 2009

1. **All are the derivatives of the neural crest *except*:**
   A. Schwann cells
   B. Cranial and spinal motor nerve
   C. Dorsal root ganglion
   D. Parasympathetic ganglion

2. **Which of the following is compound nerve?**
   A. Optic nerve
   B. Olfactory nerve
   C. Trigeminal nerve
   D. Hypoglossal nerve

3. **The modiolus represents the origin, insertion or decussation of many fibres of various muscles, which of the following muscle is not represented?**
   A. Levator labi superioris aleque nasii
   B. Zygomaticus major
   C. Orbicularis oris
   D. Buccinator

4. **Patient jaw is kept open with the bite block, which of the following muscles will be activated?**
   A. Elevator and retractor muscles
   B. Depressor and retractor muscles
   C. Depressor and protractor muscles
   D. Elevator and protractor muscles

5. **Incubation period of measles is:**
   A. 25-35 days
   B. 14-21 days
   C. 7-14 days
   D. 2-5 days

6. **Which is most antigenic?**
   A. Lipid
   B. Haptens
   C. Proteins
   D. Nucleic acids

7. Acetone is used for the fixation of which of the following?

A. Glycogen B. Enzymes
C. Lipid D. Polysaccharide

8. Contact point between the maxillary central incisor is located in:

A. Incisal 3rd B. Middle 3rd
C. Cervical 3rd D. Variable

9. What is the number of dentinal tubules present at DEJ (1 mm^2)?

A. 5000-10000 B. 15000-20000
C. 50000-70000 D. 30000-45000

10. Which of the following is true statement when comparing intertubular and peritubular dentin?

A. Peritubular dentin is hypomineralised as compared to intertubular dentin
B. Intertubular dentin is hypomineralised as compared to peritubular dentin
C. Intertubular is hypermineralized
D. Both are same mineralized

11. Which of the following is true about the salivary peroxidase enzyme present in the saliva?

A. Secreted by acinar cells of sublingual salivary gland
B. Secreted by acinar cells of minor salivary gland
C. Secreted by acinar cells of parotid and submandibular gland
D. None of these

12. Proteins present in saliva are:

A. Creatinine and albumin
B. Mucin and amylase
C. Albumin and bicarbonate
D. Albumin and calcium

13. Purine that is present in relatively high concentration in saliva:

A. Uric acid B. Adenosine
C. Thymine D. Amino acid

14. Hyperthermia resulting from an injury can be due to:

A. Fluid imbalance B. Infection
C. Drug reaction D. Not recalled

15. Which of the following is true about a patient suffering from AIDS?

A. Cause destruction of B. lymphocytes along with CD4 reduction
B. Contain DNA genome
C. Pneumocystis carnii is most common infection in AIDS patient
D. Bacteroid meningitis is most common cause of meningeal involvement in AIDS patient

16. Gene for leucocyte adhesion defect is present on:

A. Chromosome 1
B. Chromosome 5
C. Chromosome 21
D. Chromosome X

17. What is non fibrillar collagen?

A. Type III
B. Type V
C. Type IX
D. Type XI

18. Syndrome associated with gustatory sweating:

A. Eagle syndrome
B. Trotter syndrome
C. Frey's syndrome
D. Reiter's syndrome

19. Absence of one or more teeth is seen in all *except*:

A. Down's syndrome
B. Ehlers-Danlos syndrome
C. Reiger's syndrome
D. Gardner syndrome

20. Goltz Gorlin syndrome is associated with:

A. Multiple teratoma
B. Multiple osteoma
C. Multiple fibroma
D. Multiple papilloma

21. Defect in which collagen type causes dystrophic epidermolysis bullosa?

A. IV
B. II
C. VII
D. V

22. Ventilation-perfusion ratio test would be most required in case of which of following disease?

A. Eosinophilic pneumonia
B. Pulmonary embolism
C. Chronic bronchitis
D. Pneumonia

23. All of the following are true about pseudomembranous candidiasis *except*:
A. Involves surface of tongue, buccal mucosa and palate
B. It is rare and idiopathic
C. Also known as oral thrush
D. Commonly occurs in immune compromised patient

24. Which is true about papule?
A. Flat pigmented area of 1 cm diameter
B. Solid raised area with less than 1 cm diameter
C. Solid raised area with more than 1 cm diameter
D. Fluid filled raised area

25. The cell predominantly present in Stage III gingivitis:
A. Plasma cells
B. PMNs
C. Lymphocytes
D. Macrophage

26. Specific plaque hypothesis was given by:
A. Listgarten
B. Glickmann
C. Loesche
D. Socranky

27. Perimylosis is:
A. Tooth wear due to acid secretion
B. Tooth wear due to bruxism
C. Tooth wear due to dentifrices
D. Peripheral red cell destruction

28. Width of attached gingiva is:
A. From base of sulcus to mucogingival junction
B. From gingival margin to base of sulcus
C. From gingival crest to free margin
D. From gingival margin to mucogingival junction

29. Disuse atrophy of periodontal ligament is seen in all *except*:
A. Herpangina
B. SLE
C. Erythema multiforme
D. Chicken pox

30. Main causative organism in pregnancy gingivitis is:
A. B. Fosythus
B. P. gingivalis
C. P. intermedia
D. Fusobacterium

31. Destruction of the periodontal ligament without inflammation is known as:

A. Gingivitis
B. Periodontitis
C. Peridontosis
D. ANUG

32. Total arch length reduced due to mesial migration of teeth:

A. 1 cm
B. 3 cm
C. 0.5 cm
D. 0.15 cm

33. Rubber dam was introduced by:

A. G.V.black
B. S.C. Barnum
C. MacConkey
D. W. Clark

34. Type 1 acid etching pattern for composite restoration:

A. Dissolution of core prism without periphery involvement
B. Dissolution of periphery without core prism involvement
C. Dissolution of both core prism as well as periphery
D. Irregular and indiscriminate pattern

35. What is the wavelength of Er : YAG laser (um)?

A. 2.94 mm
B. 3.84 mm
C. 6.80 mm
D. 10.6 mm

36. Which of the following laser acts same as in visible light range?

A. ArF
B. ND. YAG
C. Co2
D. HeNe

37. Most radiopaque among the following is:

A. Enamel
B. Dentin
C. Cementum
D. Amalgam

38. Indication of MTA is one of the following:

A. Pulp capping
B. Root fracture
C. Apexification
D. Internal resorption

39. The critical pH of caries ranges from:

A. 3.5-5.5
B. 4.5-5.5
C. 5.0-5.5
D. 4.0-5.0

40. Caries is characterized by destruction and dissolution of inorganic and organ in portion of tooth enamel, which is the true statement regarding caries?

A. It is infectious and transmissible
B. It is multifactorial but not infectious

C. It is non-infectious but transmissible
D. It is neither multifactorial nor transmissible

41. Hard dark brown and cleanable caries which is also difficult to remove?

A. Acute caries
B. Chronic caries
C. Rampant caries
D. Eburnated caries

42. Covert caries is also known as:

A. Root caries
B. Arrested caries
C. Pit and fissure caries
D. Rampant caries

43. Pore volume in dark zone is:

A. 1%
B. 2-4%
C. 5-25%
D. 30%

44. Which of the following could be the best reason for enamel caries development?

A. Due to imbalance of Ca/PO_4 ratio of tooth
B. Due to super saturation of Ca and PO_4 of the saliva
C. Due to imbalance of pH between dental plaque and saliva
D. Due to disturbed equilibrium of Ca and PO_4 ion between saliva and plaque

45. Dentocult test in the clinics is done for detection of which of the following microorganisms?

A. Streptococcus Mutans
B. Streptococcus Sobrinus
C. Streptococcus Mitis
D. Lactobacillus

46. For how much time, the fluoride varnish should be left over the teeth in completely controlled clinical condition?

A. 2 hours
B. 6 hours
C. 8 hours
D. 12 hours

47. Number of teeth examined for PHP-index are:

A. 6
B. 12
C. 18
D. 24

48. Safely tolerated dose (STD) of fluoride:

A. 8-16 mg/kg body wt.
B. 16-32 mg/kg body wt.
C. 32-64 mg/kg body wt.
D. 1-4 mg/kg body wt.

49. Probable toxic dose of fluoride is:
A. 32-64 mg/kg body wt.
B. 8-16 mg/kg body wt.
C. 16-32 mg/kg body wt.
D. 15 mg/kg body wt.

50. Case control study is also known as:
A. Incidence study
B. Prospective study
C. Retrospective study
D. Cross-sectional study

51. A disease affecting a large population in an area with in a short period of time is called as:
A. Endemic
B. Epidemic
C. Sporadic
D. Pandemic

52. Which study is used to study large country survey?
A. Random sampling
B. Multistage sampling
C. Multiphase sampling
D. Stratified sampling

53. What is the level of fluoride present in the dental plaque?
A. 50-100 ppm
B. 8-13 ppm
C. 1-5 ppm
D. 0.1-0.5 ppm

54. Concentration of fluoride in human milk is:
A. 6-12 mg/ml
B. 3-6 mg/ml
C. 12-16 mg/ml
D. 16-20 mg/ml

55. First fluoride tooth paste approved by ADA:
A. 1931
B. 1960
C. 1964
D. 1984

56. Concentration of fluoride in ppm present in 0.05% NaF:
A. 225
B. 900
C. 9000
D. 500

57. According to WHO, fluoride mouthwash is not recommended below the age of:
A. 2 years
B. 4 years
C. 6 years
D. 10 years

58. First country to acquire fluoride varnish was:
A. Germany
B. USA
C. UK
D. India

59. Surgery of which anatomical structure results in increased perspiration and flushing while eating food?

A. Parotid gland
B. Submandibular gland
C. Both the above
D. Sublingual gland

60. The nerve injury associated with parasthesia with complete recovery is known as:

A. Neuropraxia
B. Axonemetesis
C. Neurometesis
D. None

61. True about acute osteomyelitis of mandible are all *except*:

A. Severe pain
B. Show radiolucency on the radiograph
C. Purulent exudates
D. Paraesthesia of lower lip

62. All are true about submucosal palatal cleft *except*:

A. Mainfest as defect in the underlying musculature of soft palate with notch like depression
B. Covered by mucosa but shows discontinuity in the bone from incisive foramen to posteriorly
C. Can be palpated with blunt instrument
D. False cleft

63. First sensation lost after L.A. administration:

A. Touch
B. Temperature
C. Pain
D. Proprioception

64. The sequential stage of distraction osteogenesis are:

A. Osteotomy/latency period/distraction/consolidation/remodelling
B. Distraction/osteotomy/ latency/consolidation/remodelling
C. Consolidation/latency period/distraction/osteotomy/remodelling
D. Latency period/osteotomy/distraction/remodelling/osteotomy

65. Osteo radionecrosis is due to the involvement of:

A. Blood vessels
B. Lymphatics
C. Nerves
D. All of these

66. What could be the cause of otorrhoea (bleeding from ear)?
A. Fracture of petrous part of parietal bone
B. Fracture of mastoid process
C. Rupture of tympanic membrane
D. Fracture of anterior cranial fossa

67. For cheatle forceps sterilization, which concentration of solvent is used?
A. 100%
B. 20%
C. 10%
D. 1%

68. A cyst present in the midline of neck of 6 years child:
A. Brachial cyst
B. Ranula
C. Thyroglossal cyst
D. Sternal cyst

69. According to malignant melanoma classification of tumour invasion the level III is:
A. Tumour confined to epidermis and present above basement membrane
B. Confined to papillary epidermis and is in radial growth phase
C. Throughout papillary dermis and impingement on reticular dermis and is in vertical phase
D. Tumour cells seen clearly in reticular dermis

70. Which is most severe complication of open fracture?
A. Bleeding
B. Infection
C. Non union
D. Fibrous union

71. Which is the most common cause of epistaxis?
A. Nose prick
B. Bleeding disorders
C. Hypertension
D. Nasal polyp

72. All are early complication of tracheostomy *except*:
A. Pneumothorax
B. Mediastenitis
C. Aerophagia
D. Arterial fistula/erosion

73. What is the percentage of occurrence of supernumerary teeth in maxilla?
A. 80%
B. 85%
C. 90%
D. 95%

74. Which is the true statement about change in mandibular arch circumference in a child between 5 and 18 years of age?

A. Increases by 0-1 mm
B. Decreases by 0-1 mm
C. Decreases by 3-4 mm
D. Increases by 3-4 mm

75. Mayne's appliance is a modification of:

A. Lingual arch
B. Nance palatal arch
C. Transpalatal arch
D. Band and loop

76. What could be the reason for a semicircular radiopaque present in an IOPA?

A. Artifact
B. Contamination
C. Cone cutting
D. Eburnation

77. Which of the following will give best view of articular disc?

A. Plane CT
B. Cone beam CT
C. Spiral CT
D. MRI

78. Cervical burn out is due to the presence of:

A. Proximal caries
B. Occlusal caries extending to cervical region
C. Enamel hypomineralisation
D. Thin cervical enamel

79. When comparing the digital X-ray technique to conventional X-ray; the true statement is:

A. Exposure time is slightly more than normal X-ray
B. Exposure time is nearly same
C. Exposure time is half of the normal X-ray
D. Exposure time is less than 1/3 of normal X-ray

80. The flux used for the soldering of stainless steel differ from the gold alloy is:

A. Sodium nitrate
B. Stanneous fluoride
C. Potassium fluoride
D. Calcium carbonate

81. Which of the following is least surface detail producing impression material?

A. Reversible hydrocolloid
B. Polyether

C. ZOE
D. Irreversible hydrocolloid

82. Inhibitors are added to the acrylic resins in order:
A. Initiate polymerization reaction
B. Increase the time of tough stage before the polymerization
C. Decrease the polymerization shrinkage
D. Increases the self life

83. All of the following are used as accelerator in zinc oxide eugenol *except*:
A. Acetic acid
B. Zinc acetate dehydrate
C. Calcium chloride
D. Bromoglycerine

84. Thermal conductivity of impression compound is low. What is clinical significance of this when used as an impression material?
A. The material should be immediately removed after impression
B. Heat when ethanol flame from below the tray and directly placing impression in patient mouth
C. Wait for complete cooling of the material and then suddenly remove the impression
D. Heating in hot water and immediately quenching in water for 20 minutes

85. Pantograph is used to record:
A. Jaw movement
B. Maxillary movement
C. Orientation of jaw
D. Radiographic view for maxilla and mandible

86. Primary support of a clasp is due to:
A. Occlusal rest
B. Shoulder
C. Minor connector
D. Shaddle area

87. Immediate Bennet side shift is used to define the shift when it occurs:
A. Immediately after the forward movement is completed
B. In the first 5-6 mm of forward movement
C. Before any forward movement of the orbiting condyle
D. Throughout the range of motion

88. What will be change in teeth setting for a patient with class II?

A. No alteration is required
B. Increase the freeway space
C. Decrease the freeway space
D. Teeth settling is not possible

89. What is true statement regarding ideal anterior teeth (maxillary) selection in the women for perfect smile line?

A. Width of lateral incisor should be 42% of central incisor and of canine should be 42% of lateral incisor
B. Width of lateral incisor should be 62% of central incisor and of canine should be 62% of lateral incisor
C. Width of lateral incisor should be 52% of central incisor and of canine should be 52% of lateral incisors
D. Width of lateral incisor should be 32% of central incisor and of canine should be 32% of lateral incisors

90. Interpupillary width is equal to:

A. Width of nose
B. Width of eyes
C. Distance between gonial angle
D. Width of mouth

91. Which of the following is true about, i.e., fort-1 fracture?

A. Bleeding from antrum
B. Ecchymosis and oedema around eyes
C. CSF rhinorrhea
D. Open bite

92. The maximum safe dose of 1:2,00,000 lignocaine with adrenaline is:

A. 4 mg/kg body wt
B. 5 mg/kg body wt
C. 7 mg/kg body wt
D. 10 mg/kg body wt

93. Respiratory obstruction due to tongue falling back occurs in fracture of:

A. Symphysis
B. Bilateral parasymphyseal fracture
C. Condyle
D. Angle

94. Normal chin throat angle is (in degree):

A. 70°
B. 80°
C. 90°
D. 100°

95. What is a feature of Type-A growth pattern?

A. Maxillary excess or midface grows more than the lower face
B. Mandibular excess or lower face grows more than the midface
C. Angle ANB remains same
D. Prognosis is poor

96. Direction of growth of alveolus in maxilla is:

A. Downward only
B. Downward and outward
C. Downward and inward
D. Upward and outward

97. Direction of growth of alveolar bone in mandible is by:

A. Upward and inward
B. Upward and outward
C. Upward only
D. Outward only

98. First parameter used in Steiner's analysis:

A. Facial angle
B. SNA
C. SNB
D. ANB

99. Which is the best radiograph for the estimation of gonial angle?

A. OPG
B. Lateral oblique
C. Lateral ceph
D. PA view

100. Which of the following is first of modern analysis?

A. Down's analysis
B. Rickett's analysis
C. Steiner's analysis
D. Tweed's analysis

Answers

1.	B	2.	C	3.	A	4.	D
5.	C	6.	C	7.	B	8.	A
9.	B	10.	B	11.	C	12.	B
13.	A	14.	B	15.	C	16.	C
17.	D	18.	C	19.	D	20.	D
21.	C	22.	B	23.	B	24.	B
25.	A	26.	C	27.	A	28.	A
29.	A	30.	C	31.	C	32.	C
33.	B	34.	A	35.	A	36.	D
37.	D	38.	C	39.	C	40.	A
41.	D	42.	C	43.	B	44.	C
45.	D	46.	D	47.	A	48.	A
49.	C	50.	C	51.	B	52.	B
53.	B	54.	A	55.	C	56.	A
57.	C	58.	A	59.	A	60.	A
61.	B	62.	D	63.	C	64.	A
65.	A	66.	C	67.	D	68.	C
69.	C	70.	B	71.	A	72.	D
73.	C	74.	C	75.	D	76.	C
77.	D	78.	D	79.	C	80.	C
81.	D	82.	D	83.	D	84.	C
85.	A	86.	A	87.	C	88.	B
89.	B	90.	A	91.	A	92.	C
93.	B	94.	C	95.	C	96.	B
97.	A	98.	B	99.	C	100.	C

PGI Paper
December 2008

---

1. **Middle conchae of nose are part of:**
   A. Vomer B. Maxilla
   C. Nasal bone D. Ethmoid
2. **All of the following is lined by stratified squamous epithelium *except*:**
   A. Lips
   B. Tongue
   C. Root of the soft palate
   D. Oropharynx
3. **All of the following are secretomotor to submandibular gland *except*:**
   A. Facial nerve B. Lingual nerve
   C. Mylohyoid nerve D. Chorda Tympani
4. **Which of the following muscle leads to protrusion of tongue?**
   A. Genioglossus B. Palatoglossus
   C. Styloglossus D. Geniohyoid
5. **In a child development the embryo period is:**
   A. 0-2 weeks B. 2-3 weeks
   C. 2-9 weeks D. 9 weeks to birth
6. **Which of the following bones ossify first?**
   A. Nasal bone B. Mandible
   C. Vomer D. Occipital
7. **All of the following are true about skeletal muscle *except*:**
   A. Have transverse striations
   B. Have multiple nuclei
   C. The nuclei are central
   D. They are cylindrical in shape

8. **True about HB is:**
   A. Have 4 heme molecules and 2 alpha and 2 beta chains
   B. Have one heme and one globin molecule
   C. Have two heme group and four polypeptide chain
   D. Consists of 4 different polypeptide chains

9. **Which of the following is most commonly missing teeth?**
   A. Maxillary molars
   B. Mandibular premolars
   C. Maxillary canines
   D. Mandibular incisors

10. **Gingiva is attached to enamel by:**
    A. Tight junction
    B. Hemidesmosomes
    C. Gap junction
    D. Desmosomes

11. **Biological zone is defined as:**
    A. It is 2.04 mm
    B. Synonym of biological width
    C. It is the total width of junctional epithelium, connective tissue attachment and sulcus depth
    D. It is the total width of junctional epithelium, connective tissue attachment

12. **The final evaluation of the root surface smoothness after root planning is done by:**
    A. Scaler
    B. Explorer
    C. Probe
    D. Curettes

13. **Gingivitis in leukemic patient resemble:**
    A. Bullous pemphigus
    B. ANUG
    C. Thrombocytopenic purpura
    D. Herpetic gingivostomatitis

14. **Which of the following salivary factor is not bactericidal?**
    A. Ca^{2+} and PO_4^{2-}
    B. Lectoperoxidase
    C. IgA
    D. Lysozymes

15. **Which of the following can lead to gnawing radiating pain?**
    A. Chronic periodontitis
    B. ANUG
    C. Herpetic gingivostomatitis
    D. None

16. **Which of the following condition if not treated, can lead to indifferent course?**
    A. Herpengina
    B. Herpetic gingivostomatitis
    C. Diphtheria
    D. ANUG

17. **Most common extra-oral cause of halitosis is:**
    A. Alcohol intake
    B. Indigestion
    C. Chronic sinusitis
    D. Diabetes mellitus

18. **Periodontal pack is least successful in the management of:**
    A. Antimicrobial properties
    B. Hemostasis
    C. Splinting
    D. Pain elimination

19. **Which PDL fibers are reconstructed soon after its destruction?**
    A. Oblique
    B. Alveolar crestal group
    C. Supracrestal
    D. Transseptal

20. **Change in arch length from mesial surface of permanent 1st molar between the ages of 6 and 18 years is:**
    A. Increased by 0-1 mm
    B. Increased by 3-4 mm
    C. Decreased by 0-1 mm
    D. Decreased by 3-4 mm

21. **Acellular cementum is present at:**
    A. Only at the apex
    B. Coronal half of the root
    C. Apical half of the root
    D. Middle third of the root

22. **Which furcation defect require only odontoplasty?**
    A. Grade-I
    B. Grade-II
    C. Grade-III
    D. Grade-IV

23. **True about pellicle is:**
    A. Derived from microorganisms
    B. Full of microorganisms
    C. Is inorganic in nature
    D. Prerequisite for plaque

24. **CADIA system is used to check:**
    A. Furcation involvement
    B. Bleeding sites

C. Mobility of teeth
D. Progression of periodontal disease

25. Dewey's Modification of the Angle's Class-I type II is:
A. Anterior in labioversion
B. Posterior crossbite
C. Crowded anteriors
D. Anterior crossbite

26. Type of force used in a patient activated appliance is:
A. Interrupted
B. Intermittent
C. Continuous intermittent
D. Continuous interrupted

27. The outermost envelop in Ackermann's Proffit Classification denotes:
A. Profile
B. Alignment
C. Symmetry
D. Bite depth

28. Ideal time to start an orthodontic treatment is:
A. Early mixed dentition
B. Primary dentition
C. Late mixed dentition
D. When the malocclusion first seen

29. Which malocclusion will not lead to straining of lips?
A. Class-II Div. 1
B. Class-II Div. 2
C. Bimaxillary protrusion
D. None

30. In bimaxillary protrusion the change in intrinsical angle can be:
A. Can be normal in some cases
B. Always decreased
C. Always increased
D. Changes sometime

31. A patient is having normal SNA, but the value of ANB is 8 degree. The patient is having:
A. Mandibular retrusion
B. Mandibular protrusion
C. Maxillary protrusion
D. Maxillary retrusion

32. All of the following can lead to slow maxillary expansion, *except*:

A. Ni-Ti Expander B. Hyrax
C. Coffin spring D. W-Arch

33. Loss of tooth length of premolar in case of orthodontic treatment:

A. 1.0 mm B. 2.0 mm
C. 1.5 mm D. 2.5 mm

34. Moment: Force Ratio for bodily movement of tooth is:

A. 6 B. 14
C. 10 D. Zero

35. The ossification centers present at birth are:

A. Distal end of femur
B. Humerus
C. Proximal end of tibia
D. All of the above

36. Which of the following is a tissue borne appliance?

A. Activator B. Frankel regulator
C. Herbst appliance D. Bionator

37. Which of the following is not the contribution of E.H. angle?

A. Edgewise appliance
B. Straight wire appliance
C. E-Arch appliance
D. Pin and tube appliance

38. Russel periodontal index score ranges from:

A. 0-2 B. 0-4
C. 0-6 D. 0-8

39. Horowitz and Thylstrup index is used for:

A. Index to measure fluorosis
B. Periodontal index
C. Gingival bleeding index
D. Caries index in primary teeth

40. Prevalence is defined as:

A. Rate of disease transmission
B. Proportion of population affected by disease
C. Cumulative number of cases in an area
D. New cases of particular disease occurring during a specific period

41. Incidence of a disease is:

A. Number of cases of a disease in a population at a given time
B. Proportion of population affected by disease
C. Number of new cases occurring in a population during a period of time
D. Cumulative number of cases in an area

42. Yard-stick of detection of Synder's test is:

A. Enamel solubility
B. Acid formation
C. Count of microorganism
D. pH change

43. The CPITN probe is designed by:

A. Williams B. WHO
C. Marques D. Naber's

44. True about CPITN is:

A. Scored by a special periodontal probe of length 3 to 5 mm backward for easy visibility
B. Was observed for the first time by ADA in 1992
C. Score of 3 means the treatment involves oral hygiene instruction, scaling and curettage
D. Measure 6 representative teeth

45. Which of the following sugar substitute is bactericidal?

A. Xylitol B. Glycerol
C. Sorbitol D. Mannitol

46. Simple method to evaluate the plaque after a thorough brushing can be done by:

A. Disclosing solution B. Unwaxed floss
C. Sand paper strips D. Synder test

47. The supplementation of fluoride to get maximum cariostatic effect should start from:

A. 3 months after birth B. Birth
C. 6 months after birth D. 9 months after birth

48. 1 ppm of Fluoride means:

A. 1 mg of fluoride in 1 L of water
B. 1 gm of fluoride in 1 L of water
C. 1 mg of fluoride in 10 L of water
D. 1 mg of fluoride in 100 mL of water

49. Caries activity test measures:

A. pH B. Caries susceptibility
C. Motivational aspect D. None

50. Score of 8 in Russel periodontal index means:

A. Advanced destructive periodontal disease with loss of masticatory function
B. Beginning of the destructive periodontal disease
C. Established destructive periodontal disease
D. Irreversible terminal disease

51. Critical pH for dental caries is:

A. 5.7-5.8 B. 5.4-5.5
C. 5.8-6.0 D. 6.0-6.2

52. Double blind study, true is:

A. Only the examiner know the group to which subject belong
B. The subject and the examiner do not know the details of the study
C. The subject in the study do not know the examiner doing the study
D. The research investigator is blind to the dependent and independent variable

53. Trigeminal neuralgia after ear infection is called as:

A. Sjogren syndrome
B. Geredo Nego syndrome
C. Ramsay Hunt syndrome
D. Auriculotemporal syndrome

54. Which of the following primary teeth are most commonly ankylosed?

A. Mandibular 2nd molars
B. Mandibular incisors
C. Maxillary molars
D. Maxillary premolars

55. The pathogenesis of periapical cyst is:

A. Proliferation of epithelium
B. Immune mediated bone destruction
C. Increased pressure within the cyst
D. None

56. Hydropic degeneration of the basal cell of the stratum germinativum is a feature of:

A. Pemphigus B. Syphilis
C. Leukoplakia D. Lichen planus

57. The feature that distinguishes herpes zoster from other vesiculobullous eruptions is:

A. Severe burning pain
B. Prominent crusting vesicles
C. Sub epidermal bullous formation
D. Unilateral occurrence

58. The easiest impaction of mandibular molar is:

A. Vertical
B. Horizontal
C. Distoangular
D. Mesioangular

59. A patient with condylar fracture, the occlusion is normal with normal mouth opening. The best treatment is:

A. IMF for 3 weeks
B. IMF for 5-6 weeks
C. Open reduction and bore plating
D. Conservative treatment, close observation and soft diet and return to as normal function as possible

60. Which of the following is a direct interdental wiring method?

A. Ivy islet wiring method
B. Risdon's wiring method
C. Col Stout's wiring method
D. Gilmer's wiring method

61. Latency period in distraction osteosynthesis is defined as:

A. Time period for completion of distraction process
B. Time period between distraction and functional loading of the area
C. Time period between surgical osteotomy and starting a distraction
D. Time period between starting of distraction to the completion of distraction

62. Which treatment plan will lead to rigid fixation of the fracture site?

A. IMF
B. Direct interdental wiring
C. Miniplate osteosynthesis
D. Eccentric Compression Plate Osteosynthesis

63. **A 2 cm squamous Cell CA of retromolar region invading the mandible and medial pterygoid muscle, do not show any lymph node enlargement and metastasis to distant site, it is at what TNM stage?**
A. Stage-I
B. Stage-II
C. Stage-III
D. Stage-IV

64. **In a patient of syncope the pupils are:**
A. Constricted and non-reacting to light
B. Dilated and fixed
C. Constricted
D. Dilated-fixed and non-reacting to light

65. **In CPR, the sternum should be depressed at a rate of:**
A. 1 inch per 5 second
B. 1 inch per 1 second
C. 2 inch per 5 second
D. 2 inch per 1 second

66. **Hydrocortisone acetate is injected in a painful arthritic TMJ to:**
A. Decrease the inflammatory response
B. Anesthetize the nerve supply
C. Lubricate the synovial joint
D. Increase the blood supply

67. **A patient is having displaced fracture of angle of mandible, treatment indicated is:**
A. Closed reduction and IMF
B. Open reduction and bone plating
C. Closed reduction and inter-tooth traction
D. External pin fixation

68. **Cardiac condition requiring antibiotic prophylaxis for infective endocarditis:**
A. Hypertensive heart disease
B. Rheumatic heart disease
C. Cardiac pacemakers
D. Coronary heart disease

69. **The manufacturing unit of surgical needle and sutures are sterilized by:**
A. Autoclaving
B. Boiling
C. X-rays
D. Gamma rays

70. Protein content of OKC is:

A. > Serum content B. < 4 gm/dl

C. 4-6 gm/dl D. Equals serum content

71. The color of oxygen cylinder is:

A. Black B. Blue

C. White D. Yellow

72. The sub-conjunctival hemorrhage remains bright red in color for a long time because:

A. Lack of drainage of the pooled blood

B. Natural color of blood

C. Permeability of the conjunctiva to oxygen

D. None

73. LA acts by:

A. Decreasing the inflow of Na^+ from exterior to interior

B. Decreasing the K^+ ion movement across membrane

C. Increasing the permeability of the membrane to K^+ ions

D. Decreasing the outflow of Na^+ from interior to exterior

74. A 55-year-old patient is on anticoagulants for last 6 months. He has to undergo extraction of carious tooth. What the dentist should do?

A. Stop aspirin for 3 days prior to extraction

B. Stop aspirin for 7 days prior to extraction

C. Extraction can be done as this dose of aspirin does not lead to marked bleeding during extraction

D. Give platelet infusion and then do the extraction

75. Which radiographic view is least helpful in detecting incipient caries?

A. Bite-wing radiograph

B. Occlusal view

C. Panoramic radiograph

D. IOPA

76. When using a tilted mandibular 2nd molar as an FPD abutment, the best method to compensate for the tilt is to:

A. Prepare the molar abutment for mesial half crown

B. Upright the tooth orthodontically

C. Use a non-rigid connector in the bridge

D. Modify the preparation by making a knife edge finish line on the mesial axial wall

77. Compared to cast circumferential clasp, the main disadvantage of a combination clasp, is that, it:

A. Makes greater surface contact with the tooth
B. Can flex in all spatial planes
C. Is less acceptable esthetically
D. Is more prone to breakage and damage

78. Elderly patients whose health contraindicates the lengthy and at times physically tiring appointment needed to construct fixed replacements for missing teeth, should be treated with:

A. Interim Partial Denture
B. Spoon Partial Denture
C. Transitional Partial Denture
D. Treatment Partial Denture

79. For porcelain fused to metal crowns, the porcelain should have:

A. Linear coefficient of thermal expansion less than that of metal
B. High fusion temperature
C. High fusion expansion
D. Liner coefficient of thermal expansion more than the metal

80. The green discoloration present at the margin of porcelain and metal margin is due to:

A. Oxygen B. Silver
C. Zinc D. Nickel

81. In the treatment plan of a conventional immediate complete denture, the anterior teeth are extracted:

A. After making the immediate denture
B. Before making the immediate denture
C. Before extracting the posterior teeth
D. At the first appointment

82. The Apex of the Bonwill's Triangle is located at the:

A. Lower central incisor's contact point
B. Upper central incisor's contact point
C. Anterior tip of the incisive papilla
D. Anterior most point on the chin

83. How far from gingival crevices of the teeth should the border of mandibular major connector be located?

A. 3-4 mm B. 0-2 mm
C. 6-8 mm D. 8-12 mm

84. When designing an RPD for Kennedy Class-II arch, the clasp configuration usually employed is:

A. Bilateral
B. Unilateral
C. Quadrilateral
D. Tripod

85. The so called resin retained FPDs or Maryland Bridges depend upon:

A. Indirect retention
B. Micromechanical retention
C. Chemical retention
D. Mechanical retention

86. Most recent form of MTA used as an intracanal irrigant:

A. MTA-D
B. MTA-E
C. MTA-A
D. MTA-C

87. Incipient caries was covered accidentally by pit and fissure sealant, which is correct about its progression?

A. Will not progress at all
B. Progression cannot be predicted
C. Progress at a slower rate
D. Progress at a faster rate

88. Mutans can be implicated in the etiological agent for dental caries, because it can produce:

A. α-1, 5 Intracellular Polysaccharide
B. α-1, 4 Intracellular Polysaccharide
C. α-1, 3 Extracellular Polysaccharide
D. α-1, 6 Extracellular Polysaccharide

89. Single sitting RCT is indicated in all *except*:

A. Tooth with pulpal exposure because of trauma
B. In a patient who require sedation for the management of involved tooth
C. Severe anatomic and procedural difficulty
D. An anterior single rooted tooth where esthetics is of more concern

90. Which of the following is the emergency treatment of choice in case of traumatic injury to tooth?

A. A pin retained composite restoration
B. A stainless steel or performed orthodontic band around the tooth
C. An acid etched composite restoration
D. Full veneer crown preparation with stainless steel crown

91. Which of the following is the main reason for resistant of enamel surface, to demineralization?

A. Decreased carbonate content of surface layer
B. Decreased magnesium content of surface layer
C. Increased phosphate conent of surface layer
D. Increased fluoride content of surface layer

92. Blood supply of ameloblast for most of its life cycle comes from:

A. Dental sac
B. Dental pulp
C. Dental papilla
D. Reduced enamel origin

93. Maximum growth of brain takes place in:

A. Infancy
B. Puberty
C. School
D. Preschool

94. In which of the following condition the space loss is most difficult to manage?

A. A 5 years old child with loss of a primary mandibular 2nd molar
B. A 7 years old child with loss of a primary maxillary 2nd molar
C. A 6 years old child with loss of a primary mandibular 1st molar
D. A 9 ½ years old child with loss of a permanent maxillary 1st molar

95. Traumatic injury to primary tooth leads to intrusion, after how much time the teeth usually re-erupts?

A. 30 days
B. 2 months
C. 6 months
D. 12 months

96. To prevent mesial migration of permanent 1st molar tooth, what is the ideal time to give space maintainer in case of premature loss of primary 2nd molar?

A. Immediately after extraction of the tooth
B. After healing the extraction socket
C. After the permanent 2nd molar has erupted
D. After the tooth pierces the gingival tissue

97. According to Finn the best method of brushing in mixed dentition and young adult dentition phase is:

A. Modified Stillman's method
B. Horizontal scrub method
C. Fone's method
D. Bass sulcular method

Answers

1.	D	2.	C	3.	C	4.	A
5.	C	6.	B	7.	C	8.	A
9.	B	10.	B	11.	C	12.	B
13.	B	14.	A	15.	B	16.	D
17.	C	18.	D	19.	D	20.	C
21.	B	22.	A	23.	D	24.	D
25.	A	26.	B	27.	B	28.	D
29.	B	30.	B	31.	A	32.	B
33.	C	34.	C	35.	D	36.	B
37.	B	38.	D	39.	A	40.	B
41.	C	42.	D	43.	B	44.	D
45.	A	46.	A	47.	B	48.	A
49.	B	50.	A	51.	B	52.	B
53.	B	54.	A	55.	A	56.	D
57.	D	58.	D	59.	D	60.	D
61.	C	62.	D	63.	D	64.	B
65.	D	66.	A	67.	B	68.	B
69.	D	70.	B	71.	A	72.	C
73.	A	74.	C	75.	C	76.	B
77.	D	78.	A	79.	A	80.	B
81.	A	82.	A	83.	A	84.	D
85.	B	86.	A	87.	A	88.	C
89.	C	90.	C	91.	D	92.	A
93.	A	94.	A	95.	C	96.	A
97.	C						

PGI Paper June 2008

1. **Which of the following structures is absent on the face?**
   A. Loose connective tissue
   B. Lymphatics
   C. Superficial fascia
   D. Deep fascia

2. **Structures which passes through the Sigmoid notch are:**
   A. Auriculotemporal nerve
   B. Masseteric nerve and vessels
   C. Superficial temporal vessels
   D. None

3. **Which out of the following nerve does not supply the scalp?**
   A. Greater occipital
   B. Zygomaticotemporal
   C. Auriculotemporal
   D. Infratrochlear

4. **The pharyngeal muscle attached to the mandible is:**
   A. Middle constrictor
   B. Inferior constrictor
   C. Superior constrictor
   D. None

5. **Which type of nerve cells are present in trigeminal ganglion?**
   A. Multiple polar B. Non-polar
   C. Bipolar D. Pseudo-unipolar

6. **Disease characterized by normal platelet count but increased bleeding time:**
   A. Aplastic anemia B. Glanzmann disease
   C. Hemophilia-B D. Hemophilia-A

7. **Endocrinal disturbance affecting eruption timing without causing hypoplasia:**
   A. Hyperthyroidism
   B. Hypoparathyroidism
   C. Rickets
   D. None

8. **The neurotransmitter present in postganglionic parasympathetic nerves:**
   A. Nor-Adr
   B. Dopamine
   C. Ach
   D. Adr

9. **Which of the following is the feature of iron deficiency anemia?**
   A. Increased MCH
   B. Decreased MCV
   C. Increased MCV
   D. Increased MCHC

10. **Rickettsiae causes which disease?**
    A. Relapsing fever
    B. Scrub typhus
    C. Q-fever
    D. Weil's disease

11. **Which of the following is most radioresistant tumor?**
    A. Ameloblastoma
    B. Carcinoma alveolus
    C. Ewing's carcinoma
    D. Carcinoma maxillary sinus

12. **Patient present with cotton-wool appearance of bone. Hypercementosis of the teeth, loss of visual acuity. The diagnosis is:**
    A. Cleidocranial Dysostosis
    B. Osteogenesis Imperfecta
    C. Fibrous dysplasia
    D. Paget's disease

13. **The etiology of Mickulicz disease is:**
    A. Viral infection
    B. Inflammatory disease
    C. Autoimmunity
    D. Heredity

14. **Which of the following condition do not manifest xerostomia?**
    A. Vitamin C chewing gum
    B. Atrophy of glandular tissue
    C. Sjogren syndrome
    D. Radiation around head and neck region for neoplasm

15. Rumpel Leede Test is used to measure:

A. Capillary fragility
B. Factor IX deficiency
C. Clotting time
D. Blood pressure

16. Rhabdomyoma is the neoplasm of:

A. Malignant, neoplasm of striated muscles
B. Malignant, neoplasm of smooth muscles
C. Benign neoplasm of smooth muscle
D. Benign neoplasm of striated muscle

17. Concentration of chlorhexidine used in mouth wash:

A. 0.2%
B. 0.12%
C. 2.0%
D. 0.25%

18. In Turku Study sucrose is replaced by:

A. Xylitol
B. Saccharine
C. Aspartame
D. Mannitol

19. Salt fluoridation is:

A. 0.25 gm/kg of salt
B. 0.20 gm/kg of salt
C. 0.50 mg/kg of salt
D. 2.00 gm/kg of salt

20. According to WHO the DMF index criteria for 12 years age by year 2012 and 2025:

A. 2 and 1
B. 1 and 0
C. 3 and 2
D. 4 and 3

21. The effectiveness of systemic fluoridation in caries reduction is:

A. 20%
B. 30%
C. 40%
D. 60%

22. Ideal dentist : population ratio recommended by WHO is:

A. 1:5500
B. 1:7500
C. 1:9500
D. 1:20000

23. In a normal distribution curve the (SD + 2) excludes how much values?

A. 4.3%
B. 99.7%
C. 95.7%
D. 93.4%

24. Which of the following synonym indicate caries incidence?

A. Caries activity
B. Caries increment
C. Caries attack rate
D. All of the above

25. What is true about case control study?

A. Measure incidence
B. Prospective study
C. Retrospective study
D. None

26. A group which is being studied during a study is called as:

A. Controls
B. Cohort group
C. Panel group
D. None

27. Antidote to fluoride in toxicity is:

A. Vinegar
B. $NaSO_4$
C. Milk
D. Water

28. Prevalence of defined as:

A. Rate of disease transmission
B. Cumulative number of cases in an area
C. Proportion of population affected by disease
D. New cases of a particular disease occurring during a specified period

29. Oral health status index in 1980 given by:

A. Greene and Vermillion
B. Marcus and Gershen
C. Rosebraun
D. WHO

30. Prevention of onset of risk factor is:

A. Tertiary prevention
B. Primordial prevention
C. Primary prevention
D. Secondary prevention

31. Which out of the following is true?

A. Growth of maxilla occurs in downward and forward direction
B. Alveolus is growth centre
C. Condylar cartilage is the primary cartilage
D. None

32. At 2 months of intrauterine life Head: Body ratio is:

A. 1 : 2
B. 1 : 8
C. 1 : 4
D. 1 : 16

33. Which of the following orthodontic wire can be heat treated?

A. Elgiloy
B. Ni-Ti
C. Beta-Titanium
D. Stainless steel

34. Sassouni analysis is used to describe skeletal disturbance in which plane?

A. Transverse
B. Horizontal
C. Vertical
D. Dentoskeletal

35. Malocclusion prevalence in people of Australian aborigines:

A. Class-II
B. Class-III
C. Cross bite
D. Scissor bite

36. Air sinus which can be used as skeletal maturity indicator?

A. Sphenoidal sinus
B. Ethamoidal sinus
C. Maxillary sinus
D. Frontal sinus

37. Teeth least commonly extracted for orthodontic reason:

A. Canines
B. Molars
C. Incisors
D. Premolars

38. The sound which is most affected in a patient of Class-III malocclusion:

A. Linguoalveolar Fricatives
B. Linguoalveolar consonents
C. Sibilant sounds
D. Labiodentals Fricatives

39. A 9-year-old child has Class-II Div. 1 malocclusion. What will be the treatment option?

A. High pull head gear
B. Reverse twin block
C. Face mask therapy
D. Chin cap therapy

40. Cases of hemangioma are present most commonly in which region?

A. Gastrointestinal tract
B. Head and neck
C. Liver
D. Bones

41. Non-union of fracture is due to:
A. Early mobilization
B. Bone loss due to infection
C. Mobility of fracture site
D. None

42. The type of carcinoma develop in marjolin ulcer is:
A. Adeno carcinoma
B. Fibrogenic sarcoma
C. Basal cell carcinoma
D. None

43. PTT is prolonged in case of:
A. Hemophilia-A
B. Hyperfibrinogenemia
C. Heparin therapy
D. Warfarin therapy

44. Prothrombin time is used to check out:
A. Status of anticoagulant therapy
B. Hemophilia-A
C. Hemophilia-B
D. Hemophilia-C

45. What is the maximum distance between the nasal vestibule and implant?
A. 1 mm B. 2 mm
C. 2.5 mm D. 3 mm

46. Inverted -L- shaped osteotomy, what is true?
A. To correct maxillary deformities
B. Used in mandibular prognathism cases
C. Done on the mandible portion not involving the occlusion
D. Used for treating mandibular retrognathism

47. In latency period after mandibular distraction is:
A. 5 days B. 15 days
C. 1 month D. 2 months

48. During inferior alveolar nerve block the needle is inserted in which space?
A. Pterygomandibular space
B. Masseteric space
C. Submandibular space
D. Infratemporal space

49. Floating fracture of maxilla is seen in:

A. Pyramidal fracture of maxilla
B. Fracture of alveolar process
C. Horizonal fracture of maxilla
D. None

50. Drug which can cause the osteonecrosis of the jaw is:

A. Bisphosphonate B. Calcitonin
C. Corticosteroids D. None

51. Drug which can cause the osteonecrosis of the jaw is:

A. Alendronate B. Calcitonin
C. Corticosteroids D. None

52. Concentration of N_2O used to produce dissociative sedation and analgesia:

A. 20-45% B. 15-30%
C. 50-70% D. > 70%

53. Trismus can result from the infection of which space?

A. Submasseteric space
B. Buccal space
C. Sublingual space
D. Submandibular space

54. The recommended time gap between the radiation and surgery to avoid osteoradionecrosis:

A. Immediately after radiotherapy
B. 4-6 weeks after radiotherapy
C. 6-12 months after radiotherapy
D. Any time during the course of radiotherapy

55. Topical anesthesia used are effective upon the depth of:

A. 0.5-1.0 mm B. 1.0-2.0 mm
C. 2.0-3.0 mm D. 3.0-3.5 mm

56. Ludwig's angina, untrue is:

A. Bilateral Submandibular, Sublingual, Submental space along with salivary gland enlargement
B. Involves bilateral mandibular spaces and lymphadenopathy
C. Involves submandibular, sub lingual and submental space
D. None

57. **During exodontia the force applied firstly in which direction?**
A. Lingual
B. Buccal
C. Apical
D. Coronal

58. **A pier abutment is:**
A. Abutment tooth away from the edentulous space
B. Edentulous space on one side of the abutment
C. With edentulous space on both sides of the abutment
D. Periodontally weak abutment

59. **During jaw relation protrusion records are used for:**
A. Records centric relation
B. Condylar inclination measurement of both sides
C. Record retruded contact position
D. Condylar inclination measurement of one side

60. **The patient experiencing pain at the appointment of jaw relation, which may be used as the treatment option for the condition?**
A. Using bite plane
B. Manual manipulation of the jaw
C. Using the jaw handle movement of the jaw
D. Both A and C

61. **The Partial Maxillectomy Defect Classification was given by:**
A. Jackson and Callon Fote
B. Butler
C. Aramany
D. None

62. **What is the value of condylar inclination?**
A. 10-15 degree
B. 15-20 degree
C. 20-25 degree
D. 30-40 degree

63. **How much variation in eruption of the permanent molar is considered normal?**
A. 0-6 months
B. 6-12 months
C. 12-18 months
D. 18-24 months

64. **Maximum part of Leeway space is provided by which tooth?**
A. Primary first molar
B. Primary canine
C. Primary second molar
D. All contribute equal space

65. Cariogram is given by:

A. Brathall
B. Blatterfeir
C. Aramari
D. Klevin Allen

66. Partial pulpotomy technique is given by:

A. Clark in 1976
B. Cvek in 1978
C. Bowen in 1974
D. Willet in 1980

67. Startle reflex disappear at the age of:

A. 1 year
B. 2 years
C. 3 years
D. 4 years

68. An 18-year-old female patient with swelling and pain in the mandibular third molar area will most likely to have:

A. Pericoronitis
B. Pregnancy euplis
C. Plasma cell gingivitis
D. Juvenile periodontitis

69. Green stains present on the tooth of child is due to:

A. Food debris
B. Plaque
C. Chromogenic bacteria
D. None

70. Free gingival graft during periodontal surgery is placed on:

A. Periosteum
B. Cementum
C. PDL
D. Bone

71. Disease atrophy of periodontium leads to all *except*:

A. Recession of gingiva
B. Alveolar bone become porous
C. Thinning of periodontal ligament width
D. Rearrangement of periodontal fibers

72. Trauma from occlusion leads to all *except*:

A. Angular bone loss
B. Infrabony pocket
C. Widening of periodontal ligament
D. Tooth mobility

73. Gingival bleeding index is used to assess:

A. Measures periodontal health
B. Cumulative effect of last 7 days oral hygiene
C. Cumulative effect of last 15 days oral hygiene
D. State of oral hygiene on the day of examination

74. The best way to prevent exposure of dehiscence during surgical procedure is:

A. Elevate Partial Thickness Flap
B. Elevate Coronally Repositional Flap
C. Elevate Full Thickness Flap
D. Elevate Double Flap

75. The probing force used during periodontal examination is:

A. 7.5 N
B. 25 gm
C. 0.25 N
D. 7.5 N

76. The advantage of natural tooth bristles over nylon bristle is:

A. Causes less tooth abrasion
B. Susceptible to fraying
C. Easy to clean
D. Flex more than nylon bristle

77. Width of attached gingiva:

A. Increased with age
B. Remain same
C. Decreases with age
D. None

78. Which of the following is osteoinductive material?

A. Tricalcium phosphate
B. Hydroxyapatite
C. Decalcified Freeze Dried bone
D. Dura

79. Which one of the following condition indicates a periodontal rather than an endodontic lesion?

A. A deep narrow sulcular pocket to the apex with exudates
B. Pain to palpation of the buccal mucosa near the tooth apex
C. Pain to lateral percussion with wide sulcular pocket
D. Acute pain on percussion with no swelling

80. Actinobacillus actinomycetemcomitans attachment on tooth surface can be prevented by:

A. Collagenase
B. Lactoperosidases
C. Myeloperoxidase
D. None

81. A splint can be defined as:

A. Appliance to be used during flap procedure
B. Appliance to prevent movement of mobile teeth
C. A prosthesis to keep graft in place
D. None

82. Which of the following is true regarding acute rheumatic fever?

A. Sydenham chorea is usually present
B. It follows streptococcal skin infection
C. Earliest symptom is painful migratory arthritis
D. Invariably associated with mitral valve

83. Which cardiac condition is associated with highest risk for infective endocarditis?

A. Ventricular septal defect
B. Coronary artery disease
C. Previous history of endocarditis
D. Mitral valve prolapsed without regurgitation

84. Hypokalemia is not present in which condition?

A. Patient on diuretics
B. Diarrhea
C. Chronic renal failure
D. Vomiting

85. All of the following drugs are excreted in bile:

A. Diazepam
B. Cephalosporins
C. Theophyllines
D. Amikacin

86. The tooth preparation for laminates extend to:

A. At contact point
B. Lingual to contact
C. Labial to contact
D. None

87. The acid used for microabrasion technique recommended by CROLL is:

A. H_2SO_4
B. HCl 18%
C. Citric acid 10%
D. None

88. Type of incision for periodontal surgery mainly depends on:

A. Width of attached gingiva
B. Frenal attachment
C. Presence of bony defect
D. Probing depth

89. In a Class –II cavity preparation, the gingival seat will be:

A. Left unbeveled
B. Beveled to increase retention
C. Beveled as in permanent teeth
D. None

90. Ormocers are:

A. Organically modified ceramics
B. Organically modified glass ionomers
C. Glass ionomer modifier composites
D. Composites modified glass ionomers

91. Golden preparation is:

A. 1:1.618
B. 1:0.620
C. 1:1.018
D. 2:1.618

92. Pulp vitality test usually used check:

A. Afferent nerve fibers
B. Pulp blood supply
C. Efferent nerve fibers
D. None

93. Latent period in radiology is defined as:

A. Cell rest and cell mitosis
B. Time gap between radiation exposure and radiation induced effects
C. The first and last dose in radiotherapy
D. Time gap between taking radiograph and development of image

94. Which of the following material can be confused with caries?

A. Composite
B. ZoE
C. Gutta Percha
D. Amalgam

95. For stainless steel crown the tooth surface requiring least amount of reduction is:

A. Occlusal
B. Proximal
C. Lingual
D. Buccal

96. Sunday bite is present in:

A. Class-I
B. Class-II Div.1
C. Class-II Div. 2
D. Bimaxillary protrusion

Answers

1.	D	2.	B	3.	D	4.	C
5.	D	6.	B	7.	A, B	8.	C
9.	B	10.	B, C	11.	A	12.	D
13.	C	14.	A	15.	A	16.	D
17.	A	18.	A	19.	A	20.	A
21.	D	22.	B	23.	A	24.	D
25.	C	26.	B	27.	C	28.	C
29.	B	30.	B	31.	A	32.	A
33.	A	34.	C	35.	C	36.	D
37.	A	38.	D	39.	A	40.	B
41.	B	42.	C	43.	A	44.	A
45.	A	46.	D	47.	A	48.	A
49.	C	50.	A	51.	A	52.	A
53.	A	54.	B	55.	C	56.	A
57.	C	58.	C	59.	B	60.	D
61.	C	62.	C	63.	D	64.	C
65.	A	66.	B	67.	B	68.	A
69.	C	70.	A	71.	A	72.	B
73.	D	74.	A	75.	B	76.	A
77.	A	78.	C	79.	C	80.	C
81.	B	82.	C	83.	C	84.	C
85.	D	86.	C	87.	B	88.	A
89.	A	90.	A	91.	B	92.	A
93.	B	94.	A	95.	C	96.	B

PGI Paper
December 2007

1. **Modiolus at the corner of the mouth is formed by all of the following muscles, *except*:**
   A. Orbicularis oris B. Buccinators
   C. Triangularis D. Alaqual Nasi

2. **Cartilage differ from bone in that it grow by:**
   A. Growth of the cells in lacunae
   B. Interstitial growth pattern
   C. Appositional growth pattern
   D. None

3. **Epithelium of nasal, nasopharyngeal mucosa is:**
   A. Pseudostratified columnar
   B. Stratified columnar
   C. Pseudostratified ciliated columnar
   D. Stratified squamous

4. **Anterior ethmoidal sinus drains into:**
   A. Inferior meatus B. Hiatus semilunaris
   C. Superior meatus D. None

5. **Foramen rotundum is present in which bone?**
   A. Sphenoid B. Occipital
   C. Ethmoid D. Temporal

6. **Transfer of Immunoglobulin from mother to child across placenta is example of:**
   A. Natural active immunity
   B. Natural passive immunity
   C. Acquired passive immunity
   D. Acquired active immunity

7. **True about Hb is:**
   A. Have two heme group and four polypeptide chains
   B. Have one heme and one globin molecule

C. Have 4 heme molecules and 2 alpha and 2 beta chains
D. Consists of 4 different polypeptide chains

8. **For a complete denture patient with Class II ridge relation, the freeway space:**
A. No alteration required
B. Must be decreased
C. Must be increased
D. None

9. **The minimum width of keratinized gingiva for restoration of a tooth with a crown:**
A. 2 mm B. 3 mm
C. 5 mm D. 7 mm

10. **Primary support of a clasp is due to:**
A. Shoulder B. Minor connector
C. Occlusal rest D. Saddle area

11. **Which impression material have poor surface reproduction?**
A. Irreversible Hydrocolloid
B. Polyether
C. Reversible Hydrocolloid
D. ZoE

12. **Epoxy resin for die preparation cannot be used with which impression material?**
A. Polyether B. Addition silicone
C. Polysulphide D. Hydrocolloids

13. **Pantograph tracing utilizes how many styli?**
A. 1 B. 3
C. 6 D. 12

14. **Cavernous sinus thrombosis following infection of maxillary teeth spread most often along:**
A. Ophthalmic vein B. Angular artery
C. Pterygoid plexus D. Facial artery

15. **The skin of a patient undergoing radiotherapy will show what sign in oral cavity after 2 weeks?**
A. Depigmentation of oral cavity
B. Radiation induced carcinoma
C. No change in oral cavity
D. Erythema of oral cavity

16. **The most difficult impaction of mandibular molars is:**
    A. Vertical
    B. Horizontal
    C. Distoangular
    D. Mesioangular

17. **The repair cleft palate primarily done for:**
    A. Induce the growth of maxilla
    B. Induce the growth of mandible
    C. Correction of speech
    D. Correction of esthetics

18. **In a 10-year-old child with TMJ ankylosis, the treatment of choice is:**
    A. Gap arthroplasty with costochondral graft
    B. Interpositional gap arthroplasty
    C. Gap arthroplasty
    D. None

19. **Which of the following is the radiographic feature of TMJ ankylosis?**
    A. Increased mandibular plane angle
    B. Deep antegonial notches
    C. Increased gonial angle
    D. Mandibular prognathism

20. **Best incision to expose the TMJ without dividing temporal fascia for ankylosis surgeries:**
    A. Root incision
    B. Alkayat Bramley incision
    C. Preauricular incision
    D. Risdon incision

21. **During parotid gland surgery injury to auriculotemporal nerve leads to:**
    A. Facial palsy
    B. Frey syndrome
    C. Trigeminal neuralgia
    D. Horner syndrome

22. **Lefort I fracture is characterized by:**
    A. Anterior open bite
    B. Bleeding from the maxillary antrum
    C. Bleeding from the ear
    D. Angle class II skeletal relationship on fracture site

23. Type of nerve injury in which there is only paresthesia of nerve with complete recovery?

A. Neurotmesis
B. Neuropraxia
C. Axonotmesis
D. None

24. 6 years old child's fear of dentistry is:

A. Subjective
B. Objective
C. Both subjective and objective
D. Psychological

25. The diet modification in a patient of rampant caries requires:

A. Allow no sugar for 7 days
B. Restrict sugar for meal time only
C. Allow no sugar for 21 days
D. Restrict intake of sugar only

26. Which of the following is least cariogenic?

A. Fructose
B. Glucose
C. Sucrose
D. Xylitol

27. Slot size most commonly used in orthodontics is:

A. 0.017 × 0.021
B. 0.010 × 0.020
C. 0.014 × 0.024
D. 0.018 × 0.028

28. Movement of tooth with digital pressure with hand was proposed by:

A. Celsius
B. Bakers
C. Angle
D. Hippocrates

29. Which of the following is an example of fixed functional appliance?

A. Frankel regulator
B. Activator
C. Herbst appliance
D. Bionator

30. The AO and BO in Wits appraisal is responsible of:

A. Maxilla to mandible
B. Mandible to cranium
C. Maxilla to cranium
D. Maxilla and mandible to face

31. The orthodontic wire which exhibits shape memory?

A. Stainless steel
B. Beta titanium (TMA)
C. Cobalt-chrome
D. Ni-Ti

32. **The type of anchorage used in maxillary expansion by Quad-Helix:**
A. Reciprocal anchorage
B. Complex anchorage
C. Reinforced anchorage
D. Simple anchorage

33. **The chemical mediators in orthodontic tooth movements is:**
A. Histamine
B. Serotonin
C. Prostaglandins
D. Interleukins

34. **Fracture of zygoma is best seen in:**
A. PA-view
B. Occipitomental view 30 degree
C. Panoramic view
D. Submentovertex view

35. **The distance of 5 feet in cephalometrics is between X-rays source and:**
A. Cassette on the left side of patient
B. Mid-Sagittal plane of patient
C. Right side of patient
D. None

36. **Which of the following is most radiopaque?**
A. Co-Cr crown
B. Lamina dura
C. Enamel
D. $ZnPO_2$

37. **The first step in developing of a film is:**
A. Developing of film
B. Fixing of film
C. Stirring of developer
D. Checking the level of developer

38. **Minimum depth of lesion to be visible on radiograph is:**
A. 40 mm
B. 50 mm
C. 100 mm
D. 500 mm

39. **How many teeth are present in radiograph of a new-born?**
A. 18
B. 20
C. 24
D. 26

40. **Most penetrating X-ray is:**
A. Grenz rays
B. Hard rays
C. Soft rays
D. None

41. IL-1 and TNF-α during inflammation are secreted by:
A. PMNs
B. Activated macrophages
C. Fibroblasts
D. Lymphocytes

42. The most commonly used fixatives after biopsy is:
A. Gluteraldehyde
B. 10% formalin
C. Phenol
D. Formocresol

43. True about incidence of cleft palate is:
A. There are equal incidence in both boys and girls
B. There is predilection for girls
C. These are more common in boys
D. None

44. Which of the following can lead to gnawing radiating pain?
A. Chronic periodontitis
B. ANUG
C. Herpetic gingivostomatitis
D. None

45. Hydropic degeneration of the basal cell of the stratum germinativum is a feature of:
A. Syphilis
B. Lichen planus
C. Pemphigus
D. Leukoplakia

46. Which of the following is the most likely to turn malignant?
A. Pemphigus
B. Junctional Nevus
C. Papilloma
D. Interdental Nevus

47. The low thermal conductivity of impression compound is overcome by:
A. By heating with ethanol flame and directly placing in patient's mouth
B. Heating in hot water and immediately quenching in water for 20 minutes
C. By melting it in boiling water at 50°C for one hour
D. Impression is placed in mouth till it gets cold and sudden removal of the impression

48. Solders in stainless steel differ from that of gold in:

A. KF
B. Calcium carbonate
C. Strontium fluoride
D. Silver nitrate

49. All of the following is used as accelerator in zinc oxide eugenol cement *except*:

A. Calcium chloride
B. Bromoglycerine
C. Zinc acetate dehydrate
D. Acetic acid

50. The inhibitor is added in monomer of heat cure acrylic resin to:

A. Increase the time of dough stage
B. Prolong the shelf life
C. Decrease the shrinkage of acrylic resin
D. Prevent the porosity of acrylic resin

51. Minimum concentration of chlorhexidine required for plaque control:

A. 0.2%
B. 0.12%
C. 0.4%
D. 0.25%

52. Concentration of fluoride in dentifrices:

A. 1000 ppm
B. 700 ppm
C. 1200 ppm
D. 1300 ppm

53. Plaque does not have which carbohydrate moiety?

A. Levans
B. Glucose
C. Rhamnose
D. Dextran

54. Epidemic is defined as:

A. The occurrence of any health related event in excess of the expected
B. Disease imported into the country
C. Scattered cases of a disease
D. Constant finding of a disease in a population

55. Dental fluorosis is not associated with skeletal fluorosis is:

A. 1 ppm
B. 3 ppm
C. 8 ppm
D. 10 ppm

56. The most remineralized zone in the histology of enamel caries is:

A. Surface zone
B. Body of lesion
C. Dark zone
D. Translucent zone

57. **Primary consideration in any preventive program is:**
A. Diet control
B. Pit and fissure sealant
C. Plaque control
D. Fluoride application

58. **In a large country survey the sampling method of choice is:**
A. Cluster sampling
B. Multistage sampling
C. Multiple sampling
D. Multistage random sampling

59. **Advanced Bell stage in tooth development corresponds to stage of:**
A. Apposition
B. Morpho differentiation
C. Histo differentiation
D. Initiation

60. **Von Ebner's glands are:**
A. Pure serous glands
B. Pure mucous glands
C. Mixed glands with predominant serous acini
D. Mixed glands with predominant mucous acini

61. **Cells responsible for resorption of dental hard tissue is:**
A. Giant cells
B. Osteoclast
C. Odontoclasts
D. Fibroclasts

62. **Tooth start erupting during which Nolla's stage?**
A. 4
B. 5
C. 6
D. 7

63. **Numbers of developmental lobes for primary central incisors are:**
A. 1
B. 2
C. 3
D. 4

64. **Pathologic migration of tooth occurs:**
A. Inciso-occlusal direction
B. Away from the bone resorption area
C. Towards the bone resorption area
D. Axio-incisal direction

65. Sulcular epithelium is:

A. Keratinized always
B. Non-keratinized always
C. Keratinized but become non-keratinized on removal of inflammation
D. Non-keratinized but become keratinized on removal of inflammation

66. The gingival crevicular fluid is increased in all *except*:

A. Periodontal pocket
B. Smoking
C. Trauma from occlusion
D. Gingivitis

67. McCall's Festoon occurs due to:

A. Physiological resorption
B. Inflammatory disease
C. Poor oral hygiene
D. Trauma from occlusion

68. Which of the following condition if not treated, can lead to in different course?

A. Herpetic gingivostomatitis
B. Herpangina
C. ANUG
D. Diphtheria

69. Radiopaque irregularity associated with the roots of mandibular central incisors most likely represent:

A. Subgingival pellicle
B. Hyperplastic cementum
C. Subgingival calculus
D. Root caries

70. Flow rate of unstimulated saliva is:

A. 0.1-0.2 ml/min B. 0.5-0.6 ml/min
C. 0.25-0.35 ml/min D. 0.05-0.5 ml/min

71. Which of the following salivary factor is not bactericidal?

A. IgA B. Lectoperoxidase
C. Lysozymes D. Ca^{2+} and PO_4^{2-}

72. In a 3-year-old child which of the following is the most common cyst located in the midline of neck?

A. Lymphangioma B. Brachial cyst
C. Cystic hygroma D. Thyroglossal cyst

73. Group of lymph nodes involves maximally in tubercular lymphadenitis is:

A. Supraclavicular
B. Jugulodigastric
C. Submandibular
D. Cervical

74. Which muscle is responsible for anterior and medial movement of fracture condyle?

A. Masseter
B. Medial pterygoid
C. Lateral pterygoid
D. Temporalis

75. Teeth that are extracted last in full mouth extraction are:

A. Canines
B. Molars
C. Incisors
D. Premolars

76. In which mandibular fracture the tongue fall backwards?

A. Bilateral parasymphysis fracture
B. Bilateral mandibular body fracture
C. Symphysis fracture
D. Bilateral angle fracture

77. CSF otorrhoea is due to fracture of:

A. Fracture of occipital bone
B. Fracture of ethmoid bone
C. Fracture of cribriform plate
D. Fracture of petrous part of temporal membrane

78. Which of the following suture material will lead to maximum tissue response?

A. Silk
B. Catgut
C. Nylon
D. Linen

79. Hematoma formation during or immediately following a posterior superior alveolar nerve block anesthesia is most likely a result of damage to the:

A. Pterygoid venous plexus
B. Internal maxillary artery
C. Facial artery
D. Small capillaries and the arterioles

80. The value of normal prothrombin time is:

A. 6-10 seconds
B. 11-15 seconds
C. 15-20 seconds
D. 20-30 seconds

81. Most common complication that occur in open reduction of fracture is:

A. Non-union
B. Fibrous union
C. Hemorrhage
D. Infection

82. Ammonia inhalation used during syncope acts by producing:

A. Sedation
B. Bronchodilation
C. Vasoconstriction
D. Respiratory stimulation

83. Sialography cannot be used in which condition?

A. Contracture of duct
B. Salivary duct stone
C. Viral parotitis
D. None

84. Proportion of population affected by disease at a given point of time:

A. Point prevalence
B. Prevalence
C. Ratio
D. Incidence

85. Standard deviation is a measure of all *except*:

A. Variation
B. Deviation
C. Central tendency
D. Dispersion

86. Standard deviation and variance is a measure of:

A. Deviation
B. Distribution
C. Variation
D. Dispersion

87. In which formula to calculate child dose, weight is the parameter?

A. Clark Rule
B. Dilling's Formula
C. Cowling Formula
D. Young's Formula

88. Orthodontic decompensation is done prior to orthognathic surgery to correct inclination of which tooth?

A. Canines
B. Incisors
C. Premolars
D. Molars

89. Which of the following best described combination clasp?

A. It is unesthetical and cannot be adjusted easily
B. It has retentive arm of wrought gold and reciprocal arm of cast metal

C. It has retentive arm of cast metal and reciprocal arm of wrought gold
D. None

90. Which of the following structures is absent on the face?
A. Lymphatics
B. Superficial fascia
C. Loose connective tissue
D. Deep fascia

91. Demilunes of Guazzini are defined as:
A. Serous terminals capped by mucous caps in submandibular glands
B. Mucous terminals capped by serous caps in submandibular glands
C. Mucous terminals capped by serous caps in sublingual glands
D. Serous terminals capped by mucous caps in sublingual glands

92. Which of the following is hypocalcified dentin?
A. Incremental lines
B. Predentin
C. Interglobular dentin
D. Mantle dentin

Answers

1.	D	2.	B	3.	C	4.	B
5.	A	6.	B	7.	C	8.	C
9.	C	10.	C	11.	A	12.	D
13.	C	14.	C	15.	D	16.	C
17.	C	18.	A	19.	B	20.	B
21.	B	22.	B	23.	B	24.	A
25.	C	26.	D	27.	D	28.	A
29.	C	30.	A	31.	D	32.	A
33.	C	34.	B	35.	B	36.	A
37.	D	38.	D	39.	C	40.	B
41.	B	42.	B	43.	B	44.	B
45.	B	46.	B	47.	D	48.	A
49.	B	50.	B	51.	B	52.	A
53.	C	54.	A	55.	B	56.	A
57.	C	58.	D	59.	B	60.	A
61.	C	62.	C	63.	A	64.	C
65.	D	66.	C	67.	D	68.	C
69.	C	70.	B	71.	D	72.	D
73.	D	74.	C	75.	A	76.	A
77.	D	78.	B	79.	A	80.	B
81.	D	82.	D	83.	C	84.	A
85.	C	86.	D	87.	A	88.	B
89.	B	90.	D	91.	B	92.	C

PGI Paper
June 2007

1. **The anterior displacement of articular disc is by which muscle?**
   A. Masseter
   B. Temporalis
   C. Medial Pterygoid
   D. Lateral Pterygoid

2. **Tongue on protrusion is deviated to left, the nerve injured is:**
   A. Left Hypoglossal
   B. Right Hypoglossal
   C. Left Glossopharyngeal
   D. Right Glossopharyngeal

3. **In beta thalassemia major the blood picture show:**
   A. Normocytic-Normochromic Anemia
   B. Microcytic-Hypochromic Anemia
   C. Normocytic-Hypochromic Anemia
   D. Microcytic-Normochromic Anemia

4. **Which of the following is not a part of complete blood examination?**
   A. Hematocrit
   B. WBC count
   C. Hb estimation
   D. ESR

5. **Which is incorrect?**
   A. UV rays helps in formation of Vitamin-D in skin
   B. Renal failure leads to increase in parathormone secretion
   C. 25-Hydroxycholecalciferol goes into hydroxylation in kidney
   D. 25-Hydroxycholecalciferol is used in treatment of renal failure

6. **Which of the following is most antigenic?**
   A. Haptens
   B. Nucleic Acids
   C. Lipids
   D. Proteins

7. **Which bacteria will not cause food borne infection?**
A. E. coli
B. Salmonella
C. Campylobacter
D. Pseudomonas

8. **Bacterial exotoxins are:**
A. Lipopolysaccharides
B. Proteins
C. Small polypeptides
D. Proteoglycans

9. **Hydatid cyst is due to:**
A. Bacterial infection
B. Parasitic infestation
C. Fungal infection
D. Viral infection

10. **Botulism toxin manifests as:**
A. Tachycardia
B. Bilateral cranial nerve involvement
C. Fever
D. Hypertension

11. **For uncontrolled tipping the center of rotation is at:**
A. Infinity
B. Root Apex
C. Center of Resistance
D. Incisal Edge

12. **Most posterior point on the mandible is:**
A. Gonion
B. Menton
C. Pogonion
D. Gnathion

13. **FMPA is used to assess:**
A. Mandibular vertical growth pattern
B. Mandibular horizontal growth pattern
C. Mandibular prognathism
D. Mandibular retrognathism

14. **Tooth movement requiring least amount of force is:**
A. Extrusion
B. Intrusion
C. Rotation
D. Bodily movement

15. **Tooth movement requiring force value greater than 100 gm is:**
A. Intrusion
B. Extrusion
C. Root up righting
D. Rotation

16. **Which is not the function of head gear?**
    A. Anchorage Augmentation
    B. Distabilization of Molars
    C. Uprighting of Tilted molars
    D. For maxillary protrusion

17. **A single tipping force is applied to the tooth, the center of rotation is:**
    A. 1/3rd the distance between apex and cervical line from apex
    B. 1/3rd the distance between the apex and incisal edge
    C. 2/3rd the distance between apex and cervical line from apex
    D. 2/3rd the distance between the apex and incisal edge

18. **Center of rotation for bodily movement is at:**
    A. Root apex
    B. Infinity
    C. Center of resistance
    D. Incisal edge

19. **The easiest tooth movement in orthodontics is:**
    A. Intrusion B. Derotation
    C. Bodily movement D. Extrusion

20. **Which is not a contraindication of serial extraction?**
    A. Impacted canines
    B. Open bite
    C. Ditching
    D. Lingual tipping of incisors

21. **Most accepted sequene for extraction is:**
    A. CD4 B. D4C
    C. 4CD D. 4DC

22. **Which of the following is used for rapid maxillary expansion?**
    A. Quad Helix B. W-Arch
    C. Hyrax D. Coffin Spring

23. **The time period of growth-spurts in girls occurs during?**
    A. 3, 6-7, 11-13 years of age
    B. 3, 7-9, 11-13 years of age
    C. 3, 6-7, 13-14 years of age
    D. 3, 7-9, 13-14 years of age

24. Decrease in arch length from midline to 3rd molar with mesial migration of molars with age?

A. 1 cm
B. 0.5 cm
C. 1 inch
D. 2 cm

25. Which of the following microorganism increase in pregnancy gingivitis?

A. Porphyromonas gingivalis
B. Prevotella intermedia
C. Capnocytophaga
D. Actinobacillus

26. Width of attached gingiva is:

A. From crest of marginal gingival to mucogingival junction
B. From gingival margin to base of sulcus
C. From base of sulcus to mucogingival junction
D. None

27. Specific plaque hypothesis is given by:

A. Smith
B. Loesche
C. Glickmann
D. Socransky

28. Most common cells of connective tissues are:

A. Fibroblasts
B. Plasma cells
C. Basal cells
D. Histiocytes

29. Cells present in Stage-III Gingivitis are:

A. PMNs
B. Monocytes
C. Plasma cells
D. Lymphocytes

30. Degeneration of periodontal tissue without inflammation is called as:

A. Desquamative gingivitis
B. Chronic periodontitis
C. Periodontosis
D. Pericoronitis

31. Number of bacteria in 1 ml of saliva are:

A. 500 million
B. 600 million
C. 750 million
D. 900 million

32. ZoE is not used for permanent cementation because of:

A. Less strength
B. High solubility
C. Poor marginal seal
D. Poor pulpal protection

33. Which of the following decreases with strain hardening?

A. Hardness
B. Strength
C. Proportional limit
D. Ductility

34. In measuring vicker hardness number, which of the following is used?

A. Spherical Indenter
B. Steel Ball Indentation
C. Rhomboid Shaped Indenter
D. 136 degree Diamond Pyramid

35. Coefficient of thermal expansion of metal used for PFM crowns should be:

A. Same as porcelain
B. More than porcelain
C. Less than porcelain
D. More or equal to porcelain

36. The critical structure for bone regeneration is:

A. Periosteum
B. Vascularity
C. Bone tissue
D. None

37. Which of the following can be used to stop bleeding from extraction socket?

A. Vitamin K
B. Suturing of the wound margin
C. Bone wax
D. None

38. The radiographic appearance of Cherubism is:

A. Unilateral, Multiocular, Radiolucency
B. Unilateral, Unilocular, Radiolucency
C. Bilateral, Unilocular, Radiolucency
D. Bilateral, Multiocular, Radiolucency

39. Fracture of infraorbital margin will lead to:

A. Paralysis of muscle of cheek
B. Paralysis of muscle of lower eyelid
C. Anesthesia of upper lip
D. None

40. Atropine is used in preanesthetic preparation to:

A. Decrease bronchial secretion
B. Decrease salivary secretions and depress vagal reflex
C. To reduce pain
D. To relieve anxiety

41. The recommended position to keep a person who faints during extraction:

A. Horizontal position
B. Lateral position
C. Trendelenberg position
D. Dorsosacral position

42. Battle's sign is used in fracture of:

A. Fracture Zygoma
B. Fracture Middle Cranial Fossa
C. Fracture Occipital Bone
D. Fracture Posterior Cranial Fossa

43. Maxillary antrum dips in the region of:

A. Between 1st and 2nd premolars
B. Between 2nd premolar and 1st molar
C. Between buccal roots furcation of 1st molar
D. Between 1st molar and 2nd molar

44. Clotting time is increased in:

A. Idiopathic Thrombocytopenic Purpura
B. Scurvy
C. Pernicious Anemia
D. Hemophilia B

45. Complication of osteomyelitis includes:

A. Ludwig's angina
B. Cavernous Sinus Thrombosis
C. Parotid Gland Involvement
D. All of the above

46. Ludwig's angina involves:

A. Unilateral involvement of submandibular, sublingual, submental space infection
B. Unilateral involvement of sublingual, submental space infection
C. Bilateral involvement of submandibular, sublingual, submental space infection
D. Bilateral involvement of submandibular, submental space infection

47. Osteomyelitis is caused by which bacteria?

A. Streptococci pyogenes
B. Staphylococcus aureus
C. Prevotella
D. Bacteroids

48. After Caldwell luc Procedure, intranasal antrostomy is done through:

A. Superior Meatus
B. Middle Meatus
C. Inferior Meatus
D. Floor of the Nose

49. Most of the cases of hematoma occurs during which nerve block?

A. Inferior alveolar nerve block
B. Posterosuperior nerve block
C. Infraorbital nerve block
D. Long buccal nerve block

50. The recommended time gap between the radiation and surgery to avoid osteoradionecrosis is:

A. 4-6 weeks after radiotherapy
B. 6-12 months after radiotherapy
C. Immediately after radiotherapy
D. Any time during the course of radiotherapy

51. The retentive terminals of a clasp is normally positioned:

A. Near the labial surface of he tooth
B. At the mesiolingual or distolingual line angles
C. At the mesiofacial or distofacial line angles
D. Near the facial surface

52. In complete denture patients the graphic method of recording CR is preferred over the intraocclusal check record method, if the:

A. Ridges are excessively flabby
B. Patient has uncontrolled abnormal mandibular movements
C. Jaws are normally related and the ridges are well built
D. Jaws are abnormally related

53. All other factors being equal, an FPD with a span of 2 pontics compared to an FPD with a span of one pontic will flex:

A. 2 Times
B. 4 Times
C. 6 Times
D. 8 Times

54. The success of removable die system depends upon the:

A. Abrasion resistance of the material
B. Length of the dowel pin protruding out of the master cast
C. Time involved in die construction
D. Precise relocation of the die in the working cast

55. The sclerosis of the dentinal tubules is related to:

A. Pathological Process
B. Physiological Process
C. Aging Process
D. Due to trauma to the tooth

56. Root completion occurs after how much time of eruption in permanent dentition?

A. 5-12 months
B. 12-24 months
C. 24-36 months
D. 36-48 months

57. Hair on end appearance is seen in:

A. Pernicious Anemia
B. Iron Deficiency Anemia
C. Beta Thalassemia
D. Megaloblastic Anemia

58. Most common benign neoplasm of oral cavity is:

A. Myxoma
B. Lipoma
C. Fibroma
D. Papilloma

59. A patient aged 50 years presented with history of jaw expansion and increased size of maxilla. The diagnosis is:

A. Paget's disease
B. Fibrous dysplasia
C. Acromegaly
D. Hyperthyroidism

60. Osteomyelitis begins in:

A. Periosteum
B. Medullary bone
C. Cortical portion
D. All of the above

61. True about compound odontoma:

A. Tooth like denticles
B. Tooth within tooth appearance
C. Crown is enlarged at expense of root
D. Irregular diffuse radiopaque mass surrounded by radiolucent line

62. Most common occurrence of cleft lip is:

A. Unilateral Left
B. Bilateral
C. Unilateral Right
D. Midline Defect

63. Giant cell lesions of the peridontium are best considered as:

A. Benign Neoplasm
B. Non-neoplastic Reactive lesions

C. Malignant neoplasm
D. None

64. Bence Jones protein is present in which condition?
A. Malignant Melanoma
B. Multiple Myeloma
C. Hodgkin's Lymphoma
D. None

65. Koplik spots are seen in:
A. Measles
B. German Measles
C. Herpes
D. Vericella

66. True about syphilis is:
A. Oral lesions are seen in any stage
B. Clinical manifestations occur after few months of exposure
C. VDRL test is positive in early stages of primary syphilis
D. Penicillins are ineffective

67. Lesion with a narrow stalk is described as:
A. Pedunculated
B. Sessile
C. Papillomatous
D. Hyperplastic

68. Which of the following is radiopaque mass surrounded by radiolucent line?
A. Sialolithiasis
B. Osteomas
C. Compound odontomas
D. Osteosarcoma

69. Granulation tissue is replaced by connective tissue by:
A. 7 days
B. 14 days
C. 21 days
D. 1 month

70. Leucocytes Adhesion Deficiency Syndrome Type 1 is due to defect of which chromosome?
A. Chromosome 1
B. Chromosome X
C. Chromosome 21
D. Chromosome 5

71. Fluoride concentration in 0.05% mouth rinse is:
A. 250 ppm
B. 225 ppm
C. 900 ppm
D. 1000 ppm

72. WHO Criteria for DMFT reduction by the year 2010:
A. 4
B. 3
C. 2
D. 1

73. The type of study involving repetitive examination of the sample is:

A. Cohort study B. Panel study
C. Prospective study D. Retrospective study

74. 0.2% conc. of NaF is used:

A. Once daily B. Twice daily
C. Once weekly D. Once fortnightly

75. Least cariogenic among these is:

A. Raw sugar B. Refined sugar
C. Sucrose D. Fructose

76. A 4-year-old child living in fluoride deficient area should be given fluoride supplementation as:

A. 0.25 mg B. 0.5 mg
C. 0.75 mg D. 1.0 mg

77. Dental fluorosis not associated with skeletal fluorosis is:

A. 1 ppm B. 3 ppm
C. 8 ppm D. 10 ppm

78. How many million people in the world are using the fluoridated tooth paste?

A. 100 million B. 500 million
C. 700 million D. 900 million

79. In a sample of population maximum observations are concentrated around:

A. Mean B. Mode
C. Median D. Arithmetic mean

80. Antibiotic prophylaxis is required for:

A. Cirrhosis of liver B. Bronchial asthma
C. Angina Pectoris D. Valvular Heart disease

81. Antibiotic prophylaxis is given to prevent infective endocarditis in case of:

A. Extraction of teeth
B. Scaling and curettage
C. Gingivoplasty
D. Open reduction of fracture by intra-oral route

82. Paradoxical respiration occurs in:

A. COPD
B. Upper Respiratory Obstruction

C. Guillain-Barré Syndrome
D. None

83. Steroids cause:
A. Delayed wound healing
B. No effect on wound healing
C. Rapid wound healing
D. None

84. In SIRS (Systemic Inflammatory Response Syndrome), there is all *except*:
A. Temperature < 36 or > 38 degree C
B. Blood pressure > 110/70
C. Respiratory rate > 20 per minute
D. Abnormal white blood cell count (>12,000/ml or <4,000ml)

85. A flat, circumscribed discoloration of the skin or mucosa that may very in size and shape is:
A. Epulis
B. Macule
C. Papule
D. Nodule

86. Disuse atrophy of periodontium occurs in all *except*:
A. Erythema Multiforme
B. Lupus Erythematosus
C. Herpangina
D. Chicken pox

87. Radiographically sequestrum appears as:
A. Less radiopaque than normal bone
B. More radiopaque than normal bone
C. Same radiopacity as that of normal bone
D. None

88. Bevels are given for restoration with cast gold inlay and onlay for:
A. To enhance edge strength
B. To remove unsupported enamel rods
C. Thin margins are easily adaptable
D. To prevent fracture of tooth

89. Carisolv is used for:
A. Staining carious dentin
B. Softening of dentin for removal of carious part
C. Enamel caries detection
D. Study histologic section of tooth

90. Single most reliable diagnostic criteria for squamous cell CA:
A. Invasion
B. Degeneration
C. Pleomorphism
D. Encapsulation

91. Tracheostomy is done through:
A. 1st Tracheal Ring
B. 2nd-4th Tracheal Ring
C. Cricothyroid membrane
D. Thyrohyoid ligament

92. In haemophilia pre-treatment management includes:
A. Fresh Frozen Plasma replacement
B. Thrombin Replacement
C. Factor–VIII replacement
D. Factor– VIII and IX replacement

93. Teeth present in the oral cavity on the date of first birthday of a child are:
A. Ghost teeth
B. Natal teeth
C. Neonatal teeth
D. Enamel pearls

94. Foolproof method to check the appropriateness of diet counseling is:
A. Lactobacilli count
B. Synder test
C. S. Mutans count
D. Latest dietary history

95. Drug of choice for penicillinase producing (penicillin resistant) infective microorganism:
A. Ampicillin
B. Amoxicillin
C. Erythromycin
D. Cloxacillin

96. Which of the following is best way of caries prevention?
A. Oral prophylaxis
B. Oral hygiene with fluoridated paste
C. Systemic water fluoridation
D. Diet counselling

97. Flow rate of unstimulated saliva is:
A. 0.25-0.35 ml/min
B. 0.5-0.6 ml/min
C. 0.1-0.1 ml/min
D. 0.05-0.5 ml/min

98. Drug to be contraindicated during orthodontic treatment:
A. NSAIDs
B. Corticosteroids
C. Antibiotics
D. Anesthetics

Answers

1.	D	2.	A	3.	B	4.	D
5.	D	6.	D	7.	D	8.	B
9.	B	10.	B	11.	C	12.	A
13.	A	14.	B	15.	C	16.	C
17.	A	18.	B	19.	D	20.	D
21.	A	22.	A	23.	B	24.	B
25.	B	26.	C	27.	B	28.	A
29.	C	30.	C	31.	C	32.	A
33.	D	34.	D	35.	D	36.	A
37.	C	38.	D	39.	C	40.	B
41.	C	42.	B	43.	B	44.	D
45.	D	46.	C	47.	B	48.	C
49.	B	50.	A	51.	C	52.	C
53.	D	54.	D	55.	B, C	56.	D
57.	C	58.	C	59.	A	60.	B
61.	A	62.	A	63.	B	64.	B
65.	A	66.	A	67.	A	68.	C
69.	C	70.	C	71.	B	72.	D
73.	B	74.	D	75.	A	76.	D
77.	B	78.	B	79.	C	80.	D
81.	D	82.	C	83.	A	84.	B
85.	B	86.	C	87.	B	88.	C
89.	B	90.	A	91.	B	92.	D
93.	C	94.	D	95.	D	96.	C
97.	B	98.	A				

PGI Paper December 2006

1. **Nerve supply of Lateral Pterygoid muscle is from:**
   A. Mandibular Nerve
   B. Masseteric Nerve
   C. Deep Temporal Nerve
   D. Auriculotemporal Nerve

2. **Root of tongue is attached to:**
   A. Styloid, hyoid and mandible
   B. Hyoid and mandible
   C. Mandible
   D. Hyoid bone

3. **Tooth develop from:**
   A. Endoderm and Mesoderm
   B. Ectoderm and Endoderm
   C. Ectoderm and Mesoderm
   D. All of the three germ layers

4. **Head shaped formation start as early as:**
   A. 11 days B. 31 days
   C. 21 days D. 41 days

5. **Deficiency of potassium leads to:**
   A. Muscle weakness
   B. Lethargy
   C. Muscle excitability
   D. Dry and cold skin

6. **Most antigenic among following is:**
   A. Haptens B. Nucleic acid
   C. Lipids D. Proteins

7. **Tuberculin test injection utilises:**
   A. BCG vaccine
   B. Dead strains of tubercle bacilli

C. Purified protein derivative
D. Live strains of tubercle bacilli

8. **Untrue about fungal infection is:**
A. Less virulent in pathogenicity
B. Indolent growth is a characteristic feature
C. Necrotic Foci are common
D. More common in immunocompromised individuals

9. **The condition is characterized by Butterfly Distribution on Face is:**
A. Herpangia
B. Lupus erythematosus
C. Herpes infection
D. Psoriasis

10. **Serum alkaline phosphatase level > 200 Bodansky unit is a characteristic feature of:**
A. Fibrous dysplasia
B. Osteogenesis imperfecta
C. Osteopetrosis
D. Paget's disease

11. **Charcot's Triad is a feature of:**
A. Migraine syndrome
B. Multiple sclerosis
C. SLE
D. Meiner disease

12. **Another name of Cooley's anemia is:**
A. Beta Thalassemia
B. Pernicious anemia
C. Aplastic anemia
D. Polycythema vera

13. **Which of the following is not a feature of Tertiary syphilis?**
A. Gumma
B. Tabes Dorsalis
C. Paresis
D. Hebra Nose

14. **Fluoride which is being used for Fluoridated amalgam is:**
A. NaF
B. Stannous fluoride
C. Yetterbum fluoride
D. Amine fluoride

15. Untrue about Cariosolv is:
A. Has a pH of 7.0
B. Has Leucine, lysine, glutamic acid as its component
C. Contain sodium hypochlorite
D. It is chemico-mechanical mean of canines removal

16. Radiographic view least useful in detecting incipient carious lesion:
A. IOPA with bisecting angle technique
B. Bitewing radiograph
C. Panoramic radiograph
D. IOPA with paralleling technique

17. S. mutans is a:
A. Obligate anaerobe
B. Facultative aerobe
C. Obligate aerobe
D. Facultative anaerobe

18. What is the concentration of Fluoride present in Breast Milk?
A. 3-6 mg/ml
B. 8-12 mg/ml
C. 12-16 mg/ml
D. 16-20 mg/ml

19. Epidemic is defined as:
A. The occurrence of any health related event in excess of the expectant
B. Disease imported into the country
C. Scattered cases of a disease
D. Constant finding of a disease in a population

20. Nephrotoxic concentration of fluoride is:
A. 650 nanogram F/ml
B. 500 nanogram F/ml
C. 750 nanogram F/ml
D. 850 nanogram F/ml

21. Galgan's formula used for water fluoridation is:
A. 0.34/E where E is -0.038 + 0.62 × °F
B. 0.34/E where E is -0.038 + 0.0062 × °F
C. 0.38/E where E is -0.038 + 0.062 × °F
D. 0.34/E where E is -0.38 + 0.0062 × °F

22. Primary age groups used in a WHO survey are:
A. 5, 10, 15, 30, 60 to 70 years
B. 5, 12, 15, 35 to 44, 65 to 74 years

C. 5, 15, 25, 35, 65 to 70 years
D. 5 to 10, 15, 35 to 40, 65 years

23. Test to be used for checking the effectiveness of diet counseling to reduce sugar intake:
A. Lactobacilli count test
B. S. mutans count test
C. Salivary reductase test
D. Synder's test

24. Amount of Fluoride in 1.1 mg NaF is:
A. 0.25 mg
B. 0.50 mg
C. 0.75 mg
D. 1.1 mg

25. Chi Square test is used to measure the significance of:
A. Difference between two variables
B. Relationship between exposure and effect
C. Correlation between two variables
D. Difference between two proportions

26. In a large country survey the sampling method of choice is:
A. Cluster sampling
B. Multistage sampling
C. Multiple sampling
D. Multistage random sampling

27. In a small population group with homogenous distribution, the type of sampling method used is:
A. Multistage sampling
B. Stratified sampling
C. Cluster sampling
D. Simple random

28. Radiographic view in children with require radiation exposure to be reduced by:
A. 25%
B. 50%
C. 60%
D. 75%

29. In which of the following condition of premature loss of primary teeth, the space loss is maximum?
A. Mandibular molars, closing within 6 months
B. Maxillary molars, closing within 6 months
C. Mandibular molars, closing within 3 months
D. Maxillary molars, closing within 3 months

30. **Rate of space loss after extraction of mandibular second molars is:**
A. 2.0 mm/year
B. 1.5 mm/year
C. 1 mm/year
D. 2.6 mm/year

31. **Untrue about difference between primary and permanent teeth is:**
A. Pulp chambers are wide in primary teeth
B. Pulp horns are high
C. Enamel thickness is less in primary teeth
D. Dentin is thicker in primary teeth

32. **Chronological age is defined as:**
A. Age of physiological development
B. It is the age from the birth of the child
C. Age of skeletal maturation
D. All of the above

33. **Dose of Midazolam for conscious sedation by oral route:**
A. 0.15 to 0.25 mg/kg
B. 0.25 to 1.0 mg/kg
C. 1.0 to 2.0 mg/kg
D. 2.0 to 5.0 mg/kg

34. **Change in arch length from mesial surface of Permanent 1st molars between the ages of 6 to 18 years is:**
A. Increased by 0-1 mm
B. Decreased by 0-4 mm
C. Increased by 3-4 mm
D. Decreased by 3-4 mm

35. **Untrue about pit and fissure sealant is:**
A. Not used in teeth with well coalesced pit and fissures
B. Not used in tooth is caries free for 4 years or more
C. Depth of penetration does not matter, full length application is more important
D. Indicated in teeth with depth pit and fissure with interproximal lesion

36. **Which of the following microorganism establishes itself firstly in the oral cavity of a newborn?**
A. S. mutans
B. S. salivarius
C. Lactobacilli
D. S. mitis

37. **Atraumatic Restorative treatment was given by:**
A. Smith
B. J.E. Frecknen
C. McLevan
D. McDonald

38. **Which of the following is not a true indicator of pulpal status in a primary tooth?**
A. Electric pulp testing
B. Percussion
C. Swelling
D. All of the above

39. **MTA is used for all *except*:**
A. Perforation of tooth
B. Apexification of immature teeth
C. Restoration of Class II, III cases
D. Pulpotomy procedures

40. **The treatment of Herpangina includes:**
A. High dosage of acyclovir and idoxuridine
B. Supportive and symptomatic
C. Antibiotic and analgesics
D. Application of an antiviral ointment

41. **Radiographic view most suitable to visualize zygomatic arch fracture is:**
A. Occipitomental view
B. PA view
C. Reverse Towne and view
D. Submentovertex view

42. **Which of the following muscle is involved in displacement of Fractured Condyle?**
A. Temporalis
B. Masseter
C. Lateral Pterygoid
D. Medial Pterygoid

43. **Hematoma formation around the posterior auricular region is suggestive of:**
A. Temporal bone fracture
B. Mandibular fracture
C. Parietal bone fracture
D. Lefort I fracture

44. **A 7-year-old child with slightly displaced parasymphysis fracture should be managed by:**
A. Risdon wiring
B. Intermaxillary fixation

C. Cap splint with circummandibular wiring
D. Transosseous wiring

45. Regarding Cleft Lip, maximum prevalence is seen in:
A. Bilateral
B. Unilateral right side
C. Unilateral left side
D. Midline detect

46. Neutral zone concept for arrangement of prosthetic teeth was introduced by:
A. Fish
B. Boucher
C. Bell
D. Smith

47. Which of the following case is contraindication for FPD?
A. Where esthetic requirement is high
B. Abutment teeth are endodontically treated
C. Patients with high caries index
D. Short span bridge

48. Type of finish line used for all ceramic restoration:
A. Heavy chamfer
B. Shoulder
C. Chamfer
D. Feather edge

49. True about articulator is:
A. They determine incisal guidance
B. They are laboratory analogue to stimulate jaw movements
C. They are used to determine physiologic test space
D. None

50. J aws can be related to skull by:
A. Pantogram
B. Intraoral tracing
C. Face Bow
D. Extraoral tracing

51. Mid-palatine region in complete denture case is:
A. Primary Stress Bearing area
B. Secondary Stress Bearing area
C. Primary Relief area
D. Peripheral Seal Area

52. Implant supported teeth should contact:
A. During protrusion
B. Only in centric occlusion
C. During lateral excursion
D. Eccentric positions of mandible

53. Minimum number of implants required for mandibular denture:

A. 2 B. 3
C. 4 D. 6

54. Temperature which should not exceed while implant placement:

A. 37° B. 47°
C. 59° D. 67°

55. Specific plaque hypothesis for the etiology of periodontal disease was proposed by:

A. Jenco B. Listgarten
C. Loesche D. Glickman

56. Type of cells which predominate in the Stage III lesion of Gingivitis are:

A. Macrophages B. PMN's
C. Plasma cells D. Lymphocytes

57. Diagnosis test for ANUG is:

A. Animal inoculation
B. Tissue culture
C. Complement fixation
D. Darkfield microscopy

58. Destruction of periodontium without inflammation is:

A. Periodontitis B. Periodontosis
C. Pericoronitis D. None

59. Microorganism increased in number during pregnancy gingivitis:

A. Prevotella intermedia
B. Eichenella corrodens
C. Porphyromonas melaninogenicus
D. Porphyromonas gingivalis

60. Most unreliable feature during the diagnosis of gingivitis is:

A. Color of gingiva
B. Contour of gingiva
C. Stippling of gingiva
D. None

61. **Width of attached gingiva is:**
A. From the crest of gingiva to the mucogingival junction
B. From the free marginal groove to mucogingival junction
C. From crest of gingiva to the distance apical to mucogingival junction
D. None of the above

62. **Untrue about saliva is:**
A. Function is lubrication during mastication
B. The stimulated amount to 2.0-3.0 ml/minutes
C. K^+ion concentration is increased in stimulated saliva
D. The resting amount is 0.3-0.5 ml/minute

63. **Purine present in the saliva is:**
A. Thymine
B. Uric acid
C. Adenosine
D. Cytosine

64. **The term ugly Duckling stage was coined by:**
A. Broadbent
B. McDonald
C. Brodie
D. Leeway

65. **Sutural theory of growth was given by:**
A. Enlow
B. Brodie
C. Sicher
D. Melvin and Moss

66. **Square shaped dental arch form is seen in:**
A. Class II Div.1 Malocclusion
B. Class II Div. 2 Malocclusion
C. Class III Malocclusion
D. Class I Malocclusion

67. **Y-axis is used to orient the growth tendency of:**
A. Mandible
B. Maxilla
C. Skull
D. All of the above

68. **All of the following are a feature of Complex Tongue Thrust *except*:**
A. The occlusion of teeth may be poor
B. This tongue thrust is characterized by teeth together swallow
C. Contraction of the circumoral muscles during swallowing
D. The anterior open bite can be diffused or absent

69. **A child is having bilateral distal step and proclined lateral in mixed dentition. The type of malocclusion which may develop in permanent dentition is:**

A. Class- I Malocclusion
B. Class-II Malocclusion
C. Class II Div. 2 Malocclusion
D. Class III Malocclusion

70. With the growth of dentoalveolar structure axial inclination of permanent teeth:

A. Decreases
B. Increases
C. Remain same
D. None

71. Growth of craniofacial complex occurs in which sequence?

A. Transverse-Vertical-Sagittal Direction
B. Transverse-Sagittal-Vertical Direction
C. Sagittal-Transverse-Vertical Direction
D. Sagittal-Vertical-Transverse Direction

72. True measurement of Gonial Angle can be done most accurately on which radiograph?

A. Panoramic radiograph
B. Lateral oblique view
C. Lateral cephalometrics
D. Reverse Towne's view

73. Workload Elongation of an arch wire can be increased by:

A. Increasing the thickness of wire
B. Decreasing the length
C. Increasing the length of wire by using loops
D. Decreasing the interbracket distance

74. Rate of distraction, in a case of distraction osteo-synthesis:

A. 1.0 mm/day
B. 0.5 mm/day
C. 1.5 mm/day
D. 2.0 mm/day

75. A patient is taking oral anticoagulant, INR ratio is 3.1, the treatment plan for extraction is:

A. Avoid extraction as INR is much higher
B. Proceed with normal extraction with the use of local hemostatic measures
C. Stop the oral anticoagulant for 7 days and do the extraction
D. None of the above

76. **In anaphylactic shock, the drug which is to be administered first is:**
A. Adrenaline
B. Antibiotics
C. Antihistaminic
D. Hydrocortisone

77. **Bleeding time is increased in which disease?**
A. Hemophilia-B
B. Sickle cell anemia
C. Von Willebrand's disease
D. Hemophilia-A

78. **Material of choice for implants is:**
A. Titanium
B. Vitreous carbon
C. Stainless steel
D. Ceramics

79. **Implant of choice to be widely used these days is:**
A. Endosseous screw from implant
B. Blade and vent implant
C. Transosteal implant
D. Endosseous cylindrical implant

80. **A female patient requiring mandibular advancement by 8.0 mm. What is the procedure of choice?**
A. Oblique sub condylar osteotomy
B. Extraoral vertical ramus osteotomy
C. Sagittal split osteotomy with mandibular advancement
D. None

81. **Descending Mediastenitis is a most common complication of:**
A. Space infection of the neck
B. Apical periodontitis
C. Pericoronitis
D. Danine abscess

82. **Concentration of Bupivicaine used in dentistry is:**
A. 0.5%
B. 2.0%
C. 4.0%
D. 5.0%

83. **25 years healthy patient require extraction of grossly decayed third molar, the treatment indicated is:**
A. Extraction of tooth without any need of medication
B. Extraction under antibiotic cover and analgesics
C. Extraction of tooth under antibiotic cover
D. None

84. Treatment of choice for OKC present in the ramus of mandible:

A. Enucleation
B. Marsupialization
C. Surgical excision
D. Enucleation and peripheral ostectomy

85. Type of MTA used as a root canal irrigant:

A. MTA-B B. MTA-A
C. MTA-D D. MTA-E

86. Clinical significant of sclerotic dentin is:

A. It is soft in consistency
B. It is dark brown in color
C. Resistant to decay
D. None

87. Which of the following is not a safe procedure during rubber dam isolation?

A. Visual inspection of the oral cavity after procedure
B. Using suction along with rubber dam
C. Ask the patient to continuously swallow this saliva
D. Ask the patient to collect the saliva and spit at the end of procedure

88. All of the following are recent caries diagnostic aids *except*:

A. Infrared Crystallography
B. Optical Coherence Tomography
C. Terahartz imaging
D. Infrared Thermography

89. The highest percentage of lateral canals occurs:

A. In the middle third of the root
B. In the coronal third of the root
C. In the apical third of the root
D. Anywhere along the root, depending on the tooth in question

90. The technique of choice for removing poorly condensed gutta-percha is:

A. Hand instrumentation
B. Automated instrumentation
C. Ultrasonic instrumentation
D. Rotary instrumentation

91. **Endodontic retreatment:**
A. Has a poorer prognosis than original treatment
B. Is performed only in endodontic failures
C. Has different objects lives than primary treatment
D. Is a technically challenge as original treatment

92. **Primary function of MTA is:**
A. Restorative in deciduous anterior teeth
B. Apexification in an immature traumatized pulpless teeth
C. Root canal restorative material in deciduous teeth
D. None

93. **Which of the following is 1st generation injectable Cephalosporin?**
A. Cefadroxil
B. Cephalothin
C. Ceftrixone
D. Cefotaxime

94. **Corticosteroids are useful in case of:**
A. Rheumatoid arthritis
B. Pemphigus
C. Graft patients
D. All of the above

95. **Leukocyte adhesion deficiency syndrome Type I is because of defect of which chromosome?**
A. X-chromosome
B. Chromosome 21
C. Chromosome 11
D. Chromosome 8

96. **Matrix Metalloproteinase are active during which stage of Amelogenesis?**
A. Protective
B. Formative/secretory
C. Organizing
D. Desmolytic

97. **Main cells of connective tissue are:**
A. PMNs
B. Fibroblasts
C. Macrophages
D. Basal cells

98. **Skin margins while suturing on face are:**
A. Inverted
B. Edge to edge
C. Everted
D. Overlapped

Answers

1.	A	2.	B	3.	C	4.	C
5.	A	6.	D	7.	C	8.	C
9.	B	10.	D	11.	B	12.	A
13.	D	14.	B	15.	A	16.	C
17.	D	18.	B	19.	A	20.	D
21.	B	22.	B	23.	D	24.	B
25.	D	26.	D	27.	D	28.	B
29.	B	30.	C	31.	D	32.	B
33.	B	34.	B	35.	D	36.	B
37.	B	38.	A	39.	C	40.	B
41.	D	42.	C	43.	A	44.	C
45.	C	46.	A	47.	C	48.	B
49.	B	50.	C	51.	C	52.	B
53.	A	54.	B	55.	C	56.	C
57.	D	58.	B	59.	A	60.	C
61.	B	62.	C	63.	B	64.	A
65.	C	66.	B	67.	A	68.	B
69.	C	70.	B	71.	B	72.	C
73.	C	74.	A	75.	B	76.	A
77.	C	78.	A	79.	A	80.	C
81.	A	82.	A	83.	A	84.	D
85.	C	86.	C	87.	B	88.	A
89.	A	90.	A	91.	A	92.	B
93.	B	94.	D	95.	B	96.	B
97.	B	98.	C				

PGI Paper June 2006

1. **The nerve emerges from the two superficial heads of lateral pterygoid muscle is:**
   A. Masseteric nerve
   B. Nerve to pterygoid muscle
   C. Inferior alveolar nerve
   D. Buccal nerve

2. **The anterior two-thirds of the tongue is supplied by:**
   A. Glossopharyngeal nerve
   B. Vagus nerve
   C. Chorda tympani nerve
   D. Lingual nerve

3. **The tongue:**
   A. Contains foramen cecum which is present on the dorsum of frenulum
   B. Contains 6-10 circumvallate papilla located posterior to sulcus terminalis
   C. Embryologically derives from first brachial arch only
   D. Separated from the epiglottis by both lateral side of vallecula

4. **Which of the following is correct?**
   A. Hard palate is formed by maxilla, palatine and vomer bone
   B. All the constrictors of pharynx are inserted into a median raphae on the anterior wall of the pharynx
   C. The posterior wall of pharynx, the lower part of thyropharyngeus is a multiple sheet of muscle and is overlapped by the upper and middle constrictors
   D. Tensor palatine forms a dedicated tendon which winds round the pterygoid hamulus and flattens out to form the palatine aponeurosis

5. During removal of submandibular gland which of the following nerve gets injured?

A. Glosspharyngeal nerve
B. Vagus nerve
C. Accessory spinal nerve
D. Hypoglossal nerve

6. Lacrimal gland is located in a groove overlapped by:

A. Levator palpebrae supreoris
B. Levator palpebrae inferioris
C. Orbicularis oculi
D. Orbicularis oris

7. The muscle which is resected in classical radical neck dissection is:

A. Sternomastoid
B. Sternothyroid
C. Sternocricoid
D. Sternohyoid

8. Which of the following is the best site of absorption of calcium?

A. Ascending colon
B. Ileum
C. Middle segment of small intestine
D. Proximal segment of small intestine

9. The fuel value of fat is:

A. 4
B. 7
C. 9
D. 5

10. Which of the following correctly indicates the infectivity of hepatitis virus in human?

A. HBcAg
B. HBeAg
C. Anti-HBC
D. Anti-HBS

11. Which of the following is not associated with dentino-genesis imperfecta?

A. Osteopetrosis
B. Obliteration of pulp
C. Osteogenesis imperfecta
D. Hereditary opalscent dentin

12. A painful, depapillated and atrophic tongue is associated with:

A. Atrophic glossitis of syphilis
B. Sideroblastic anemia
C. Nutritional deficiency anemia
D. Aplastic anemia

13. Smooth tongue is associated with:

A. Nutritional deficiency anemia
B. Sideroblastic anemia
C. Hemolytic anemia
D. Aplastic anemia

14. Enlarged tongue is associated with:

A. Syphilis
B. Thyrotoxicosis
C. Tuberculosis
D. Amyloidosis

15. A 36-year-old female complains of asymptomatic bilateral striation of white lines on buccal mucosa. The histologic examination shows hyperkeratosis, degeneration of basal layer of cells and infiltration of T-lymphocytes in papillary layer of connective tissue. The most probable diagnosis is:

A. Lichen planus
B. Leucoedema
C. Squamous cell carcinoma
D. Candidiasis

16. Rhabdomyoma is:

A. Tumour of striated muscle
B. Tumour of smooth muscle
C. Tumour of bone
D. Tumour of unstriated muscle

17. The "Cotton-wool" appearance, hypercementosis along with enlargement of maxillary tuberosity bone is characterized by:

A. Fibrous dysplasia
B. Osteosarcoma
C. Hyperparathyroidism
D. Paget's disease

18. All of the following is the extraglandular manifestation of primary Sjogren's syndrome *except*:

A. Arthritis
B. Lymphadenopathy
C. Thrombocytopenia
D. Raynaud's phenomena

19. Teratoma is best described as:

A. Harmatomus development manifestation consisting of three different layers

B. Originates from mesodermal tissue
C. Associated with very painful condition
D. Occurs most commonly in stomach and lungs

20. The most cariogenic bacteria is:
A. S. Mutans
B. Lactobacillus
C. Actinomycetes
D. Both A and B

21. 1 part per million F is equal to:
A. 0.1 mg of F in 1 liter of water
B. 10 mg of F in 10 liter of water
C. 1 mg of F in 1 liter of water
D. 100 mg of F in 10 liter of water

22. "Duraphat" is:
A. NaF
B. CaF_2
C. APF
D. SnF_2

23. Fluoride application is most effective for prevention of:
A. Pit and fissure caries
B. Occlusal caries
C. Smooth surface caries
D. Deeply caviated caries

24. The blood is:
A. Continuous variable
B. Simple variable
C. Simultaneous variable
D. Discrete variable

25. The "Variable" is best described as:
A. Coefficient of variability
B. Root square standard deviation
C. Simple standard deviation
D. Independent of standard deviation

26. Incidence is:
A. Number of cases of a non-specific disease within a defined population over a period of time
B. Number of cases of a specific diseases within a defined population over a period of time
C. That portion of population affected by a disease or other condition at a given time
D. Number of all cases of specific diseases within a defined population over a period of time

27. The treatment needs of a periodontal disease is measured by:

A. CPITN
B. Loe and stillness index
C. Periodontal Russel index
D. Ramfjord periodontal index

28. Among the following fluoride is found in maximum concentration:

A. Tea leaves
B. Sea fish
C. Coconut water
D. Pineapple

29. The foolproof method to check the diet counselling is:

A. Patient diet history
B. Synder test
C. Lactobacillus count test
D. Patient oral hygiene

30. The last primary tooth to be replaced by a permanent tooth is?

A. Maxillary incisor
B. Maxillary canine
C. Mandibular molar
D. First molar

31. A distal shoe space maintainer is indicated when a primary:

A. First molar is prematurely lost
B. Second molar is lost after the eruption of permanent first molar
C. Second molar is lost prior to eruption of permanent first molar
D. Canine is in cross bite

32. Anatomical structure injured in excision of ranula:

A. Submandibular duct
B. Parotid duct
C. Lingual artery
D. Lingual nerve

33. All of the following causes excessive bleeding during tooth extraction *except*:

A. Hemophilia-A
B. Hemophilia-B
C. Von-Willebrand disease
D. Anti thrombin III deficiency

34. The most common tumor of oral cavity is:

A. Osteosarcoma
B. Malignant melanoma
C. Squamous cell carcinoma
D. Basal cell carcinoma

35. Most commonly Sialolith is found in:

A. Ductis of rivinus
B. Gland's of mohl
C. Wharton's duct
D. Stensen's duct

36. Mucocele most commonly occur because of:

A. Trauma
B. Viral infection
C. Bacterial infection
D. Sialodentitis

37. The most difficult extraction of impacted tooth is:

A. Vertical
B. Mesioangular
C. Horizontal
D. Distoangular

38. The low thermal conductivity of impression compound is overcome by:

A. By heating with ethanol flame and directly placing in patient's mouth
B. Heating in hot water and immediately quenching in water for 20 minutes
C. By melting in boiling water at 50°C for one hour
D. Impression is placed in mouth till it get cold and sudden removal of impression

39. The inhibitor is added in monomer of self cure acrylic resin to:

A. Decrease the shrinkage of acrylic resin
B. Prevent the porosity of acrylic resin
C. Increase the time of dough stage
D. Prolong the shelf life

40. Age hardening is a process done at:

A. Heating above 700°C for 30 minutes and quenching in water
B. Heating at 700°C for 1 hour and quenching in water
C. Heating upto 200-450°C for 15 to 30 minutes and quenching in water
D. Heating at 700°C for 10 to 15 minutes and quenching in water

41. Immediate Bennet side shift is used to define the shift when it occurs?

A. Immediately after the forward movement is completed
B. In the first 5-6 mm of forward movement
C. Before any forward movement of the orbiting condyle
D. Throughout the range of motion

42. The cuspal inclines of the maxillary buccal cusp and the mandibular lingual cusp should be grounded if they are in deflective occlusal contact is:

A. Balanced position
B. Working position only
C. Both working and balancing position
D. Central position

43. Group function of the occlusion is characterized by:

A. Absence of bilateral balanced occlusion
B. Cuspid rise in protrusion
C. Working side contacts from canine to all posterior teeth, without balancing side contacts
D. Disocclusion of posterior teeth when mandible is protruded

44. Which of the following is utmost important factor considered in balanced occlusion with little change in esthetics and change in inclination or amplitude leads to the loss of facial appearance?

A. Inclination of incisal guidance
B. Compensating curve of spee
C. Inclination condylar guidance
D. Cuspal height and angulation

45. Which of the following configuration is used in designing an RPD with Kennedy-Class II edentulous teeth?

A. Tripod
B. Quadrilateral
C. Unilateral
D. Bilateral

46. Which of the following is disadvantage of combination clasp in comparison to circumferential clasp?

A. More tooth is covered with a bar clasp arch because of its occlusal direction of approach
B. It is easily distorted by handling of the patient
C. It can flex in any spatial plane
D. Avoid the use of extraarticular occlusal record

47. All of the following are protective agent in periodontal disease *except*:

A. V. Provella B. C. Ochracea
C. S. Sanguis D. B. Oralis

48. The group of periodontal fibres which resist the masticatory forces:

A. Horizontal B. Oblique
C. Transseptal D. Alveolar

49. The width of attached gingiva with age:

A. Increases
B. Decreases
C. Remains unchanged
D. Unpredictable

50. The most common periodontal fiber which regenerate after injury is:

A. Horizontal fibers B. Oblique fibers
C. Transseptal fibers D. Apical fibers

51. McCall's festoon occurs due to:

A. Periodontal disease
B. Poor oral hygiene
C. Physiological resorption
D. Trauma from occlusion

52. The gingival crevicular fluid is increased in all *except*:

A. Smoking
B. Gingivitis
C. Trauma from occlusion
D. Periodontal pocket

53. Transgingival probing is a clinical procedure:

A. Used in determination of underlying bony topography
B. To measure the periodontal pocket depth
C. To determine the clinical attachment
D. To detect the transformation bony defect

54. Gingival enlargement in pregnancy is termed as:

A. Granuloma pyogenicum
B. Gingivitis
C. Angiogranuloma
D. Pyogenic granuloma

55. The gingival enlargement in leukemia mainly results from:

A. Hormonal disturbances
B. Poor oral hygiene
C. As an inflammatory reaction of plaque
D. Leukemic cellular infiltration

56. Pathologic migration of tooth occurs:

A. Axioinclined direction
B. Always from the bone resorption area
C. Towards the bone resorption area
D. Inciso/occlusal direction

57. The most common brushing technique used in preschool child is:

A. Charter's method
B. Bass method
C. Modified Stillman technique
D. Fone's technique

58. The flap technique procedure which does not increase the width of attached gingiva:

A. Free gingival graft
B. Undisplaced flap
C. Apically positioned flap
D. Fenestration procedure

59. Stainless steel contains:

A. 8% chromium and 8% Nickel
B. 18% chromium and 18% Nickel
C. 18% chromium and 8% Nickel
D. 8% chromium and 18% Nickel

60. The "Anatomic" type of mouth breathing is characterized by:

A. Enlarged tonsil
B. Enlarged adenoids
C. Short upper lip
D. Enlarged tonsil and adenoids

61. Which of the following treatment is not done in mixed dentition period?

A. Distobuccal rotation of teeth
B. Anterior cross bite
C. Posterior cross bite
D. Class II malocclusion

62. The teeth considered in classification of malocclusion is:

A. Permanent lower first molar
B. Permanent upper first molar
C. Permanent lower second molar
D. Permanent upper second molar

63. The repair of cleft palate is primarily done for:

A. Correction of esthetics
B. Correction of speech
C. Induce the growth of mandible
D. Induce the growth of maxilla

64. Anterior cranial base is represented by:

A. Nasion to Bolton
B. F-H plane
C. Nasion to Basion
D. S-N plane

65. Frankfort horizontal plane is formed by:

A. Nasion to Bolton
B. Sella to Nasion
C. Porion to Nasion
D. Porion to Orbitale

66. In Ackermann-Proffit classification the outer envelop describes:

A. Alignment
B. Profile
C. Anteroposterior relation
D. Transverse relation

67. Andrew's 2nd key of occlusion states:

A. Plane of occlusion
B. Interarch relation
C. Crown angulation
D. Crown inclination

68. The three landmarks which determine the skeletal convexity is:

A. Nasion, sella and articulare
B. Glabella, prosthion and supramentale
C. Orbitale, anterior nasal pine and pogonion
D. Nasion, subspinale and pogonion

69. The normal percentage of enlargement or magnification considered normal in cephalogram is?

A. 1-2%
B. 6-7%
C. 8-10%
D. 10-13%

70. Most easiest movement during orthodontic treatment is:

A. Tipping B. Intrusion
C. Extrusion D. Bodily movement

71. A single force is applied to the crowns of the upper incisors. Tipping is around the point of rotation present at:

A. Apical 1/3rd B. Infinity
C. Middle 1/3rd D. Coronal 1/3rd

72. Edge-wise bounded brackets are used:

A. With rectangular arch wire
B. To obtain edge to edge occlusion
C. With labial arch wires at incisal and gingival edges of each bracket
D. On incisal edges of anterior teeth

73. The fracture of intracapsular articular disc of TMJ causes:

A. Dislocation B. Chronic pain
C. Arthritis D. Ankylosis

74. All of the following cyst is associated with impacted tooth *except*:

A. Keratogenic cyst
B. Primordial cyst
C. Dentigerous cyst
D. Calcifying epithelial odontogenic cyst

75. The most common tumor associated with mandible is:

A. Teratoma B. Odontoma
C. Admantinoma D. Osteoma

76. Traumatic injury of a nerve causing paresthesia is:

A. Axonometesis B. Toxolysis
C. Neurotemesis D. Neuropraxia

77. The maximum dose of lignocaine with 1:200000 adrenaline that can be admitted to a patient is:

A. 9 mg/kg body wt B. 7 mg/kg body wt
C. 11 mg/kg body wt D. 14 mg/kg body wt

78. During inferior alveolar nerve block the needle of LA syringe is penetrated into parotid gland. Which of the following structure is most likely to be penetrated?

A. Internal carotid artery

B. External carotid artery
C. Lingual artery
D. Lingual nerve

79. A child got injury in the chin 3 years ago. His intrinsical distance is 8 mm while opening the mouth mandible deviates to the left side. What is the most probable diagnosis?

A. Unilateral right side temporomandibular joint ankylosis
B. Bilateral temperomandibular joint ankylosis
C. Anterior open bite with TMJ ankylosis
D. Unilateral left side temporomandibular joint ankylosis

80. A patient with unfavourable fracture of the angle of mandible is best treated by:

A. Closed reduction with cap splint
B. Closed reduction with IMF
C. Circum-mandibular wiring
D. Open reduction with bone plate fixation

81. Post auricular ecchymosis in case of fracture of the base of skull is called:

A. Tinell's sign
B. Bell's sign
C. Battle's sign
D. Nicolky's sign

82. Following bilateral mandibular fracture in the canine region (Parasymphysis), the following muscles will tend to pull the mandible back:

A. Geniohyoid, Geniglossus and mylohyoid
B. Mylohyoid, hyoglossus and sternohyoid
C. Hyoglossus, mylohyoid and geniglossus
D. Anterior belly of digastricus, geniohyoid and geniglossus

83. Guerin fracture is:

A. Maxillary fracture
B. Maxillary and nasal bone fracture
C. Nasal bone fracture only
D. Maxillary and zygomatic fracture

84. In blow out fracture which of the following is seen?

A. Exophthalmous
B. Enophthalmos
C. Conjunctival hemorrhage
D. Bulbar hemorrhage

85. **All of the following are features of TMJ dislocation *except*:**
   A. Anterior displacement of condyles
   B. Anterior open bite
   C. Deafness
   D. Can be reduced by applying pressure on the mandible

86. **Sagittal split osteotomy is a procedure done for:**
   A. Maxillary retrognathism B. Mandibular retrognathism
   C. Maxillary prognathism D. Mandibular prognathism

87. **Intra oral vertical ramus osteotomy is done for:**
   A. Mandibular setback B. Maxillary deformity
   C. Mandibular advancement D. Anterior open bite

88. **Which of the following causes difficulty in location of progressive pulp?**
   A. Inflammation B. Ankylosis
   C. Trauma D. Periodontal disease

89. **The blue coloured reamer is number as:**
   A. 30 and 60 size of instrument
   B. 10 size of instrument
   C. 25 and 50 size of instrument
   D. 6 size of instrument

90. **Elli's classification of teeth which is non-vital with or without crown fracture is:**
   A. Class III B. Class IV
   C. Class V D. Class VI

91. **The traumatic loss of a tooth due to injury is:**
   A. Concussion B. Luxation
   C. Transplantation D. Avulsion

92. **Which of the following antibiotics is not used in the treatment of infectious mononucleosis?**
   A. Erythromycin B. Gentamycin
   C. Ciprofloxacin D. Ampicillin

93. **In a 3-year-old child which of the following is the most common cysts located in the midline of neck?**
   A. Lymphangiocele B. Cystic hygroma
   C. Branchial cyst D. Thyroglossal cyst

94. **Which of the following forms the cavity lesion of lung as clinical manifestation?**

A. Wegener's granulomatosis
B. Scleroderma
C. Systemic lupus erythematous
D. Progressive systemic sclerosis

95. All of the following is used as accelerator in zinc oxide eugenol cement *except*:
A. Calcium chloride
B. Bromoglycerine
C. Zinc acetate dehydrate
D. Acetic acid

96. Most effective radiograph for visualization of mesiodens is:
A. Periapical graph
B. Bite wing graph
C. OPG
D. Occlusal graph

97. The radiation equivalent dose of 60 Gy (Gray) is equal to:
A. 6 rad.
B. 60 rad.
C. 600 rad.
D. 6000 rad.

98. The best radiograph used to visualize the zygomatic arch fracture is:
A. Submentovertex view
B. Transcranial view
C. Lateral oblique view
D. Postero-anterior view

99. All of the following are features of mandibular fracture *except*:
A. Paresthesia of lip
B. Malocclusion
C. Fractured ends are prevented from dislocation by masticatory muscle
D. Are usually compound

100. Which of the following is true about modified Stillman brushing technique?
A. Used in patient after periodontal surgery to help in healing of wound
B. Indicated in patient with severe gingival inflammation associated with deep periodontal pocket
C. Used to stimulate the gingiva and initiate the profuse bleeding
D. Used in patient with severe gingival recession and to prevent the plaque accumulation of exposed root

Answers

1.	D	2.	C	3.	D	4.	D
5.	D	6.	A	7.	A	8.	D
9.	C	10.	B	11.	A	12.	C
13.	A	14.	D	15.	A	16.	A
17.	D	18.	A	19.	A	20.	D
21.	C	22.	A	23.	C	24.	A
25.	B	26.	D	27.	A	28.	A
29.	C	30.	B	31.	C	32.	A
33.	D	34.	C	35.	C	36.	A
37.	D	38.	D	39.	D	40.	C
41.	C	42.	B	43.	C	44.	A
45.	A	46.	C	47.	B	48.	B
49.	A	50.	C	51.	D	52.	C
53.	A	54.	C	55.	D	56.	C
57.	D	58.	D	59.	C	60.	C
61.	A	62.	B	63.	D	64.	D
65.	D	66.	A	67.	C	68.	D
69.	B	70.	C	71.	A	72.	A
73.	B	74.	B	75.	C	76.	D
77.	C	78.	B	79.	D	80.	D
81.	C	82.	D	83.	A	84.	B
85.	C	86.	B	87.	A	88.	A
89.	A	90.	B	91.	D	92.	B
93.	D	94.	A	95.	B	96.	A
97.	D	98.	A	99.	C	100.	D

PGI Paper December 2005

1. **Which one of the following is a branch of middle meningeal artery?**
   A. Petrous part of internal carotid artery
   B. Maxillary part of external carotid artery
   C. Cavernous part of internal carotid artery
   D. Cerebral part of internal carotid artery

2. **Temporalis muscle is inserted into:**
   A. Condylar process B. Coronoid process
   C. Lingula D. Ramus of mandible

3. **Which one of the following nerves supply buccinator muscle?**
   A. Trigeminal nerve
   B. Facial nerve
   C. Glossopharyngeal nerve
   D. Ansa cervicalis

4. **Massetric nerve is a branch of:**
   A. Anterior trunk of mandibular nerve
   B. Main trunk of mandibular nerve
   C. Posterior trunk of mandibular nerve
   D. Maxillary nerve

5. **Which one of the following structures passes through the centre of cavernous sinus?**
   A. Occulomotor nerve
   B. Trochlear nerve
   C. Abducens nerve
   D. Ophthalmic nerve

6. **Blood coagulation is impaired in:**
   A. Tetany B. Hyperparathyroidism
   C. Rickets D. None

7. Fructose intolerance is to:

A. Fructose only B. Fructose and glucose
C. Sucrose only D. Fructose and sucrose

8. Endotoxins differ from exotoxins, in that they are:

A. Heat stable B. Proteins
C. Can be toxoided D. Complement fixed

9. Immunity that is conferred to the foetus by transfer of IgG and IgA antibodies is called as:

A. Active acquired immunity
B. Passive acquired immunity
C. Natural active immunity
D. Passive natural immunity

10. Name the disease that results due to surgery of the parotid gland:

A. Tic doloureux B. Meniere's syndrome
C. Bell's palsy D. Frey's syndrome

11. Respiratory obstruction due to tongue falling back occurs in:

A. Bilateral condylar neck fracture
B. Bilateral angle fracture
C. Symphysis menti fracture
D. Bilateral parasymphysis fracture

12. Orthognathic decompensation is done:

A. Is done at the time of surgery
B. Is done before the surgery
C. Is done after the surgery
D. Nature itself decompensates for dental compensation

13. LA toxicity complications *except*:

A. Cardiac depression
B. CNS depression
C. Paresthesia
D. Respiratory depression

14. KHN of enamel is close to:

A. Pure gold
B. Amalgam
C. Porcelain
D. Composite

15. Which one of the following increases the strength of agar hydrocolloid impression material?

A. Borax
B. Water
C. Sulfates
D. Carbonates

16. The least accurate impression material is:

A. Impression compound
B. Reversible hydrocolloid
C. Elastomers
D. Irreversible hydrocolloid

17. The advantage of composite restoration over silicates is that it:

A. Least soluble in oral fluids
B. Chemical retention to tooth structure
C. Fluoride release
D. Antibacterial action or cement

18. Bonding in pit and fissure sealants is:

A. Mechanical interlocking due to acid etching of enamel
B. Chemical bonding to tooth structure
C. Physical bonding to the tooth structure
D. All of the above

19. The metal that acts as anti-corrosive agent is:

A. Chromium only
B. Nickel only
C. Cobalt
D. Molybdenum

20. Galavanic (or) electrolytic corrosion occurs in:

A. Between amalgam and composite restoration
B. Between similar metal
C. Between amalgam and metal restoration
D. All

21. Which of the properties of an alloy decreases on age hardening?

A. Strength
B. Ductility
C. Hardness
D. Proportional limit

22. Zinc oxide eugenol becomes hard by formation of:

A. Zinc eugenolate
B. By evaporation of eugenol
C. By evaporation of hydrogen
D. By formation of water by product

23. A cool glass slab is used in mixing zinc phosphate cement:

A. To increase working time
B. To increase setting time
C. To decrease setting time
D. To decrease strength

24. The alloy that exhibits the shape-memory effect is:

A. Chrome-cobalt alloy
B. Nickel-titanium alloy
C. Stainless steel
D. Beta-titanium

25. Wits appraisal (Ao-Bo) represents:

A. Mandibular and maxillary anterior posterior relation
B. Mandibular and maxillary sagittal relationship
C. Mandibular and maxillary vertical relationship
D. All of the above

26. The anchorage utilized by quad helix is:

A. Simple
B. Reinforce
C. Extraoral
D. Reciprocal

27. Maximum amount of incisor retraction achieved is:

A. 7 mm
B. 16 mm
C. 9 mm
D. 26 mm

28. An example of fixed functional appliance is:

A. Activator
B. Bionator
C. Frankel
D. Herbst

29. When a disease spreads rapidly from one person to another, it is known as:

A. Pandemic
B. Endemic
C. Epidemic
D. Sporadic

30. NaF is applied:

A. Once daily
B. Once in two days
C. Twice in a week
D. Once a week

31. What is the dosage of fluoride for a 2-3 years old child residing in an area with fluoride conc. < 3 ppm?

A. 1.4 mg
B. 0 mg
C. 1 mg
D. 2 mg

32. Deflouridating material is:

A. Duraphat
B. Brudevold's solution
C. Fluorprotector
D. Alumina

33. Gingival index is:

A. Sillness and loe
B. Loe and sillness
C. Green and vermillion
D. Russel

34. Which of the following conditions require prophylactic antibiotic coverage?

A. Rheumatic heart disease
B. Mitral valve disease
C. Mitral regurgitation
D. Aortic valve disease

35. Group of viruses that inhabit the alimentary tract of children below 2 years age:

A. Coxsackie virus
B. Paramyxovirus
C. Varicella zoster virus
D. Herpes simplex virus

36. Emphysema is collection of:

A. Pus
B. Air
C. Liquid
D. Blood

37. Syndrome associated with ear infection:

A. Ramsay hunt syndrome
B. Grimspan syndrome
C. Eagle's syndrome
D. Plummer-Vinson syndrome

38. Calcification of deciduous incisors is completed at:

A. 1 ½ month
B. 2 months
C. 5 months
D. 4 months

39. Green stains on the teeth in children are due to:

A. Chromogenic bacteria
B. Nasmyth's membrane
C. Amalgam staining
D. Internal resorption

40. Type of fear of child on his first dental visit is:

A. Fear of unknown
B. Fear of dentist
C. Fear of pain
D. Fear of injection

41. When blood is present at the end of paper point it indicates?

A. Haematoma formation
B. Incomplete removal of pulp
C. Periapical infection
D. Perforation of root

42. Working length of a root canal is:
A. Equal to radiographic length
B. 0.3 mm short of radiographic length
C. 0.3 mm more than radiographic length
D. Not related to radiographic length

43. Instrument no. 40 represents:
A. Diameter at D1
B. Diameter at D2
C. Diameter at D1 + D2
D. Diameter at D2-D1

44. K. File differs from reamer in:
A. Flexibility and cutting efficiency
B. Manufacture and design
C. Amount of force application
D. Material use

45. H.file is used to:
A. Locate the canal orifice
B. Flare the root canal
C. For irrigation of root canal
D. All of the above

46. Minimum concentration of chlorhexidine present in mouth wash is:
A. 0.12 % B. 0.2 %
C. 0.4 % D. 0.02 %

47. Which of the following is true about plaque?
A. Visible to the naked eye
B. Without plaque calculus formation does not occur
C. Mechanical irritant to cause gingivitis
D. Without plaque periodontitis may occur

48. Which of the following is contraindicated in ANUG?
A. Chlorhexidine B. Corticosteroids
C. H_2O_2 D. Betadine

49. Which of the following is not a periodontal emergency?
A. Periodontal disease

B. ANUG
C. Pericoronitis
D. Desquamative gingivitis

50. CADIA is:
A. Prognosis of periodontal disease
B. Computer aided densitometric image analysis
C. Periodontal probe
D. None

51. Recently advanced diagnosis of periodontal organism is:
A. Dipslide method
B. Nucleic acid probes
C. Roentzem method
D. None

52. Initial dental caries occur as a:
A. Brown area resistant to explorer tip
B. White chalky area
C. Black spot
D. Red line

53. Initiation of smooth surfaces caries occurs by:
A. Streptococcus mutans
B. Actinomycetes
C. Lactobacillus
D. Velionella

54. The distance between source and object in lateral cephalogram is:
A. 5 feet (or) 60 inches
B. 5.5 feet
C. 6.5 feet
D. 6 feet

55. RPD prime support on:
A. Rest
B. Retention
C. Reciprocal arm
D. Auxillary arm

56. Temporary restorations or crowns which match natural teeth in colour is:
A. Celluloid
B. Porcelain
C. Gold restoration
D. ZOE restoration

Answers

1.	B	2.	B	3.	B	4.	A
5.	C	6.	A	7.	D	8.	A
9.	D	10.	D	11.	D	12.	B
13.	C	14.	C	15.	A	16.	D
17.	A	18.	A	19.	A	20.	C
21.	B	22.	A	23.	A	24.	B
25.	A	26.	D	27.	A	28.	D
29.	C	30.	D	31.	B	32.	D
33.	B	34.	A	35.	A	36.	B
37.	A	38.	D	39.	A	40.	A
41.	B	42.	B	43.	A	44.	B
45.	B	46.	D	47.	B,D	48.	B
49.	D	50.	B	51.	B	52.	B
53.	A	54.	A	55.	A	56.	A

PGI Paper June 2005

1. **Amount of magnification possible with panoramic radiograph may be:**
   A. 5-10% B. 10-15%
   C. 20-25% D. 30-35%

2. **The width of bracket most commonly used are:**
   A. 0.014 and 0.024 B. 0.018 and 0.028
   C. 0.017 and 0.021 D. 0.010 and 0.020

3. **A child presents with an injury that left the crown displaced lingually and root facially. What should be done?**
   A. Extraction B. Leave it
   C. Observe D. None

4. **Amount of salt in salt fluoridation is:**
   A. 5 mg of potassium iodine
   B. 10 mg of potassium iodide
   C. 70 mg of sodium fluoride
   D. 80 mg of sodium fluoride

5. **Muscle arising above and below the alveolar process is supplied by which motor nerve?**
   A. Inferior alveolar nerve
   B. Greater palatine nerve
   C. Masseteric nerve
   D. Lower buccal branch of facial nerve

6. **Film badge worn by X-ray technician should be changed:**
   A. Every one month
   B. Every two months
   C. Every three months
   D. Every four months

7. **A swelling behind the ear suggest fracture of:**
   A. Zygomatic complex
   B. Condylar fracture
   C. Temporal bone
   D. Orbital floor fracture

8. **Masseter is supplied by which sensory nerve?**
   A. Olfactory nerve
   B. Maxillary nerve
   C. Mandibular nerve
   D. Ophthalmic nerve

9. **Which point is not seen on mandible?**
   A. Porion
   B. Gnathion
   C. Submentale
   D. Pogonion

10. **Line of treatment of unfavourable fracture of angle of mandible is**
    A. Miniplates with screws
    B. Not treatment, observe
    C. Cap splint fixation
    D. Circumferential wiring

11. **Vertical section of ramus of mandible is done in which condition?**
    A. Maxillary prognathism
    B. Mandibular protrusion
    C. Mandibular retrusion
    D. Maxillary retrognathism

12. **Xerostomia is not seen in**
    A. Vitamin 'C' chewing
    B. Surgical removal of gland
    C. Post-radiation
    D. Sjögren's syndrome

13. **Major connector is placed at what distance from gingival?**
    A. 4-6 mm
    B. 2-4 mm
    C. 6-8 mm
    D. 1-2 mm

14. **Flush terminal plane is drawn joining the distal surface of:**
    A. Permanent 1st molars
    B. 1st deciduous molars
    C. Deciduous 2nd molars
    D. Permanent 2nd molars

15. The concentration of stannous fluoride is:

A. 8% SnF B. 3% SnF
C. 2% SnF D. 1.23% SnF

16. A double blind study refers to:

A. Giving drug to control group and place to population
B. Individual and control does not know identity of study
C. Drug and placebo given to population
D. Giving drug to population and placebo to control group

17. WHO day is:

A. 8th May B. 7th April
C. 7th May D. 8th May

18. Which is the enzyme that prevents the adhesion of actinomyces to adhere to the tooth structure?

A. Xanthine oxidase B. Myeloperoxidase
C. Enolase D. Glucosyl transferase

19. Specific oral lesion seen in infectious mononucleosis is:

A. Multiple bruises
B. Haemorrhagic palatal petechiae
C. Palatal
D. Multiple draining ulcers

20. In β-thalassemia the RBC are:

A. Microcytic, hypochromic
B. Normocytic, normochromic
C. Macrocytic, hypochromic
D. Normocytic, hypochromic

21. Which is not a polysaccharide sugar?

A. Maltose B. Lactose
C. Galactose D. Sucrose

22. Bonwill's equilateral triangle the apex of triangle is located at:

A. At the anteriormost part of lower central incisor
B. At the prominent part of chin upper central
C. The anterior part of incisive papilla
D. At the anteriormost part of incisor

23. In peck and peck analysis the mesiodistal dimension of which teeth is taken into consideration?

A. Upper incisors B. Lower incisors
C. Canines D. Premolars

24. Intraepithelial bullae that peels off on application of pressure is seen in:

A. Pemphigus
B. Leukoedema
C. Lichen planus
D. Erythema multiforme

25. The EDTA used as anticlotting agent when blood:

A. Not an anticoagulant
B. When it is to be tested in test tube
C. Be transfused immediately through IV

26. Greening of porcelain metal interface is due to:

A. Copper
B. Tin
C. Oxygen
D. Silver

27. The tooth which undergoes relapse most commonly is:

A. Derotated teeth
B. Teeth involved during space closure
C. Retroclined teeth
D. Intruded teeth

28. The anatomical cause of mouth breathing is:

A. Enlarged tonsils
B. Enlarged adenoids and tonsils
C. Enlarged adenoids
D. Short upper lip

29. Trephination is the process which is used to:

A. Surgical procedure to remove teeth
B. Rescue the pus entrapped between two cortical plates
C. It is a type of root canal treatment
D. All of the above

30. The classification of malocclusion in mixed dentition state depends on:

A. Deciduous 1st molar relation
B. Canine relation
C. Deciduous 2nd relation
D. Angle's classification

31. In herpes zoster the infection is characterized as:

A. Bilateral lesions
B. Desquamation lesions
C. Unilateral lesions
D. Bizarre pattern

32. The severe gnawing pain is seen in:

A. Pemphigus
B. Desquamative gingivitis
C. PHGS
D. ANUG

33. The increase in caries incidence is seen when the salivary flow is:

A. < 8 ml/min B. < 6 ml/min
C. < 5 ml/min D. < 7 ml/min

34. Baume spaces are seen between:

A. Between upper lateral and canine
B. Upper canine and first molar, lower lateral and canine
C. Between lower lateral and canine
D. Upper lateral and canine, lower canine and first molar

35. In rampant caries, which tooth is mostly affected?

A. Maxillary first molars
B. Mandibular incisors
C. Maxillary incisors
D. Mandibular first molars

36. Most sensitive cells to X-rays are:

A. Neurons
B. Germ cells of reproductive system
C. Cells of skin
D. Muscles

37. Trauma to the nerve with paraesthesia is called:

A. Neurotmesis B. Axonotmesis
C. Neuropraxia D. None

38. The free gingival graft is placed:

A. Bone B. On the periosteum
C. Gingiva D. Periodontal pocket

39. The factors which does not determine occlusal disturbances is:

A. TMJ pain B. Pain during chewing
C. Mobility of teeth D. Wear facets

40. The last solution in root canal treatment before dressing is:

A. Hydrogen peroxide
B. Sodium hypochloride
C. Normal saline
D. EDTA

41. At pH 4.5, the:

A. Dissolution of hydroxyapatite occurs
B. Dissolution of hydroxyapatite decreases

C. Dissolution of fluorapatite occurs
D. Dissolution of fluorapatite increases

42. The sugar that causes least decrease in pH is:
A. Inulin B. Glucose
C. Lactose D. Maltose

43. The percussion test is used to determine:
A. Vitality of pulp B. Periodontal disease
C. Periapical lesion

44. In construction of immediate denture, anterior teeth that are extracted:
A. After posterior teeth
B. After denture construction
C. In first appointment
D. Before construction of denture

45. In patients where long produce are not recommended and require fixed prosthesis the mode of treatment is:
A. Transitional denture
B. Transitional RPD
C. Interim denture
D. Treatment denture

46. Sign of irreversible pulp, it is:
A. Pain with cold water
B. Dull pain
C. Spontaneous pain
D. All of the above

47. Traumatic occlusion will have all *except*:
A. Wear facets
B. Infrabony pockets
C. Migration of teeth
D. Widening of periodontal ligament

48. The amount of 1:200,00 epinephrine that can be given safely to an average adult is:
A. 7mg/kg body wt B. 10 mg/kg body wt
C. 12 mg/kg body wt D. 14 mg/kg body wt

49. Filler particles in composite resin is:
A. Quartz B. Colloidal silica
C. Aluminium

Answers

1.	C	2.	B	3.	C	4.	A
5.	D	6.	A	7.	B	8.	B
9.	A	10.	A	11.	C	12.	A
13.	C	14.	C	15.	A	16.	B
17.	B	18.	B	19.	B	20.	A
21.	C	22.	A	23.	B	24.	A
25.	A	26.	A	27.	A	28.	D
29.	B	30.	C	31.	C	32.	D
33.	C	34.	D	35.	C	36.	B
37.	C	38.	A	39.	C	40.	B
41.	A	42.	A	43.	B	44.	B
45.	B	46.	D	47.	B	48.	A
49.	A						

PGI Paper

2004

1. **All of the following are anatomically related to mandibular nerve *except*:**
   A. Inferior alveolar nerve
   B. Lingual nerve
   C. Chorda tympani nerve
   D. Auriculotemporal nerve

2. **Deltoid ligament is seen in:**
   A. Shoulder B. Knee
   C. Hip D. Ankle

3. **Which of the following muscles separates the carotid triangle from the submandibular triangle?**
   A. Superior belly of the omohyoid
   B. Sternothyroid
   C. Posterior belly of the digastric
   D. Anterior belly of the digastric

4. **The numbers of essential amino acids are:**
   A. 8 B. 6
   C. 12 D. 16

5. **Semi-essential amino acids are:**
   A. Proline and tyrosine
   B. Ornithine and citrulline
   C. Valine only
   D. Arginine and histidine

6. **Purine bases are:**
   A. Adenine, Guanine
   B. Cytosine, Guanine
   C. Adenine, Cytosine
   D. Cytosine, Thymine, Uracil

7. Following would give biuret test positive:

A. Lipids B. Glycine
C. Carbohydrates D. Proteins

8. In hema group, Fe is present as:

A. Ferric ion B. Ferrous in Hb end Fe^{+++} in Hb
C. Ferrous form D. None of the above

9. Each haemoglobin molecule contains:

A. 2 heme group + 2 globin chains
B. 1 heme group + 1 globin chains
C. 4 heme group + 4 globin chains
D. 4 heme group + 2 globin chains

10. The average mesiodistal diameter of the crown is:

A. 8 mm B. 10 mm
C. 9 mm D. 11 mm

11. The fifth cusp on the crown of the first maxillary molar is related to which cusp?

A. Mesiobuccal B. Mesiolingual
C. Distolingual D. None of the above

12. A heart-shaped outline from the occlusal aspect is seen in:

A. Mandibular first molar
B. Maxillary first molar
C. Maxillary second molar
D. Mandibular second molar

13. From the occlusal aspect the mandibular first molar is:

A. Hexagonal B. Trapezoidal
C. Rhomboidal D. Rectangular

14. The root completion of the mandibular second molar takes place by:

A. 6-7 years B. 9-10 years
C. 12-13 years D. 14-15 years

15. The tooth which usually has the largest pulp chamber in the mouth is the:

A. Maxillary canine
B. Maxillary central incisor
C. Mandibular first molar
D. Maxillary first molar

16. **The most important additive to the powder of poly-carboxylate cement is:**
   A. Stannous oxide B. Magnesium oxide
   C. Aluminium oxide D. Stannous flouride

17. **The average life of silicate cement restoration is:**
   A. 2 years B. 4 years
   C. 6 years D. 8 years

18. **The principal constituent of set silicate cement matrix is:**
   A. Hydrated aluminium phosphate with calcium fluoride
   B. Hydrated aluminium phosphate crystals, CaF2 aluminosilicate gel
   C. Hydrated aluminosilicate gel
   D. Hydrated aluminium phosphate

19. **Secondary caries found to be less when cavity restoration is done with:**
   A. Zinc phosphate cement
   B. Silver amalgam
   C. Silicate cement
   D. Gold inlays

20. **The powder of glass ionomer cement is:**
   A. Aluminosilicate glass
   B. Aluminosilicate with $Al_2O_4^-$ and silica oxide
   C. Hydrated aluminium phosphate with silica particles
   D. Aluminosilicate glass with fluoride fluxes

21. **All of the following cements has anticariogenic property *except*:**
   A. Glass ionomer cement
   B. Zinc silicophosphate
   C. Polycarboxylate cement
   D. Silicate cement

22. **The cavity varnish applied reduces postoperative sensitivity in amalgam restoration by:**
   A. By altering the chemical composition of restoration materials
   B. Minimize marginal leakage around restoration
   C. By preventing penetration of corrosion products into the dentinal tubules
   D. Decreasing conduction of heat to pulp

23. Stage recognised in the firing of dental porcelain given below. Which of the state is not correct?

A. Low bisque B. Medium bisque
C. Cold stage bisque D. High bisque

24. In low bisque stage of firing, which of the following statement is not correct?

A. Lacks complete cohesion
B. The fired article exhibits rigidity but is porous
C. Negligible amount of firing shrinkage is present
D. Exhibits smoother surface

25. The process of changing the rubber base product or liquid polymer, to a rubber like material is generally known as:

A. Vulcanization B. Chain lengthening
C. Condensation D. Boiling

26. Linear contraction of elastomeric impression with passage of time is highest in:

A. Polyether B. Condensation silicone
C. Polysulphide D. Addition silicone

27. Thickness of lead apron to prevent radiation:

A. 1 mm B. 0.5 mm
C. 7 mm D. 3 mm

28. The atom which scatters X-rays more is:

A. Lead B. Mercury
C. Carbon D. Hydrogen

29. The following is not an ionizing radiation:

A. CT B. USG
C. MRI D. All are ionising

30. Not a source of neutrons:

A. Linear accelerator B. Betatron
C. Cyclotron D. All of the above

31. Used in both teletherapy and brachytherapy:

A. Iridium B. Pallidium
C. Radium D. Cobalt

32. Radioactivity was discovered by Becqueral in:

A. 1901 B. 1796
C. 1896 D. 1996

33. Medusa lock appearance in X-ray is seen in:

A. Hookworm
B. Tapeworm
C. Ascaris and tapeworm
D. Ascariasis

34. Shortest acting local anesthetic:

A. 2-chloroprocaine
B. Dibucaine
C. Procaine
D. Tetracaine

35. Best analgesic is:

A. Trilene
B. Halothane
C. Ether
D. Chloroform

36. Site of action of anesthetic muscle relaxant is:

A. Central
B. Myoneural junction
C. Red nucleus
D. Ascending reticular activating system

37. Drugs which does not cross blood brain barrier:

A. Hyoscine
B. Physostigmine
C. Atropine
D. Neostigmine

38. Adrenaline is contraindicated during .... anesthesia.

A. Trilene
B. Ether
C. Halothane
D. Thiopentone

39. Liquefactive necrosis is common in:

A. Liver
B. GIT
C. Heart
D. Brain

40. Which is not a complication of blood transfusion?

A. DIC
B. Hyperthermiac
C. Tetany
D. Hyperkalemia

41. Autoimmune haemolytic anemia is seen in:

A. ALL
B. AML
C. CLL
D. CML

42. All are true of Hodgkin's lymphoma *except*:

A. Osteolytic metastasis
B. Contiguous spread
C. Females less common
D. Bimodal age pattern

43. Streptococci are morphologically arranged in:

A. Pairs B. Chains
C. Clusters D. None of the above

44. Metachromatic granules or Babes-Ernst granules are characteristic of:

A. Neisseria B. Clostridia
C. Corynebacterium D. Pneumococci

45. The characteristic morphological arrangement of corynebacterium is in:

A. Cuneiform B. Stellate form
C. Drumstick pairs D. Chains

46. The clinical manifestations of tetanus are due to:

A. Neurolysin
B. Haemolysin
C. Tetanolysin
D. Tetanospasmin

47. Pulpotomy is indicated if:

A. When pulp does not respond to vitality test
B. When pulp is grossly infected
C. Root apex is not completely developed
D. When pulp exposure has occurred for more than 48 hours

48. The seepage into the canal can be decreased by:

A. Sealing the canal with zinc phosphate
B. Sealing the canal with formocresol dressing
C. Sealing the canal with GIC
D. Sealing the canal with zinc-iodine solution

49. Splinting of fracture teeth can be done by:

A. Solid facial bonding of crown of teeth adjacent to each other
B. Acid etch technique, cementation of bonded resin with ligation
C. Acid etch technique, cementation of plastic orthobrackets in composite
D. All of the above

50. Splint should be removed in:

A. 1 week B. 2 weeks
C. 3-6 weeks D. 2 months

51. Which of the following is wrong?

Root repair following treatment of a fracture occurs by:

A. Calcified tissue
B. Fibrous tissue
C. Granulomatous tissue
D. Connective tissue

52. In concussion:

A. Tooth is loose and displaced
B. Tooth has abnormal motility but is not displaced
C. Tooth is sensitive to percussion but is not displaced
D. All of the above

53. If a tooth gets a blow parallel to its long axis, it is likely to get:

A. Intruded
B. Extruded
C. Avulsed
D. Luxated

54. Haemorrhage is the gingival sulcus indicates:

A. Fracture of bone
B. Tooth displacement
C. Trauma to gingiva
D. Torn gingiva

55. Thermal and electrical tests indicates:

A. Sensitivity tests for nerve function
B. Absence of blood circulation within the pulp
C. Presence of blood circulation within the pulp
D. None of the above

56. Thiersch's graft is a:

A. Pedicle graft
B. Partial thickness skin graft
C. Pinch skin graft
D. Small full thickness skin graft

57. Today the most common cause of a true aneurysm is:

A. Syphilitic
B. Atherosclerosis
C. Congenital
D. A gunshot wound

58. An overdose of heparin is treated by:

A. Prostigmine
B. Prostaglandins
C. Protamine sulphate
D. Phenindione

59. A green stick fracture:
A. Is a fatigue fracture
B. Occurs chiefly in the elderly
C. Is a spiral fracture of tubular bone
D. Is a fracture where part of the cortex is intact and part is crumpled or cracked

60. A giant cell tumour of bone will be shown on X-ray:
A. Codman's triangle
B. A soap-bubble appearance
C. Sun-ray spicules
D. Spotty calcification

61. Dead bone is recognised on X-ray because:
A. It is more radiopaque
B. It is more radiolucent than normal
C. It has a soap-bubble appearance
D. Osteophytes grown out from it

62. Muscles of mastication are derivatives of:
A. 1st arch
B. 2nd arch
C. 3rd arch
D. 6th arch

63. Anterior 2/3rd of the tongue is formed from:
A. Hypobranchial eminence
B. Lateral lingual swellings and tuberculum impar
C. Tuberculum impar
D. Copula lateral lingual swellings

64. Warfarin impairs the conversion of vitamin-K to its active form thereby affecting clotting factors:
A. IX, XII, X, VII
B. I, II, IX, X
C. II, VII, IX, X
D. II, III, X, IX

65. The variant of ameloblastoma which has the best prognosis is:
A. Plexiform
B. Desmoplastic
C. Follicular
D. Unicystic

66. Odontogenic keratocysts has a predilection for occurring in the:
A. 3-4th decade and 7th decade
B. 2-3rd decade and 5th decade
C. 2-3rd decade and 6th decade
D. 3-4th decade and 6th decade

67. The odontogenic tumor which is the most common is?
A. Ameloblastoma
B. Enameloma
C. Ameloblastic fibroma
D. Odontoma

68. Relative to a heterogeneous population, the incidence of malocclusion in a homogeneous population generally is:
A. Slightly higher
B. Lower
C. About the same
D. Significantly higher

69. Which of the following antibiotics is most frequently associated with pseudomembranous colitis?
A. Clindamycin
B. Cephalosporins
C. Penicillin G
D. Ampicillin

70. Which of the following is correct about treatment of facial nerve palsy?
A. In initial stages includes systemic corticosteroid therapy
B. Involves non-steroidal anti-inflammatory drugs only
C. Is carried out by oral anti histaminics
D. Involves resection of extracranial portion of nerve

71. Chronic respiratory infection, steatorrhea and disturbance in electrolyte balance is in:
A. Hepatitis
B. Cystic fibrosis
C. Amoebiasis
D. Colon carcinoma

72. Fracture of 8-year-old circumandibular at symphysis is mostly reduced by:
A. Risdon wiring
B. Erich arch bar
C. No treatment
D. Cap splint circumandibular wiring

73. Vitamin B_{12} acts as coenzyme to which one of the following enzymes?
A. Glycogen synthase
B. Hormocysteine methyl transferase
C. Isocitrate dehydrogenase
D. G-6-P dehydrogenase

74. Best view of space of TMJ is by:
A. Transcranial view
B. Transorbital view
C. Lateral oblique
D. Transpharyngeal view

75. A fracture of eye by a ping pong ball is:

A. Orbital fracture B. Blow in fracture
C. Blow out fracture D. Compound fracture

76. After CPR acidosis can be heart counteracted by:

A. Oxygen
B. IV bicarbonate solution
C. Ringer lactate
D. All of the above

77. Lateral pharyngeal space is not connected directly by:

A. Submandibular space
B. Sublingual space
C. Buccal space
D. Parapharyngeal space

78. Which of them is not rigid osteosynthetic fixation?

A. Wiring B. Microplating
C. Osteosynthesis D. Screw plating

79. The supervision of a child's development of occlusion is most critical at ages:

A. 7-10 years B. 14-17 years
C. 11-14 years D. 3-6 years

80. Hilton's method deals with:

A. Biopsy removal
B. Preanesthetic check-up
C. Drainage of an abscess
D. Decompression of a cyst

81. The plane of occlusion is measured from the most prominent cusp of lower:

A. First permanent molar to lower central incisors
B. First permanent molar to lower canine
C. Second permanent molar to lower canine
D. Second permanent molar to lower central incisors

82. The distal surface of the distobuccal cusp of upper first permanent molar contacts the mesial surface of mesiobuccal cusp of lower:

A. First permanent premolar
B. First permanent molar
C. Second permanent premolar
D. Second permanent molar

83. The mesiolingual cusp of upper first permanent molar seats in the central fossa of the lower:

A. First permanent molar
B. Second permanent molar
C. First permanent premolar
D. Second permanent premolar

84. Examination for prematurely lose teeth, extracted or congenitally missing teeth can be best done with the help of:

A. Orthopantomograph
B. Intraoral periapical radiographs
C. Facial photograph
D. Study models

85. A radiopaque line is observed is the dentin underlying a three-month-old class-II amalgam restoration. Which of the following bases was used in this restoration?

A. Zinc oxide eugenol
B. Zinc phosphate cement
C. Calcium hydroxide
D. Zinc oxide eugenol and formocresol

86. When the tooth is rotated on its long axis, the condition is known as:

A. Perversion
B. Axiversion
C. Torsiversion
D. Transposition

87. When a tooth is impacted, the condition is known as:

A. Transposition
B. Axiversion
C. Torsiversion
D. Perversion

88. Class-I canine relationship means that:

A. The lower canine is placed forward to the upper canine and there is no overlapping
B. Upper canine is in edge to edge contacts with lower canine
C. Distal incline of upper canine contacts the mesial incline of lower canine
D. Mesial incline of the upper canine overlaps the distal incline of the lower canine

89. The first community water fluoridation was carried out in:

A. 1945, Oak Park
B. 1945, Evanston

C. 1945, Grand Rapids
D. 1945, Colorado

90. When the distal incline of upper canine contacts the mesial incline of lower canine, the canine relationship is termed as:

A. Class I B. Class II
C. Class III D. Class IV

91. Angle's classification is based on which tooth as stable landmark and guideline for occlusion?

A. Maxillary first permanent molar
B. Maxillary second permanent molar
C. Mandibular first permanent molar
D. Mandibular second permanent molar

92. Malocclusion is classified according to Angle considering the irregularity of teeth in the:

A. Vertical plane
B. Transverse plane
C. Lateral direction
D. Anteroposterior plane

93. The absorbed fluoride ions are mainly eliminated by the:

A. Kidney B. Intestines
C. Lungs D. Liver

94. Topical preparation of acidulated phosphate fluoride:

A. 1.25% of F ions B. 1.23% of F ions
C. 1.37% of F ions D. 2% of F ions

95. Rampant caries is most commonly caused by:

A. Lack of calcium intake
B. Improper brushing technique
C. Excessive bottle feeding
D. Excessive sweet intake

96. Chlorohexidine, a chemotherapeutic agent used for treating plaque, calculi and gingivitis is a:

A. Antibiotics
B. Quaternary ammonium compounds
C. Bis-guanide
D. Organic compound

97. The human plasma lipoprotein containing the highest percentage of triacylglycerol by weight is:

A. HDL
B. Chylomicrons
C. LDL
D. VLDL

98. For optimum results topical fluoride application should be administered:

A. Prophylactic odontomy
B. Every three months
C. Topical fluoride restoration
D. All of the above

99. For optimum results topical fluoride application should be administered:

A. Every three months
B. Every twelve months
C. Every six months
D. Every eighteen months

100. To achieve caries reduction diet modification must be directed towards:

A. Foods that will buffer saliva
B. High calcium and vitamin intake
C. Reduction of carbohydrate intake
D. Detergent foods

Answers

1.	C	2.	D	3.	C	4.	A
5.	D	6.	A	7.	D	8.	C
9.	C	10.	B	11.	B	12.	C
13.	A	14.	D	15.	A	16.	D
17.	B	18.	B	19.	C	20.	D
21.	C	22.	B	23.	C	24.	D
25.	A	26.	B	27.	B	28.	D
29.	D	30.	B	31.	A	32.	C
33.	D	34.	A	35.	C	36.	B
37.	D	38.	C	39.	D	40.	B
41.	C	42.	A	43.	B	44.	C
45.	A	46.	D	47.	C	48.	D
49.	D	50.	C	51.	A	52.	C
53.	D	54.	B	55.	A	56.	B
57.	B	58.	C	59.	D	60.	B
61.	A	62.	A	63.	B	64.	C
65.	D	66.	C	67.	D	68.	B
69.	A	70.	A	71.	B	72.	D
73.	B	74.	D	75.	C	76.	B
77.	C	78.	A	79.	A	80.	C
81.	D	82.	D	83.	A	84.	A
85.	C	86.	B	87.	D	88.	D
89.	C	90.	B	91.	A	92.	D
93.	A	94.	B	95.	C	96.	C
97.	B	98.	A	99.	C	100.	C

PGI Paper May and Nov. 2003

1. **The primate spaces are related to the position of the diastema that are:**
   A. Distal to the maxillary primary canines and mesial to the mandibular primary canines
   B. Mesial to the maxillary primary canines and distal to the mandibular primary canines
   C. Distal to the maxillary and mandibular primary canines
   D. Mesial to the maxillary and mandibular primary canines

2. **Spacing in anterior teeth in deciduous dentition:**
   A. Common and desirable
   B. Uncommon and undesirable
   C. Common and undesirable
   D. Uncommon

3. **A 9 years old child came to the dental clinic with spacing in anterior teeth. The line of treatment is:**
   A. Fixed appliance
   B. Removable appliance
   C. Inclined plane
   D. No treatment, observation of the patient

4. **Breathing is termed anatomic breathing if:**
   A. Short upper lip
   B. Enlarged adenoid
   C. Enlarged tonsil
   D. Both A and B

5. **ANB angle refers to:**
   A. Skeletal relation
   B. Transverse discrepancy
   C. Dental malocclusion
   D. None of the above

6. **Which of the following is anti-flux?**
   A. Borax
   B. Boric acid
   C. Carbonate
   D. Graphite

7. **The first tissue to react when orthodontic forces are applied in:**
   A. PDL
   B. Cementum
   C. Dentine
   D. Alveolar bone

8. **Anterior inclined plane should not be used for prolonged period because it causes:**
   A. Growth discrepancy
   B. Supra eruption of posterior teeth
   C. Deep bite
   D. Cross bite

9. **Prolonged retention is usually needed in:**
   A. Diastema
   B. Mild crowding
   C. Anterior cross bite
   D. Deep bite

10. **Enlow's 'V' principle of growth of found in:**
   A. Cranial base
   B. Maxilla and mandible
   C. Maxilla only
   D. None of the above

11. **Oral and nasal capsule of functional growth related to:**
   A. Periosteal matrix
   B. Sutural matrix
   C. Capsular matrix
   D. None of the above

12. **In Sicher's theory, sutures act as:**
   A. Has independent growth potential
   B. Dependent on cranial base
   C. Used for growth adjustment
   D. None of the above

13. **Best time to see a 3 years old child in the dental office:**
   A. Early in the morning
   B. Just before lunch
   C. Just after lunch
   D. Anytime

14. N_2O more than 30-40% causes:

A. Diffusion hypoxia B. Anoxia
C. Amnesia D. Ataxia

15. The pulp horn that is most likely to be exposed during cavity preparation on deciduous molars is:

A. Mesiobuccal of first molar
B. Distobuccal of first molar
C. Mesiobuccal of second molar
D. Distobuccal of second molar

16. In formocresol, ratio of formalin to cresol:

A. 3 : 2 B. 2 : 3
C. 1 : 2 D. 2 : 1

17. Face Bow measures relationship of maxilla to:

A. Opening and closing axis
B. Mandible
C. Zygomatic bone
D. None of the above

18. When notching condylar guidance, incisal pin should be:

A. In contact with guidance table
B. Out of contact
C. Not at all related
D. None of the above

19. Over dentures used to:

A. Preserve alveolar bone
B. Maintain proprioception from periodontal ligament
C. Retention
D. All of the above

20. Number of swallowing per day:

A. 300 B. 400
C. 1500 D. 600

21. Intra enamel depth preparation in porcelain laminate veneer:

A. 0.5 mm B. 0.75 mm
C. 1 mm D. 2 mm

22. Which of the following is not indicated for maxillary anterior pontic?

A. Ridge lap

B. Modified ridge lap
C. Hygienic
D. Ovate

23. Impurities in casting is removed by:
A. Annealing
B. Degassing
C. Pickling
D. Conditioning

24. RPD is indicated in all *except*:
A. Long edentulous spaces
B. Multiple edentulous spaces
C. Excessive loss of alveolar bone
D. Distal abutment loss

25. If severe bony undercut exists, best treatment:
A. Remove both undercuts so that no undercuts exists
B. Remove undercut on one side
C. Nothing but do only alveolar ridge contouring
D. None of the above

26. When a forcep is to be utilized for removal of a tooth, the first direction for the force to be applied is:
A. Occlusally
B. Buccally
C. Lingually
D. Apically

27. Inferior alveolar nerve block is given in:
A. Retromolar area
B. Pterygomandibular space
C. Submandibular space
D. Submental space

28. Floating maxilla is found in:
A. LeFort I or guerin fractures
B. LeFort II or pyramidal fractures
C. Cranimandibular dysjunction
D. All of the above

29. Diplopia after fracture results from entrapment of:
A. Inferior rectus
B. Inferior oblique
C. Lateral rectus
D. Superior oblique

30. For an 8-year-old child with TMJ ankylosis, the treatment of choice is:
A. Gap arthroplasty
B. Condylectomy
C. Gap arthroplasty with costochondral grafting
D. Treatment not required

31. Odontogenic tumors just 1cm away from lower border:

A. Enbloc resection
B. Hemimandibulectomy
C. Ennucleation
D. None

32. Palatal abscess most commonly results from infection of:

A. Maxillary centrals
B. Maxillary laterals
C. Maxillary canine
D. Maxillary premolars

33. The incision for drainage in Ludwig's Angina extends:

A. Upto the neck
B. To the angle of mandible
C. Floor of the mouth
D. All of the above

34. Pericoronitis is seen in relation to:

A. Impacted third molars only
B. Around incompletely erupted crowns
C. Completely erupted crowns only
D. None of the above

35. After extraction of upper central incisor, patient develops ophthalmoplegia, meningitis, and lateral rectus paralysis. The diagnosis is:

A. Cavernous sinus thrombosis
B. Not related
C. Cellulitis
D. Ludwig's angina

36. Melanoma is:

A. Benign tumor of skin and mucous membrane
B. Malignant tumor of skin and mucous membrane
C. Malignant tumor of melanophores
D. Benign tumor of melanophores

37. Compound odontoma shows

A. Mixed tissue of dental origin with no resemblance to tooth structure
B. Numerous tooth like structure with denticles commonly found in maxillary lateral incisors

C. Haphazardly arranged calcified mass
D. All of the above

38. Least cariogenic among these:
A. Raw starch
B. Cooked starch
C. Sucrose
D. Fructose

39. Splitted papule at the corner of mouth:
A. Recurrent herpes labialis
B. Recurrent herpetic stomatitis
C. Increased vertical dimension
D. Secondary syphilis

40. Acute herpetic gingivostomatitis:
A. Occur in children and young adults
B. Occur only in young children
C. Occur in only adults
D. All of the above

41. Quantity of current can be increased by:
A. Increased milliampere
B. Increased time
C. Increased tube current
D. All of the above

42. An incipient carious lesion on an inter proximal surface is usually located:
A. At the contact area
B. Facial to contact area
C. Gingival to contact area
D. Lingual to contact area

43. Sandwich technique consists of:
A. GIC and composite
B. Amalgam and GIC
C. Amalgam and composite
D. None of the above

44. The most retentive type of pin is:
A. Cemented pin
B. Self threading pin
C. Friction locked pin
D. Amalgam pins

45. **Difference between class II amalgam and cast restoration is:**
   A. Bevels
   B. Occlusal resistance form
   C. Outline form
   D. Proximal retention

46. **The minimally acceptable restoration for an endodontically treated maxillary first premolar is:**
   A. An onlay
   B. An MOD amalgam
   C. A full cast crown
   D. An occlusal amalgam

47. **Sprue pin is attached to posterior teeth in:**
   A. Cusp tip
   B. Contact area
   C. Marginal ridge
   D. Proximal surface

48. **Fracture tooth is restored with:**
   A. Pin retained amalgam
   B. Cast gold
   C. Both
   D. Direct gold

49. **Inlay is:**
   A. Cast gold
   B. Direct gold
   C. Both
   D. None of the above

50. **Sodium nitrite is used as:**
   A. Antiplaque agent
   B. Antirust agent
   C. Desensitizing agent
   D. Bleaching agent

51. **Sequence of endodontic instrumentation:**
   A. Broach – Reamer – File
   B. Reamer – Broach – File
   C. File – Reamer – Broach
   D. File – Broach – Reamer

52. **Initial threshold of the electric test in a traumatic tooth is to:**
   A. Establish baseline of the physical status of the pulp
   B. Is positive in healthy pulp
   C. Is negative in root canal tooth
   D. Is repeated after 30 days

53. Normal depth of gingival sulcus in adult does not exceed:
A. 0.5–1 mm
B. 2–3 mm
C. 1–2 mm
D. 1–3 mm

54. Pellicle is a:
A. Salivary protein
B. Plaque
C. Microorganism
D. Calculus

55. Earliest clinical sign of gingivitis is:
A. Bleeding on probing
B. Change in colour
C. Change in contour
D. Change in size

56. Mc Calls festoon result from:
A. Normal physiological process
B. Tooth brush trauma
C. Occlusal trauma
D. Food lodgement

57. Apostrophe shaped area:
A. Stillman's cleft
B. Mc Calls festoons
C. Gingival sulcus
D. None of the above

58. Ultrasonic scaler can be used in:
A. AIDS patient
B. Asthmatics
C. Root planning
D. Heavy calculus

59. GTR is related to:
A. Gingivoplasty
B. Frenectomy
C. Mucogingival surgery
D. Gingivectomy

60. Which of the following is not a part of epidemiological triad?
A. Agent
B. Host
C. Disease
D. Environment

61. Which of the following is used as a reference for a study through a period of time?

A. Base line data
B. Prevalence
C. Incidence
D. Rate

62. **Repetitive study of individuals over successive period of time for clinical trials:**
A. Cohort study
B. Prospective study
C. Case control study
D. Panel study

63. **The occurrence of dental caries in a population at a given point of time may be termed as:**
A. Incidence
B. Point Prevalence
C. Period Prevalence
D. None of the above

64. **A group of persons given a drug and another is given similar form of inactive counterpart. This is known as:**
A. Single blind study
B. Double blind study
C. Placebo
D. Controlled trial

65. **Russel's periodontal index ranges from:**
A. 0-2
B. 0-4
C. 0-6
D. 0-8

66. **DMF teeth:**
A. 28
B. 32
C. 30
D. 26

67. **Ramjford index is used on:**
A. All permanent teeth
B. Selected six permanent teeth
C. Selected twelve permanent teeth
D. None of the above

68. **In dentrifrices concentration of fluoride is:**
A. 800 ppm
B. 2000 ppm
C. 1000 ppm
D. 600 ppm

69. **In ceramic restoration, which can be used?**
A. 1.23% APF
B. 8% SnF_2
C. 6% SnF_2
D. 2% NaF

70. **In Snyder's test, the colour of medium changes from green to yellow in 72 hours. It indicates:**
A. Highly conducive B. Slightly conducive
C. Medium D. No effect

71. **Best caries activity test used for field study is:**
A. Lactobacillus count test
B. Streptococcus mutans
C. Snyder's test
D. None of the above

72. **Albans test is an example of:**
A. Caries activity test
B. Acid producing test
C. Caries susceptibility test
D. None of the above

73. **Caries activity test is increased in:**
A. Xerostomia
B. Sugar diet
C. Taking much carbohydrate food
D. None of the above

74. **Use of pit and fissure sealants in incipient caries lesion will:**
A. Cut off nutrient supply
B. Death of microbes
C. More nutrient supply
D. None of the above

75. **Rigor mortis results after death is due to:**
A. Failure of acetylcholine to diffuse
B. Failure of ATP supply
C. Failure of breakdown of calcium bridges
D. None of the above

76. **Which is the best material for RPD impression?**
A. Impression plaster
B. Irreversible hydrocolloid
C. Reversible hydrocolloid
D. None of the above

77. **Retarder in zinc oxide eugenol is:**
A. $CaCl_2$
B. Zinc acetate

C. Alcohol
D. Glycerine

78. Cross linking of denture base resins is done to:
A. To increase solubility
B. To decrease crazing
C. To increase abrasion resistance
D. None of the above

79. Impurities in casting is removed by:
A. Annealing B. Degassing
C. Pickling D. Conditioning

80. Which of the following refractory is used to counteract most of the expansion?
A. Quartz B. Cristoballite
C. Tridymite D. Corundum

81. The effect of zinc oxide eugenol on the pulp:
A. Is irritating
B. Encourages pulpal fibrosis
C. Is sedating
D. Has no effect

82. Metastaic calcifications are seen in:
A. Hypoparathyroidism
B. Vitamin D deficiency
C. Hypercalcemia
D. All of the above

83. If patient suffered from exaggerated effect of pharmacological effect:
A. Idiosyncrasy
B. Toxicity
C. Side effect
D. None of the above

84. Highest point on skull:
A. Pterion B. Porion
C. Lambda D. Vertex

85. Origin of maxillary artery:
A. Angle of mandible
B. Neck of condyle
C. Body of mandible
D. Coronoid

86. **Paralysis of upper eyelid is due to paralysis of:**
A. III
B. IV
C. V
D. VII

87. **All of the following muscles are supplied by the mandibular nerve *except*:**
A. Masseter
B. Buccinator
C. Medial pterygoid
D. Anterior belly of digastrics

88. **The ganglion associated with lacrimal gland:**
A. Sphenopalatine
B. Otic ganglion
C. Submandibular
D. Ciliary

89. **Posterior belly of digastrics is attached to:**
A. Styloid
B. Hyoid
C. Mastoid notch
D. Thyroid

90. **All of the following muscles are supplied by accessory nerve *except*:**
A. Palatopharyngeous
B. Stylopharyngeous
C. Palatoglossus
D. Musculus Uvulae

91. **Fat provides ___ of body's calories.**
A. 40%
B. 30%
C. 50%
D. 75%

92. **Daily vitamin A intake:**
A. 1000 I.U.
B. 2000 I.U.
C. 3000 I.U.
D. 4000 I.U.

Answers

1.	B	2.	A	3.	D	4.	A
5.	A	6.	D	7.	A	8.	B
9.	A	10.	B	11.	C	12.	A
13.	A	14.	C	15.	A	16.	C
17.	A	18.	B	19.	D	20.	D
21.	A	22.	C	23.	C	24.	B
25.	A	26.	D	27.	B	28.	A
29.	A	30.	C	31.	A	32.	B
33.	C	34.	B	35.	A	36.	B
37.	B	38.	A	39.	D	40.	A
41.	D	42.	C	43.	B	44.	B
45.	A	46.	A	47.	D	48.	B
49.	A	50.	B	51.	C	52.	D
53.	B	54.	A	55.	A	56.	C
57.	A	58.	D	59.	C	60.	C
61.	B	62.	D	63.	B	64.	C
65.	D	66.	B	67.	B	68.	C
69.	D	70.	B	71.	B	72.	A
73.	A	74.	A	75.	B	76.	B
77.	D	78.	B	79.	C	80.	B
81.	C	82.	C	83.	B	84.	D
85.	B	86.	A	87.	B	88.	A
89.	C	90.	B	91.	B	92.	D

PGI Paper December 2002

1. **Muscle originating from scaphoid fossa is:**
   A. Levator palatine B. Tensor palati
   C. Palatoglossus D. Superior constrictor

2. **Nerve which hooks around Wharton's duct is:**
   A. Mylohyoid nerve
   B. Lingual nerve
   C. Auriculotemporal nerve
   D. Inferior alveolar nerve

3. **Posterior belly of digastrics is derived from:**
   A. First brachial arch
   B. First brachial pouch
   C. Second brachial arch
   D. Second pharyngeal pouch

4. **Calcination hormone from parathyroid gland function in:**
   A. Resorption of bone
   B. Deposition of bone
   C. Reabsorption of Ca^{++} from intestine
   D. Secretion of Ca^{++} in urine

5. **Enzymes involved in degradation of epinephrine:**
   A. Cholinesterases
   B. Anticholinesterases
   C. Carbamoyl O-transferase
   D. Oxidases

6. **Exotoxins are:**
   A. Lipid-polysaccharide complex
   B. Protein compound
   C. Lipoprotein
   D. None

7. **Total protein content of the body is:**
   A. 3-4 g/100 ml B. 6-8 g/100 ml
   C. 11-40 g/100 ml D. 9-10 g/100 ml

8. **Which of the organelles contain DNA?**
   A. Nucleus B. Nucleolus
   C. Golgi D. Ribosome

9. **Heat hardening is the process done at:**
   A. Heating 75°C and slowly cooling to zero degrees
   B. Heating quickly up to 45°C followed by sudden quenching
   C. Heating upto 25°C
   D. Heating at 75°C and then quenching to room temperature

10. **Annealing occurs at:**
    A. 22 °C B. 45 °C
    C. 35 °C D. Solidus temperature

11. **Si-Cu eutectic alloy has a characteristic property of that fusion temp of:**
    A. The resultant alloy is greater
    B. The resultant alloy is lesser
    C. The resultant alloy varies according to the content of Si and Cu
    D. None

12. **Trisodium phosphate in alginate act as:**
    A. Accelerator B. Retarder
    C. Fillers D. Reactor

13. **Setting time of ZOE is best controlled by:**
    A. Adding a drop of eugenol
    B. Adding a drop of water
    C. Cooling the glass slab
    D. Altering ratio of two pastes

14. **Setting time of Mercury is best controlled by:**
    A. Using spherical particles
    B. Lathe cut alloy
    C. Altering Hg-alloy ratio
    D. Triturtion time

15. **Activator in self-cured resins is:**
    A. Lead peroxide B. Tertiary amine
    C. Heat D. Hydrozuinolone

16. Subsurface porosity is due to:
A. Thermal changes
B. Thickness of the resin
C. Lack of temperature
D. Packing past the dough stage

17. Trismus during block anesthesia is a result of:
A. Massive edema
B. Damage to medial pterygoid
C. Damage to lateral pterygoid
D. Damage to IAN

18. Increase in concentration of Nitrous oxide results in:
A. Diffusion hypoxia
B. Bradycardia
C. Respiratory depression
D. All

19. Marsupilization is the procedure done in:
A. Large cyst
B. P.D.cyst
C. Aneurysmal bone cyst
D. Stafne cyst

20. In bone scintigraphy all is gussed *except*:
A. Avascular necrosis
B. Fractures
C. Osteomyelitis
D. None

21. LA with adrenaline is absolutely contraindicated in:
A. First trimester of pregnancy
B. Hyperthyroidism
C. Hemophilia
D. Hypertension

22. Sterilization and disinfection differ from that:
A. Sterilization kills spores
B. Disinfection removes bacteria from surface
C. Sterilization is temporary
D. None

23. Treatment of mucocele on lower lip:
A. Incision
B. Excision

C. Excision with adjacent glands
D. Biopsy

24. In blow out fractures:
A. Enophthalmos
B. Exophithalmous
C. Bulbar haemorrhage
D. None

25. Which of the following are not non-absorbable sutures?
A. Silk
B. Catgut
C. Metal
D. Nylon

26. First group of fibres damaged in periodontitis:
A. Dentogingival fibres
B. Transseptal fibres
C. Oblique fibres
D. Transverse fibres

27. The area which is most prone to infection:
A. Marginal gingiva
B. Sulcular epithelium
C. Interdental col
D. Attached gingiva

28. Group of fibres, which resist the masticatory forces?
A. Dentogingival
B. Transseptal
C. Oblique
D. Horizontal

29. When P.D. probing in gingivitis done, depth is measured:
A. Base of pocket to CEJ
B. Base of pocket to free marginal gingiva
C. Marginal gingiva to CEJ
D. Junctional epithelium to free gingival margin

30. Occlusal guards are given to:
A. Prevent bruxuism
B. To guard the dentition
C. To alter the muscle forces
D. None

31. Multiple teeth are splinted in FPD to:
A. Stabilize the arch form
B. To distribute the load
C. To help PD condition
D. None

32. Crater like punched appearance of gingiva seen in:
A. ANUG
B. Gingivostomatitis
C. Gingivitis
D. Periodontitis

33. Mc Call Festoons are seen in which teeth?
A. Central incisors B. Canine and premolars
C. Lateral incisors D. Molars

34. Clinical signs of gingivitis appear in:
A. Initial gingivitis B. Early gingivitis
C. Late gingivitis D. Advanced gingivitis

35. Water irrigating devices are used:
A. As an adjuct to toothbrush
B. Replaces toothbrush
C. Alters the plaque and increases gingival health
D. Kills the bacteria

36. Gracey Curretes have a characteristic feature that:
A. They are used for area of surface of the tooth
B. They have double cutting edge
C. They can be used anywhere in oral cavity
D. All

37. After PD surgery patient immediate recall is done after:
A. 1 week B. 2 weeks
C. 3 weeks D. 4 weeks

38. Objective of scaling and root planning is:
A. To obtain surface, smooth that of glass
B. To remove cementum
C. To improve gingival health
D. None

39. Pregnancy gingivitis is due to:
A. Due to plaque B. Hormonal changes
C. Due to bacteria D. None

40. ANUG is best visualized:
A. Craters like lesions
B. Severe gingivitis
C. Recession of gingiva
D. None

41. Radiographic changes in periodontitis are:
A. Relation of soft and hard lesions
B. Lamina dura is damaged
C. Pocket depth
D. None

42. Epithelial attachment is derived from:

A. Reduced enamel epithelium
B. Dental papilla
C. Junctional epithelium
D. Dental sac

43. Which of following is a rare occurrence?

A. Enamel meet cementum at a point
B. Enamel overlaps cementum
C. Cementum overlaps enamel
D. Both never meet

44. At what age half of primary and half of permanent teeth are there in the oral cavity?

A. 11 years
B. 9 ½ years
C. 8 ½ years
D. 7 years

45. Bone at forming stage has:

A. Osteoclasts, osteoblast, osteoid
B. Odontoblasts and megakaryocyte
C. Megakaryocytes, osteoblasts, osteoclasts
D. None

46. 8% SnF2 contains how much % of F2?

A. 1%
B. 2%
C. 3%
D. 4%

47. Nalgonda tech is used for:

A. Deflouridation
B. Flouridation
C. Purification of water
D. None

48. In dentifrices concentration of F is:

A. 800 ppm
B. 2000 ppm
C. 1000 ppm
D. 600 ppm

49. Non nutritive sugar is:

A. Mannitol
B. Sacharain
C. Sucrose
D. Maltose

50. Most of the values in data spread along the:

A. Mean
B. Mode
C. Median
D. Arythmatic mean

51. HOME is:

A. Aversive technique

B. Remodelling
C. Psychologic improvement
D. None

52. In diet counselling to reduce caries:
A. Sugar is restricted to meals time
B. Sugar is restricted to one time a day
C. Restricted to only liquid sugars
D. Restricted to fibrous food

53. Concentration of F in 1.23% APF gel is:
A. 22600 ppm B. 12300 ppm
C. 5620 ppm D. None

54. 0.2% NaF mouth rinse is recommended:
A. Once daily B. By weekly
C. Fortnightly D. Twice weekly

55. Parent instructions are given to take care of child's oral health since:
A. First tooth erupts in the oral cavity
B. All the 1 teeth are erupted
C. All 2 teeth are present
D. At the age of 2

56. 0.05% of NaF has concentration of F:
A. 9000 ppm B. 1000 ppm
C. 225 ppm D. 2.50 ppm

57. Repetition of a study in a given group is:
A. Panel study B. Cohort study
C. Group study D. High risk

58. Quebec counter in cause activity best is for:
A. Lactobacillus colonies
B. Streptococcus colonies
C. Areas of bacterial activity
D. None

59. Best method to deflect patient compliance:
A. Changed diet pattern
B. Improvement of oral condition that like bleeding on probing
C. Brushing technique
D. Regular follow ups

60. Caries activity increases in:
A. Xerostomia

B. Sugar diet
C. Taking much carbohydrate food
D. None

61. Minimal dentinal destruction to get evident on the radiograph:

A. 30 microns
B. 40 microns
C. 100 microns
D. 200 microns

62. Bence Jones proteins in urine are found in:

A. Multiple myeloma
B. Fibrous dysplasia
C. Peutz-Jeghers syndrome
D. Paget's disease

63. Fully set $ZnPO_4$ has pH of:

A. 3-4
B. 6-7
C. 8-11
D. 5-4

64. Purpose of cavity preparation is:

A. To receive restorating material
B. To cleanse the caries
C. To remove bacterias
D. None

65. The lip is supported by:

A. Relation of lip edge and facial surfaces of teeth
B. Labial sulcus between teeth and lip
C. Relationship of tongue and teeth
D. None

66. The edge wise technique:

A. Rectangular wire is used
B. Double slots brackets are used
C. Round wire is used
D. Double wire is used

67. In tipping of teeth the center of rotation is at:

A. Apical 1/3
B. At middle 1/3
C. Cervical 1/3
D. Infinity

68. If early surgery of cleft palate is done, the facial profile becomes:

A. Concave
B. Convex
C. Straight
D. Concavoconvex

69. Functional matrix theory was given by:

A. Scot B. Melvin Moss
C. James D. Angle

70. Langer's line on skin:

A. Parallel to collagen fibres
B. To the skin fibres
C. In the region of neck
D. None

71. Which of the following is true statement of remineralization?

A. Saliva is artificial medium for remineralization
B. Large crystals are formed
C. Crystals formed are weak
D. None

72. Exarticulation of teeth means:

A. Intrusion B. Extrusion
C. Subluxation D. Avulsion

73. Anterior mild crowding in mixed dentition. Line of treatment is:

A. Space analysis
B. Disking of canines or accommodate erupting lateral incisor
C. Extraction of all 1st premolars
D. None

74. At birth the following teeth are calcifying:

A. Primary incisors and first 4 molars
B. Primary canines and second 2 molars
C. Permanent canines
D. Permanent 3rd molars

75. Calcification of which tooth starts at birth?

A. Permanent first molar
B. Permanent second molar
C. Permanent canines
D. Permanent third molar

76. PH of Ca (OH)2 is:

A. 8-9 B. 9-11
C. 3-4 D. 6-7

77. Most effective way to control caries at home:

A. Dentifrices
B. Mouth wash
C. Disclosents
D. APF gel

78. Pulp capping and pulpotomy is contraindicated in:

A. Coronal pulp is inflamed
B. Reduction pulp is inflamed
C. Accidental exposure
D. Young permanent teeth

79. Apexification is done with:

A. $Ca(COH)_2$ at the apex
B. $Ca(COH)_2$/direct pulp capping
C. Indirect pulp capping
D. None

80. Chances of endodontic failure is maximum with:

A. Incomplete obturation
B. Inadequate BMP
C. Improper irrigation
D. None

81. Reaming action of the reamer is:

A. Pushing regenerating
B. Pushing, rotating and regenerating
C. Pushing and pulling
D. None

82. In β-thalassemia, RBC's are:

A. Microcytic hypochromic
B. Macrocytic hypochromic
C. Normocytic normochromic
D. Microcytic hyperchromic

83. Two or more teeth united by roots:

A. Concrescence
B. Dialaceration
C. Tourodontism
D. Talen's tooth

84. Failure of casting to seat on the cast is overcome by:

A. Scraping the cast to seat
B. Forcefully position the casting
C. Wash the casting with HCl
D. Discard if the discrepancy is more than 0.03 mm

85. Porcelain, metal bond in PFM is:

A. Chemical
B. Mechanical
C. Chemical Mechanical
D. Electrical

86. Badges should be worn by dental technician energy:

A. 1 man B. 2 men
C. 3 men D. 4 men

87. In children radiographic dose should be (that of adults):

A. 25% B. 50%
C. 75% D. Adult dose

88. In steps in developing film first step is to:

A. Stirring the solution
B. Washing of film
C. Dip in developer
D. Dip in fixer

Answers

1.	B	2.	B	3.	C	4.	B
5.	C	6.	B	7.	B	8.	A
9.	D	10.	D	11.	B	12.	B
13.	C	14.	D	15.	B	16.	A
17.	B	18.	D	19.	A	20.	D
21.	B	22.	B	23.	C	24.	A
25.	B	26.	A	27.	C	28.	C
29.	B	30.	C	31.	B	32.	A
33.	B	34.	B	35.	C	36.	A
37.	A	38.	C	39.	A	40.	A
41.	B	42.	B	43.	D	44.	C
45.	A	46.	B	47.	A	48.	A
49.	A	50.	A	51.	A	52.	A
53.	B	54.	C	55.	A	56.	C
57.	A	58.	A	59.	B	60.	A
61.	B	62.	A	63.	A	64.	A
65.	A	66.	A	67.	A	68.	A
69.	B	70.	A	71.	A	72.	D
73.	B	74.	A	75.	A	76.	B
77.	D	78.	B	79.	A	80.	A
81.	B	82.	A	83.	A	84.	D
85.	C	86.	A	87.	B	88.	A

PGI Paper

June 2001

1. **Nutritional supply of the ameloblasts during most of their life cycle is from the:**
   A. Dental pulp
   B. Odontoblastic processes
   C. Dental sac
   D. Reduced dental organ

2. **Epithelium of the inner surface of the gingival sulcus**
   A. Has no rete pegs
   B. Has prominent rete pegs
   C. Is keratinized
   D. Is para-keratinized

3. **Muscles which are involved in the rotation and protrusion of the mandible:**
   A. Masseter
   B. Medial and lateral pterygoid
   C. Temporalis
   D. Digastric

4. **The secretomotor supply of the praotid gland is through:**
   A. Otic ganglion
   B. Gasserian ganglion
   C. Geniculate ganglion
   D. Submandibular ganglion

5. **Streptococcus mutans is implicated in the etiology of dental caries because of its capability of produce:**
   A. 1, 3 glucose extracellular polysaccharide
   B. 1, 4 glucose extracellular polysaccharide
   C. 1, 6 glucose extracelluler polysaccharide
   D. 1, 4 glucose intracelluler polysaccharide

6. **The change in the colour of traumatic primary incisor is due to:**

A. Laceration of periodontal ligament
B. Diffusion of biliverdin in dentinal tubules
C. Development of heavy laryer of tertiary dentin
D. Internal resorption of dentin

7. **Laboratory test of ANUG is:**
A. Complement fixation
B. Darkfield examination
C. Tissue culture
D. Animal inoculation

8. **Radiographic appearance of the inferior dental canal and roots of the mandibuar third molar:**
A. Tram lines visible
B. Radiolucent band evident in relation to root of third molar which is grooved tunnelled
C. Winter's lines
D. Tram lines enhanced

9. **A 3 cm squamous cell carcinoma of the retromolar trigone and invading the mandible and the medial pterygoid muscle is at what TNM stage?**
A. Stage I
B. Stage II
C. Stage III
D. Stage IV

10. **Plummer-Vinson syndrome:**
A. Is due to folic acid deficiency
B. Common in males
C. Not associated with oral premalignancy
D. Syndrome association with post-cricoid carcinoma

11. **Common oral change seen with nutritional anemia is:**
A. Enlarged tongue
B. Atrophic glossitis
C. Generalised osteolysis
D. Focal marrow expansion

12. **"The Window period" in HIV infection means:**
A. The time lapse between the infection and detection of viral antibodies
B. The time lapse between the infection and development of AIDS
C. The time lapse between obtaining the sample and detection of virus in the lab
D. None of the above

13. Opaque porcelain is:

A. Feldspathic glass
B. Opacifiers like zirconia and titanium oxide
C. Not used to mask the colour of the cement used in placing of restoration
D. Used to produce the characteristic translucency which is an inherent aspect of the incisal edge in natural teeth

14. "Brush heap" structure is found in:

A. Zinc oxide impression material
B. Agar
C. Condensation silicone
D. Polyether

15. Score of 8 on the Russel periodontal index shows:

A. Irreversible terminal disease
B. Established destructive periodontal disease
C. Beginning destructive periodontal disease
D. Advanced destructive periodontal disease with loss of masticatory function

16. The name of the sample group of individuals when followed for successive examination to evaluate the effect of oral preventive programmes is:

A. Panel group
B. Cohort group
C. High risk group
D. Prospective group

17. A high dental caries individual is on preventive schedule the sugar exposure should be:

A. Reduced to meal times
B. Reduced to no exposure permanently
C. Reduced to no exposure for 21 days
D. Reduced to meal time exposure for 21 days

18. After diet counselling the foolproof method to monitor diet change is:

A. Lactobacillus count
B. Streptococcus mutans count
C. Snyder test
D. Patients diet history

19. Least cariogenic sugar is:

A. Fructose
B. Glucose
C. Sucrose
D. Xylitol

20. CPITN:

A. Was observed for he first time by ADA in 1992

B. Scored by a special peridontal probe of length 3 to 5 mm backward for easy visibility

C. Measure 6 representative teeth

D. Score of '3' means the treatment involves oral hygiene instructions, scaling and curettage

21. 3 D classification of orthodontia was given by:

A. Angle
B. Simon
C. Dewey
D. Baume

22. For large country surveys the sampling method of choice is:

A. Multiple sampling

B. Multistage sampling

C. Cluster sampling

D. Multistage random sampling

23. Case control studies are also called:

A. Retrospective
B. Prospective
C. Prevalence
D. Incidence

24. To achieve caries reduction in adults the diet modification should be:

A. Rich in calcium and vitamins

B. Restrict sugars to 5 times a day

C. Restrict sugars to 3 times a day

D. Restrict in between meals sugar intake

25. Dental floss is used to:

A. Remove interdental plaque

B. Remove interdental food and debris

C. Massage gums

D. Prevent gingival recession

26. Concentration of chlorhexidine gluconate in mouthwash effective for plaque control is:

A. 0.2%
B. 0.02%
C. 2.0%
D. 0.12%

27. Earliest symptom of gingivitis is:

A. Pain

B. Increased gingival fluid exudation

C. Change in the colour of gingiva

D. Bleeding from the gingival sulcus of gentile probing

28. At what concentration of fluoride in the drinking water does chronic dental fluorosis occur without skeletal fluorosis:

A. 1 ppm
B. 3 ppm
C. 8 ppm
D. 10 ppm

29. In a 9-year-old which permanent tooth surface will show greatly increased caries incidence?

A. Labial surface of central incisor
B. Occlusal surface of central incisor
C. Mesial surface of central incisor
D. Occlusal surface of lateral incisor

30. Which disclosing solution differentiates between mature and newly formed plaque?

A. Iodine
B. Erythrosine
C. Two tone dye solution
D. Mercurochrome

31. The onset of action of lidocaine is:

A. 1–2 minutes
B. 5–10 minutes
C. 3–5 minutes
D. 7–8 minutes

32. Which other factor in the Stephan's curve is related to the caries incidence and sugar intake?

A. Physical form of sugar
B. Frequency form of sugar
C. pH of paque
D. Quantity of sugar intake

33. Chronic fluoride toxicity results in:

A. Extreme arthritic changes of the spine resulting in rigidity
B. Calcifications of the sheaths of muscles and tendons
C. Osteosclerosis
D. All of the above

34. Gracy curettes are area specific instruments because:

A. They are used in the specific areas of the US
B. They adapt to specific areas of the tooth or root
C. They have more than one angle per cutting edge
D. They are used for root planning

35. While using a periodontal probe to measure the depth of the periodontal pocket the pocket is measured from?

A. Free gingival margin to the cementoenamel junction
B. Junctional epithelium to the free gingival margin
C. Base of pocket to the cementoenamel junction
D. Base of pocket to mucogingival junction

36. Which of the following is not a nonabsorbable suture material?

A. Silk
B. Wire
C. Chromic gut
D. Synthetic fibre

37. The condition which results from the rubbing of the teeth against each other is called:

A. Abrasion
B. Attrition
C. Erosion
D. Ablation

38. Least width of attached gingiva is found on the facial aspect of:

A. 1st premolar
B. 2nd premolar
C. Lateral incisor
D. Canine

39. The earliest sign of gingivitis which is of treat help for diagnostic and treatment planning is?

A. Pain
B. Increased gingival fluid exudation
C. Spontaneous bleeding
D. Bleeding from gingival sulcus on gentle probing

40. The gingiva in a patient of HIV is similar to the gingiva in:

A. Linchen planus
B. ANUG
C. Acute gingivitis
D. Chronic gingivitis

41. A radiolucency area between the maxillary central incisors is most probably:

A. Dentigerous cyst
B. Globulomaxillary cyst
C. Nasopalatine cyst
D. Primordial cyst

42. The temperature lag between the gelation temperature and the liquefaction temperature of the gel is known as:

A. Osmosis
B. Imbibition
C. Green heat
D. Hysteresis

43. How soon after a moisture contamination does a zinc containing amalgam alloy start expanding:

A. 24 horus B. 1–2 days
C. 3–5 days D. 7 days

44. A six-year molar begins to calcify at:

A. Six months IU B. At birth
C. 1 year after birth D. 3 years age

45. Which of the following does not lie on the mandible?

A. Pogonion B. Porion
C. Menton D. Gnathion

46. At which stage of tooth development does an aberration lead to congenital absence of the lateral incisor?

A. Histodifferentiation
B. Morphodifferentiation
C. Initiation
D. Apposition

47. In between which primary teeth, do primate spaces occur?

A. Primary maxillary and mandibular canine and first molar
B. Primay maxillary canine and lateral incisor and mandibular primary canine and first molar
C. Primary maxillary canine and lateral incisor and madibular primary canine and lateral incisor
D. Primary maxillary canine and first molar and mandibular primary canine and lateral incisor

48. Which primary teeth are severely involved in nursing bottle caries?

A. Maxillary primary first molars
B. Primary canines
C. Mandibular primary incisors
D. Maxillary primary incisors

49. Green stains which occur frequently in children are due to?

A. Enamel deficiency
B. Dentin deficiency
C. Materia alba
D. Chromogenic bacteria

50. Absorbed fluoride is eliminated by:

A. Kidneys B. Lungs
C. Saliva D. Intestines

51. The hypoplastic defects of the enamel appear in a radiograph as:

A. Radiolucent
B. Radiopaque
C. Sclerotic
D. Indistinguishable from the normal enamel

52. The cause of sensation of tissue tearing during local anesthesia administration is due to:

A. Passage through a cyst
B. Passage through a muscle
C. Passage through an area of infection
D. Barb on the needle

53. The failure of a calcium hydroxide pulpotomy done on a primary 1st molar is due to:

A. Internal resorption
B. External resporption
C. Pulp calcification
D. Pulp fibrosis

54. Dental age refers to:

A. Stage of dental maturation
B. Age at which a given tooth eruption occurs
C. Time period of an eruption potential
D. Number of years elapsed since a given tooth erupted

55. After the age of six the increase in the size of mandible occurs at:

A. Symphysis
B. Between canines
C. Along the lower border
D. Distal to 1st molars

56. The cranial vault increases rapidly postnatally. By the age of six what % of cranial growth is completed?

A. 50% B. 80%
C. 90% D. 100%

57. The stainless steel wires and bands used in orthodontics are composed of:

A. 18 Cr and 8 Co
B. 8 Cr and 18 Co
C. 18 Cr and 8 Ni
D. 8 Cr and 18 Ni

58. Which tooth in a mandibular arch is commonly malopposed due to arch space discrepancy?

A. 1st molars B. 2nd molars

C. 1st premolars D. 2nd premolars

59. A canine retractor is best used for moving a buccally placed canine. For moving it distally and palatally it is called:

A. Palatal canine retractor

B. U loop canine retractor

C. Reverse U loop canine retractor

D. Buccal self supported canine retractor

60. For a bodily movement of a small tooth the force required is:

A. 25–30 g B. 40–75 g

C. 120–150 g D. More than 150 g

61. When an anchor unit is allowed to tip, it is called----- anchorage.

A. Simple B. Compound

C. Complex D. Reciprocal

62. Down's cephalometric analysis uses---line as a reference plane.

A. ANS–PNS

B. SN plane

C. Porion–Orbitale

D. Gonion–Menton

63. Tweed's triangle denotes:

A. The position of maxilla and mandible to each other

B. The angle between the mandibular plane and mandibular incisors

C. Relationship between maxillary central and mandibular central incisor

D. Profile of an individual

64. Alban's test measures:

A. Soluble proteins

B. Caries activity

C. Immunoglobulins in saliva

D. Masticatory function

65. The best sustaining topical effect of fluoride is obtained by:

A. NaF
B. APFgel
C. Duraphat
D. SnF

66. The amount of recommended fluoride in a toothpaste is:

A. 700 ppm
B. 1000 ppm
C. 1200 ppm
D. 1400 ppm

67. The concentration of NaF in a daily mouth rinse is:

A. 0.02%
B. 0.5%
C. 0.03%
D. 0.05%

68. Which of the following is a contraindication for pulp capping and pulpotomy?

A. Accidental exposure in a vital tooth
B. If there is inflammation of the radicular pulp
C. Greatly curved and tortuous roots
D. None of the above

69. Root canal is flooded with antiseptic so as to:

A. Prevent the removal of the shavings from the root canal
B. Where there is an absence of instrumentation
C. Prevent infection during instrumentation
D. Avoid instrumentation

70. Caries activity:

A. Correlates with lactobacillus count in an individual
B. Increases in immunodeficiency states
C. Increases in xerostomia
D. Related to the quantity of sugar intake

71. Hard brown lesions present on the labial surfaces of cuspid teeth not painful to excavation yield few flakes of dry dentin. This type of caries is:

A. Active carious lesion
B. Arrested carious lesion
C. Local enamel hypoplasia
D. Abrasion

72. Composite restorative material in comparison with acrylic have:

A. Less compressive strength
B. More polymerisation shrinkage
C. More abrasive strength
D. More water uptake

73. The reason for localised shrinkage porosity is:

A. Overheating of alloy
B. Overheating of the investment
C. Thin sprue
D. No reservoir

74. The relationship between the working edge of the instrument and the tooth surface is:

A. Angulation
B. Access
C. Adaptation
D. Activation

75. Plaque is colonised earliest by:

A. Spirochetes
B. Gram positive rods and cocci
C. Gram negative rods and cocci
D. Actinomycetales

76. The most harmful plaque which penetrates the connective tissue and caused bone destruction is?

A. Subgingival tooth attached plaque
B. Subgingival tooth unattached plaque
C. Subgingival epithelium attached plaque
D. Subgingival plaque

77. A pocket which is 5 mm in depth and with loss of attachment is 3 mm. Total loss of attachment is:

A. 5 mm
B. 2 mm
C. 3 mm
D. 8 mm

78. In the walking bleach technique:

A. It uses a heat treatment
B. It requires the patient to report in 24 hours
C. Can be done with 35 percent hydrogen peroxide
D. It uses a mixture of sodium perborate and hydrogen peroxide

79. Recapitulation:

A. Uses large files to flare the root canal
B. Removing debris with a smaller instrument then the instrument that goes to the apex
C. Use of larger files to flare the root canal but in between use of small instruments to confirm the initial length
D. The use of various types of reamers and files to enlarge the root canal

80. Initial threshold of the electric test in a traumatic tooth is to:
A. Establish base line of the physical status of the pulp
B. Is positive in healthy pulp
C. Is negative in root canal tooth
D. Is repeated after 30 days

81. Wax pattern is ideally invested immediately to decrease the dimensional changes caused by:
A. Decreased flow
B. Continuous expansion of the wax
C. Relaxation of the internal stresses
D. Water loss

82. The best restoration for posterior tooth with an undermined cusp with caries is:
A. Cast gold
B. Silver amalgam
C. Direct gold filling
D. Pin retained amalgam restoration

83. The problem faced in a denture with supraerupted natural teeth in the other arch is:
A. Difficulty during teeth setting
B. It effects the stability of the denture
C. Difficulty during mastication
D. Abrasion of artificial teeth

84. Heel-raising movement of an RPD is prevented by:
A. Occlusal rests
B. Minor connector
C. Direct retainer
D. Indirect retainer

85. Uncontrolled diabetes poses a problem to a prosthodontist as:
A. More bone resorption
B. Increased salivary flow
C. Less bone resorption
D. Less tissue laxity

86. The powder of dental plaster and dental stone differ in:
A. Solubility
B. Shelf life
C. Chemical formulation
D. Particle porosity

87. The most important reason for retaining healthy roots and prescribing an overdenture rather than extractions and a conventional complete denture is:

A. To preserve the alveolar bone
B. An overdanture is easier to construct rather than a complete denture
C. The apparent ease with which the patient adapts to an overdenture
D. To retain some degree of proprioception form the healthy periodontal ligament of the roots

88. Secondary peripheral seal area of a mandibular complete denture is:

A. Labial border
B. Buccal border
C. Distolingual border
D. Anterior lingual border

89. Stability in an RPD is best ensured by:

A. Flat plane teeth
B. Incorporating harmonious occlusion
C. Dependents on clasping and indirect retention
D. Using prorcelain teeth

90. An FPD is indicated to replace maxillary 1st and 2nd premolar. Abutment teeth are in normal alignment that is maxillary canine and 1st molar. The connectors of choice are:

A. Precision attachments on maxillary canine and 1st molar
B. Soldered joint on canine and non-precision dovetail keyway on 1st molar
C. Soldered joint on 1st molar with a subocclusal rest on canine
D. Soldered joints on both canine and 1st molar

91. Drugs associated with gingival changes are:

A. Phenytoin, cyclosporine and nifedipine
B. Nifedipine, ibuprofen and lignocaine
C. Cyclosporin, chlorine and iodine
D. Phenytoin, hydrogen hydrogen peroxide and paracetamol

92. Infraorbital technique used in surgery anesthetises the:

A. Palatal side
B. Tuberosity area
C. Buccal side
D. Maxillary incisor to 1st premolar

93. The treatment for a mandibular fracture between the incisors is:

A. Risdon wiring
B. Essig wiring
C. Cap split with circum-mandibular wiring
D. Transosseious wiring

94. A patient who faints during extraction should be positioned in the:

A. Lateral position
B. Horizontal position
C. Trendelenburg position
D. Dorsosacral position

95. The extraoral X-ray view required for a fracture of mandible is:

A. Submentovertex
B. Posterioanterior
C. Waters'
D. Towne's

96. The action of adrenaline is potentiated in the presence of all *except*:

A. Halothane
B. Ethyl chloride
C. Cyclopropane
D. Ether

97. The following cyst is associated with impacted tooth *except*:

A. Dentigerous cyst
B. Calcifying epithelial odontogenic cyst
C. Keratocyst
D. Primordial cyst

98. The colour of a nitrous oxide cylinder is:

A. Red
B. Blue
C. White
D. Green

99. Guerin fracture is:

A. Maxillary fracture
B. Maxillary and zygomatic fracture
C. Maxillary and nasal bone fracture
D. Nasal bone fracture only

Answers

1.	D	2.	A	3.	D	4.	A
5.	C	6.	B	7.	B	8.	B
9.	B	10.	D	11.	B	12.	A
13.	B	14.	B	15.	D	16.	B
17.	A	18.	C	19.	D	20.	C
21.	B	22.	C	23.	A	24.	D
25.	A	26.	A	27.	B	28.	A
29.	C	30.	C	31.	C	32.	C
33.	D	34.	B	35.	B	36.	C
37.	B	38.	A	39.	D	40.	B
41.	C	42.	D	43.	C	44.	B
45.	B	46.	C	47.	B	48.	D
49.	D	50.	A	51.	A	52.	D
53.	A	54.	A	55.	D	56.	C
57.	C	58.	D	59.	A	60.	B
61.	A	62.	D	63.	B	64.	B
65.	D	66.	B	67.	B	68.	B
69.	C	70.	C	71.	B	72.	C
73.	D	74.	C	75.	B	76.	C
77.	D	78.	D	79.	C	80.	A
81.	C	82.	A	83.	A	84.	D
85.	A	86.	D	87.	A	88.	D
89.	B	90.	D	91.	A	92.	D
93.	A	94.	C	95.	D	96.	D
97.	D	98.	B	99.	A		

PGI Paper June 2000

1. **In a patient it is noticed that when he protrudes his tongue it deviates to the left. The nerve damaged is:**
   A. Left hypoglossal
   B. Left glossopharyngeal
   C. Right hypoglossal
   D. Right glossopharyngeal

2. **Fracture or separation of porcelain and metal occurs due to:**
   A. Increased thickness of porcelain
   B. High occlusal contact
   C. No metal conditioner used
   D. Centric occlusal contact on metal-ceramic interface

3. **The cuspal inclines of the maxillary buccal cusps and the mandibular lingual cusps are in deflective contact. Balancing has to be done in which position?**
   A. Centric
   B. Working
   C. Balancing
   D. Working and balancing

4. **Which part of the RPD resists torquing movements?**
   A. Denture base B. Clasp
   C. Major connector D. Guiding plane

5. **Recontouring and selective grinding procedures are carried out in a complete denture to:**
   A. Decrease the vertical dimension of occlusion
   B. Decrease cuspal height
   C. Enhance curve of spree
   D. Remove occlusal disharmony

6. **Which of the following may least be used in an abutment?**

A. Tooth and minimum crown
B. Tooth with short tapered crown and conical roots
C. Rotated and tipped tooth
D. Pulp treated tooth

7. **CSF rhinorrhoea is found in:**
A. Frontal bone structure
B. Zygomaticomaxillary fracture
C. Nasoethmoidal fracture
D. Condylar fracture

8. **Which of the following is not a feature of lefort II fracture?**
A. Enophthalmos
B. Malocclusion
C. Paresthesia
D. CSF rhinorrhoea

9. **Sialoliths are most commonly found in the:**
A. Parotid duct
B. Sublingual gland
C. Submandibular duct
D. Minor salivary glands

10. **Masticatory space infections are clinically characterised by:**
A. Dyspnoea
B. Trismus
C. Erythema
D. Hematemesis

11. **The local anaesthesia technique which is contra-indicated in hemophilics is:**
A. Infraorbital nerve block
B. Inferior alveolar nerve block
C. Nasopalatine nerve block
D. Mental nerve block

12. **Sedation by which of the following routes can be reversed most rapidly?**
A. Oral
B. Inhalation
C. Intravenous
D. Intramuscular

13. **The type of load on teeth that is most destructive to the periodontium is:**
A. Vertical
B. Oblique
C. Horizontal
D. Apical

14. **Oral irrigating devices act:**
A. As an adjunct to toothpaste

B. Substitute to toothbrush
C. Effective for plaque removal
D. Dilute or alters or disrupts the plaque content

15. **Materia alba is:**
A. Only visible with disclosing agents
B. Acquired bacterial coating less adherent than plaque
C. Only removed with brushing
D. Same as food debris

16. **Internal resorption in a tooth is seen as:**
A. Calcium hydroxide pulpotomy
B. Replacement resorption
C. Non-proliferating lesion
D. Desensitizing booth

17. **Which of the following is most difficult to manage?**
A. Loss of mandibular 2nd deciduous molar in 5-year-old child
B. Loss of mandibular 2nd deciduous molar in 9½-year-old child
C. Loss of mandibular 2nd deciduous molar in 8-year-old child
D. Loss of mandibular 2nd deciduous molar in 10½-year-old child

18. **Best space maintainer is:**
A. Active space maintainer
B. Passive space maintainer
C. Band and loop
D. Pulpotomised primary tooth

19. **A nine-year-old child has a lingually locked 21. Most probable cause is:**
A. Premature loss of 51
B. Premature loss of 61
C. Prolonged retention of 61
D. Pronounced facioversion on eruption of 31

20. **The deciduous canine emerges:**
A. Before lateral incisor
B. Before first molar
C. After first molar
D. After second molar

21. Order for eruption of primary teeth:

1. Central incisor
2. Lateral incisor
3. Canine
4. 1st molar
5. 2nd molar

A. 12345
B. 12435
C. 21435
D. 12453

22. Anterior diastemas close with the eruption of:

A. 1st molar
B. 3rd molar
C. Canines
D. Premolars

23. If the second deciduous molar is lost prematurely, maxillary space loss occurs in:

A. 1st 6 months
B. 3–9 months
C. 6–12 months
D. 12–18 months

24. The best form of a space maintainer to prevent the mesial drift to the first molar is:

A. To construct a space maintainer as soon as the molars pierce the gums
B. As soon as the second deciduous molar are lost
C. Distal shoe type space maintainer
D. Loop and band type space maintainer

25. Tetracycline stains appear as:

A. Yellow and brown stains in enamel and dentin
B. Yellow and brown stains only in enamel
C. Yellow and brown stains only in dentin
D. Only yellow stains in enamel

26. Stannous fluoride concentration use in topical fluoride is:

A. 8%
B. 2%
C. 1.23%
D. 12%

27. DMF(s) is defined as:

1. Irreversible index
2. Measures cumulative index
3. Morbidity index:

A. 1 only
B. 2 only
C. 3 only
D. All of the above

28. Prevalence is defined as:

A. Number of new cases in an area
B. Cumulative number of cases in an area
C. Rate of disease transmission
D. Proportion of population affected by a disease

29. **Minimum amount of chlorhexidine required in mouthwash for plaque prevention:**
A. 0.10% B. 0.12%
C. 0.2% D. 0.22%

30. **Minimum amount of fluoride needed in dentrifices to prevent caries:**
A. 1000 ppm B. 2000 ppm
C. 3000 ppm D. 4000 ppm

31. **Which of the following does not constitute the carbohydrate component of the plaque?**
A. Dextran B. Glucose
C. Levan D. Rhamnose

32. **Carious lesions are not detected till they involve the following amount of tooth:**
A. 30 microns B. 40 microns
C. 100 microns D. 200 mincrons

33. **Which of the following drug combinations are associated with gingival changes?**
A. Nifedipine, cyclosporin and phenytoin
B. Nifedipine, cyclosporin and ibuprofen
C. Nifedipine, cyclosporin and nimesulide
D. Phenytoin, quinine and cyclosporin

34. **In a tooth which has been endodontically treated there is pain on percussion and slight mobility due to:**
A. Loose crown B. Tooth fracture
C. Psychosomatic D. Eccentric contact

35. **Koplik's spots are found in:**
A. Measles B. Whooping cough
C. Herpangina D. Diphtheria

36. **A tooth which erupts in the first 30 days of infancy is called?**
A. Neonatal tooth B. Natal tooth
C. Nursing tooth D. Infant tooth

37. **Odontogenic tumour associated with unerupted tooth in a child is:**
A. Ameloblastic fibroma
B. Odontogenic myxoma
C. Odontogenic adenomatoid tumor
D. Cementifying fibroma

38. A 4-year-old child has less number of teeth and lateral incisors with bifurcated roots with two root canal is called:
A. Dilaceration
B. Concrescence
C. Fusion
D. Gemination

39. Infectious mononucleosis has:
A. Multiple draining sinuses
B. Ulcers which bruise easily
C. Palatal perforation
D. Alveolar bone loss

40. The mental foramen which appears as a rediolucency and can be mistaken for a periapical pathology lies close to the apex of which tooth?
A. Mandibular 1st molar
B. Maxillary 1st molar
C. Mandibular premolar
D. Mandibular canine

41. The roots of which of the following lie close to the sinus?
A. Maxillary 2nd premolar
B. Maxillary 1st premolar
C. Maxillary 2nd premolar
D. Maxillary canine

42. Paper points are best sterilized by:
A. Boiling in water bath
B. Flame
C. Hot air oven
D. Cold sterilization

43. Abscess of which tooth due to its anatomical location drains palatally?
A. Maxillary central incisor
B. Maxillary lateral incisor
C. Maxillary canine
D. Mandibular lateral incisor

44. A sinus associated with a periapical pathology requires:
A. Broad spectrum antibiotics
B. RCT with excision of sinus
C. RCT with periapical curettage
D. RCT with no treatment for sinus

45. A maxillary central incisor with a dowel crown shows:

A. Broad spectrum antibiotic therapy
B. Remove the down crown
C. Redo the RCT and apicoectomy
D. Perform apicoectomy with retrograde filling

46. Best method for obturating a root canal of a tooth is:

A. Thermoplastic GP
B. Silver cone
C. Resorbable paste
D. GP with sealer

47. If the pocket dept is 5 mm and the gingival recession is 3 mm, the total loss of attachment is:

A. 5 mm
B. 3 mm
C. 8 mm
D. 2 mm

48. Which of the following plaque is most harmful and causes spread of inflammation to the connective tissue leading to bone destruction:

A. Subgingival epithelial attached
B. Subgingival unattached
C. Subgingival plaque
D. Supragingival plaque

49. Benzoin methyl ether in a polymer indicates that they may be cured in the presence of:

A. UV light
B. Visible light
C. Infrared light
D. Diketones

50. A small radiolucent area at the periapical region of a non-vital root. Canal treated tooth is observed treatment is:

A. Redo RCT
B. Periapical curettage
C. Periapical curettage with apicectomy
D. RCT, periapical curettage and apicectomy

51. Increased bleeding during pulp amputation indicates:

A. Acute pulpitis
B. Arterial hyperemia
C. Passive hyperemia
D. Chronic suppurative pulpitis

52. Toothache relieved with cold water indicates:
A. Acute pulpitis
B. Arterial hyperemia
C. Irreversible pulpitis
D. Venous hyperemia

53. The most effective and least objectionable topical fluoride is:
A. Sodium fluoride
B. Strontium fluoride
C. APF gel
D. Stannous fluoride

54. Which strain of yeast is found in the root canal?
A. Candida albicans
B. Cryptococcus
C. Histoplasma
D. Actinomyces

55. Moisture contamination of amalgam can lead to:
A. Marginal breakdown
B. Shrinkage
C. Delayed expansion
D. Increased

56. Pulp horn exposure occurs most commonly with:
A. Mesiobuccal horn of the 1st molar
B. Distobuccal horn of the 1st molar
C. Mesiobuccal horn of the 2nd molar
D. Distobuccal horn of the 2nd molar

57. Desirable root canal filling material in deciduous teeth is:
A. Gutta percha
B. Calcium hydroxide
C. Silver amalgam
D. Zinc oxide and eugenol

58. Four canals are seen in:
A. Upper 1st molar
B. Lower 1st molar
C. Upper 2nd molar
D. Lower 2nd molar

59. Chin cap therapy is used for:
A. Skeletal Class III deformity
B. Dental Class III deformity

C. Skeletal Class II deformity
D. Dental Class II deformity

60. Most common malocclusion found in people is:
A. Class I with incisior crowding
B. Class II division I
C. Class II division II
D. Class III

61. Dolichocephalic facial type is:
A. Broad dental arches
B. Long and narrow dental arches
C. Paraboloid dental arches
D. Round dental arches

62. The best time to treat a cross-bite is:
A. When the roots are fully developed
B. When the roots are 2/3rd developed
C. Permanent dentition has completely erupted
D. As and when detected

63. Helix in a finger spring for mesial movement lies:
A. Mesial to the long axis of the tooth
B. Distal to the long axis of the tooth
C. In line to the long axis of the tooth
D. Perpendicular to the long axis of the tooth

64. Optimum orthodontic force should not exceed the:
A. Arterial blood pressure
B. Venous blood pressure
C. Capillary blood pressure
D. Masticatory pressure

65. Which of the following is not an example of inter-maxillary anchorage?
A. Criss-cross elastics for cross-bite correction
B. Class II elastics between maxillary and mandibular incisors
C. Baker's anchorage
D. Retraction of the upper incisors by tipping them lingually and using lower molars as anchorage

66. Highest point on the concavity posterior to the occipital condyles is:
A. Pogonion
B. Basion

C. Bolton's point
D. Gonion

67. Adult face is formed by fusion of:
A. First and second branchial arches and tissues surrounding the developing forebrain
B. Second and third branchial arches and tissues surrounding the developing forebrain
C. First and fourth branchial arches
D. First and third branchial arches

68. Severely crowded mandibular incisors are due to:
A. Mesial migration of teeth
B. Premature loss of deciduous teeth
C. Supernumerary teeth
D. Tooth size-arch length discrepancy

69. In a Class-II division 2, the most typical characteristics seen is:
A. Open bite
B. Steep mandibular plane
C. Mesio-occlusion of molars
D. Lingual inclination of maxillary central incisors

70. A radio-opaque area is seen in the dentine of a 3-month-old Class-II Silver amalgam restoration base is:
A. Calcium hydroxide
B. Zinc oxyphosphate
C. Zinc oxide and eugenol
D. Zinc oxide eugenol and formocresol

71. In a 2-year-old child maxillary deciduous central incisor is intruded by 4 mm. Treatment is:
A. Remove the intruded incisor
B. Reposition the intruded incisor
C. Make patient comfortable and observe
D. Reposition and splint

72. Retention in a stainless steel crown is achieved primarily by:
A. Chamfer
B. Cement
C. Parallel distal and mesial grooves
D. Crimping

73. Interdental spacing found in the maxillary arch of the deciduous dentition is:

A. 2 mm B. 4 mm
C. 6 mm D. 8 mm

74. Mostly common missing tooth in the permanent dentition is:

A. Maxillary canine
B. Maxillary first molar
C. Mandibular second premolar
D. Mandibular first molar

75. Eugenol is not used with zinc oxide in a periodontal dressing as it acts to:

A. Allergic reactions
B. Delays wound healing
C. Irritated the wound
D. Induces liver disease

76. The belly layer is a synonym for:

A. Protective oxide layer formed
B. Overglaze
C. Tarnish and corrosion
D. Molecular disorganized surface on a highly polished material

77. Viscoelastic substances may be defined as those which on removal of load show?

A. No recovery
B. Complete recovery
C. Slow recovery
D. Fatigue

78. Trisodium phosphate in alginate acts as:

A. Filler
B. Retarder
C. Reactor
D. Accelerator

79. Function carnauba wax:

A. To provide a smooth and glossy surface
B. Increase toughness
C. Decrease toughness
D. Decrease flow at room temperature

80. Which of the following properties of dental materials is time dependent?

A. Creep
B. Resilience
C. Elastic limit
D. Ultimate strenght

81. Which of the following amalgam alloys is least susceptible to creep?

A. Lathe cut
B. Spherical
C. Microfine
D. Dispersion with high frequency

82. Most common site of bone destruction in a pathologically involved primary second molar is:

A. Bifurcation
B. Apex
C. Lateral surface
D. Peridontium

83. Giant cell lesions of the periodontium are best considered as:

A. Benign neoplasias
B. Malignant neoplasias
C. Hypothyroidism
D. Non-neoplastic reactive lesions

84. A radiopaque mass continuous with the cemento-enamel junction attached to the distal of the first premolar is:

A. Hyperkeratosis
B. Calculus
C. Full debris
D. Epithelial attachment

85. The radiographic view of choice for zygomatico maxillary complex fractures is:

A. True lateral
B. Occipitomental 30°
C. AP skull
D. PA skull

86. While taking radiographs for children by what % should X-ray beam exposure should be reduced?

A. 25%
B. 50%
C. 75%
D. As adult

87. **Pulp tissue is:**
A. Nervous
B. Vascular
C. Granulomatous
D. Loose connective

88. **Developed hyperactivity to a drug is:**
A. Tolerance
B. Antagonism
C. Detoxification
D. Desensitization

89. **Which of the following drugs causes extra pyramidal symptoms?**
A. Antibiotics
B. Salicylates
C. Barbiturates
D. Phenothiazines

90. **Heparin, apart from releasing lipoprotein lipase in the blood exerts its anti-coagulant action by:**
A. Binding to calcium
B. Inhibiting fibrinogen synthesis
C. Inhibiting prothrombin synthesis
D. Inhibiting thrombin synthesis

91. **The organism that causes infective endocarditis is:**
A. Streptococcus mitis
B. Staphylococcus aureus
C. Streptococcus viridans
D. Staphylococcus pyogenes

92. **S. mutans is involved in dental caries initiation. Other bacteria also involved is:**
A. S. Sarcinus
B. S. Macae
C. S. Sanguis
D. S. Salivarua

93. **Hemoglobin has:**
A. Four polypeptide chains, 2 Alpha, 1 Beta, 1 Gamma chain
B. Four haeme molecules and four polypeptide chains
C. Four Haeme molecules, 2 Alpha and 2 Beta chains
D. One haeme and one globin molecule

94. **The bacteria associated with root surface caries is:**
A. Lactobacillus
B. Staphylococcus
C. Fusobacterium
D. Artrobacter

95. **Staphylococcal bacteria are:**
A. Gram negative
B. Tend to form chains

C. Found in grape like clusters
D. Associated with dental caries

96. Secretometer fibres to the submandibular salivary gland are carried in all the following *except*:

A. Facial B. Chorda tympani
C. Mylohyoid D. Lingual

97. The muscle arising from the outer surface of the alveolus of the region of the molars is supplied by which nerve?

A. Trigeminal B. Facial
C. Mandibular D. Inferior alveolar

98. Taste sensations from the posterior one-third of the tongue are carried by............cranial nerve.

A. VII B. V
C. X D. IX

Answers

1.	A	2.	D	3.	C	4.	D
5.	D	6.	B	7.	C	8.	A
9.	C	10.	B	11.	B	12.	B
13.	C	14.	D	15.	B	16.	C
17.	A	18.	D	19.	C	20.	C
21.	B	22.	C	23.	A	24.	D
25.	A	26.	A	27.	D	28.	B
29.	B	30.	A	31.	D	32.	B
33.	A	34.	D	35.	A	36.	A
37.	C	38.	B	39.	B	40.	C
41.	B	42.	D	43.	B	44.	D
45.	D	46.	D	47.	A	48.	A
49.	A	50.	C	51.	B	52.	C
53.	C	54.	A	55.	C	56.	A
57.	D	58.	A	59.	A	60.	A
61.	B	62.	D	63.	A	64.	C
65.	D	66.	C	67.	A	68.	D
69.	D	70.	A	71.	C	72.	C
73.	B	74.	C	75.	A	76.	D
77.	C	78.	B	79.	D	80.	A
81.	D	82.	A	83.	D	84.	B
85.	B	86.	B	87.	D	88.	A
89.	D	90.	D	91.	C	92.	C
93.	C	94.	C	95.	C	96.	C
97.	B	98.	D				

PGI Paper

June 1999

1. **Plaster of paris:**
   A. Is wet calcined hemihydrate
   B. Has porous and irregular
   C. Is a-hemihydrate
   D. Has a W/P of 0.2

2. **The advantage of ZOE impression paste:**
   A. Has dimensional stability
   B. Does not adhere to tissues
   C. Is easy manipulation
   D. Does not require special trays

3. **Self-cure acrylic is different from heat-cure acrylic in that self-cure acrylic:**
   A. Requires heat for polymerisation
   B. Is more porous
   C. Is dimensionally stable
   D. Has greater strength

4. **Which of the following is present in the powder of the acrylic resin?**
   A. Methyl methacrylate
   B. Benzoyl peroxide
   C. Hydroquinone
   D. D-methyl paratoloudine

5. **An 8-year-old child has end-on-end molar occlusion. The clinician should:**
   A. Observe and wait for the other permanent teeth to erupt
   B. Do the distal disking of 2nd primary molar
   C. Extract the 1st primary molars
   D. Serial extraction

6. **A radiopaque area is observed under a 3-month-old silver amalgam filling. The base used most probably was:**
   A. Calcium hydroxide
   B. ZOE
   C. Formacresol ZOE
   D. Zinc oxyphosphate

7. **A 10-year-old child with primary molar in various stages of exfoliation has a sight crowding in the lower anterior. The clinician should:**
   A. Observe him after 1 year
   B. Obtain study casts and perform arch-length analysis
   C. Observe him after 6 months
   D. Delay the treatment until all permanent teeth erupt

8. **A 9-year-old child has tooth 21 lingually locked. The most probable cause is:**
   A. Premature loss of 51
   B. Prolonged retention of 61
   C. Failure of 61 to erupt
   D. Facioversion of 31

9. **Which of the following statements best describes the relationship between fluorides and dental caries?**
   A. Children living in areas of endemic mottling lend to show a higher DMF index then those living in areas where mottling is rare
   B. Children living in areas of endemic mottling tend to show a lower DMF index than those living in areas where mottling is rare
   C. Children drinking optimal quantities of fluoridated water have about the same number of interproximal carious lesions but significantly fewer pit and fissure caries than do children who drink the same quantities of nonfluoridated water
   D. Optimal effects of fluoride can be achieved only at levels where mottled enamel also occurs

10. **A 10-year-old child reports with loss of primary lower 2nd molar. His occlusion is normal. The clinician should:**
   A. Construct a suitable RPF
   B. Place a functional space maintainer

C. Make a distal-shoe space maintainer
D. Base his choice of treatment upon X-ray findings

11. The most probable cause of crowding in lower anterior region is:
A. Prolonged retention of lower primary incisors
B. Premature exfoliation of lower primary incisors
C. Presence of supernumerary teeth
D. Tooth-size arch length discrepancy

12. Prolonged retention of primary tooth may lead to:
A. Altered path of permanent tooth eruption
B. Root resorption of adjacent tooth
C. Ankylosis of permanent tooth
D. Warping of roots of adjacent teeth

13. In a 9-year-old child the X-ray of a permanent 1st molar with early acute pulpal abscess will show:
A. Furcation involvement
B. Little change from normal
C. Widening of PDL
D. Narrowing of PDL

14. A distal shoe type of space maintainer is indicated in:
A. Loss of primary anterior tooth
B. If the primary 2nd molar is lost before the eruption of permanent 1st molar
C. If the primary 2nd molar is lost after the eruption of permanent 1st molar
D. Loss of primary 1st molar

15. Which of the following is not true of a fixed appliance?
A. Economical
B. Rotation and extrusion movements are possible
C. Paient co-operation is not required
D. Tipping and bodily movement are possible

16. Which of the following is not a procedure of preventive othodontics?
A. Topical fluoride applications
B. Serial extractions
C. Lip guard
D. Thumb sucking correction

17. The abnormal swallowing pattern with the poorest prognosis is:

A. Simple tongue thrust
B. Complex tongue thrust
C. Infantile swallow
D. Retained infantile swallow

18. A corrected anterior cross-bite is retained by:

A. Over-correction
B. Normal incisor correction
C. Hawley's retentive appliance
D. Palatal acrylic appliance with no labial arch wire

19. Which of the following is not an indication for a class II activator?

A. Mandibular retrusion
B. Horizontal/anterior type of mandibular growth
C. Crowding lower anteriors
D. Upright lower anteriors

20. On a cephalogram if FMA angle is 25° the patient is:

A. Long face
B. Short face
C. Average face
D. Mandibular growth is rotated backwards

21. If anterior cross-bite is not corrected with ice-cream spatula, then the appliance indicated is:

A. Inclined plane
B. Z-spring
C. Fixed appliance
D. Tongue blade

22. If surgery is performed on the hard palate of a 3-year-old for cleft palate which results in the inhibition of growth centre, then the facial profile will be:

A. More convex
B. More concave
C. Normal
D. Elongated

23. In a 10-year-old child the lower canines are trying to erupt in 2 mm insufficient space. The primary molars are large and firmly fixed. The 1st primolars are also erupting. The treatment of choice is:

A. Remove primary 2nd molars
B. Place a removable bite-opener
C. Remove 1st premolars
D. Mesial stripping of primary 2nd molars

24. If a normal SNA=82°. A patient has SNA=90°. This suggests:

A. Maxillary teeth protrusion
B. Maxillary protrusion
C. Mandibular protrusion
D. Mandibular retrusion

25. A carious lesion in the buccal development groove of lower 1st molar is:

A. Class I cavity
B. Class II cavity
C. Class III cavity
D. Class IV cavity

26. A polished silver amalgam will:

A. Corrode
B. Tarnish
C. Not tarnish and corrode
D. Not show secondary caries

27. Resistance form is that shape of cavity which:

A. Prevents displacement of restoration
B. Permits the restoration to withstand occlusal forces
C. Allows adequate instrumentation
D. Allows the restoration to withstand occlusal forces and prevent displacement

28. Chemical adhesion with the tooth is exhibited by:

A. Polycarboxylate cement
B. Composite resins
C. Direct filling resin
D. BIS-GMA resin

29. To avoid pulpal irritatin below a resistant metallic restoration, the minimum dentin thickness which should remain is:

A. 0.5 mm
B. 1.5 mm
C. 1.0 mm
D. 2.0 mm

30. 1% of sodium nitrite is a:

A. Disinfectant
B. Anti-rust agent
C. Bleaching agent
D. Sterilizing agent

31. The most common error sent during access cavity preparation of maxillary and mandibular incisors is:

A. Perforation of the lingual or labial walls
B. Gouging of pulpal contents

C. Tooth facture
D. All of the above

32. Which of the following is a contraindication of pulp capping and pulpotomy?
A. Accidental exposure during cavity preparation in a vital tooth
B. Bleeding during pulp extirpation
C. Inflammation and pain in a tooth
D. None of the above

33. When cementing a post of a crown:
A. The cement is applied only to the post but not in the canal
B. Same cement is applied to the post and the crown
C. ZOE-ortho-ethoxy benzoic acid is used as a cement
D. EDTA increases retention

34. The function of proximal grooves in a class II cavity is:
A. Resistance form
B. Retention form
C. Increases strength
D. Resistance and retention form

35. Most common cause of clicking in a complete denture is:
A. Posterior teeth place too horizontally on the arch
B. Excessive vertical dimension
C. Less vertical dimension
D. Poor retention

36. Splinting of several teeth together serving as abutments help in:
A. Eliminate the chances of food impaction and peridontal diseases in neighbouring teeth
B. Distribute occlusal load widely
C. To eliminate the chances of care is developing due to dental plaque formation
D. Cover the wider area for pontics

37. The cuspal inclines of maxillary buccal cusps and mandibular lingual cusps are ground if they are in deflective occlusal contact in:
A. Working side
B. Balancing side
C. Working and balancing side

38. The tilting of a cast during surveying is an RPD does not change the:

A. Position of undercuts
B. Path of insertion
C. Placement of clasps
D. Amount of undercut

39. The most common cause of fracture of porcelain at the porcelain metal interface is:

A. Occlusal trauma
B. Improper firing schedule
C. Failure to use a metal conditioner
D. Inadequately designed metal framework

40. Most common complaint of the patient with a thick-palatal bar in an RPD is:

A. Distortion under occlusal stress
B. Poor dissipation of force due to rigidity
C. Difficulty in pressing the food backward and swallowing
D. Loss of taste sensation

41. Over dentures are indicated over retained roots instead of extracting them and making complete dentures because:

A. To maintain the alveolus height
B. To allow proprioception from the PDL of remaining roots
C. Easier to contrust overdentures
D. Easy acceptance of patients

42. The coronoid process:

A. Limits the retention of maxillary posterior teeth setting
B. Limits the thickness of the distobuccal flange of the upper complete denture
C. Limits the thickness of the distobuccal flange of the lower complete denture
D. Determines PPS

43. Pink tooth is:

A. Chronic hyperplastic pulpitis
B. Internal resorption
C. Pulpal hyperaemia
D. Periapical abscess

44. Leutics glossitis can occur in connection with:

A. Vitamin B deficiency
B. Vitamin C deficiency
C. Iron deficiency
D. Syphilis

45. Proximal caries can be detected best with:

A. Intra-oral periapical radiographs
B. Bitewing radiographs
C. Occlusal radiographs
D. Orthopantomographs

46. The right age to begin visitis of a child to a dentist is:

A. 1 year
B. 2 years
C. 3 years
D. 4 years

47. An 11-year-old child has discomfort in tooth. On examination his gums are slightly inflamed but the tooth is mobile. There is a big class II filing but no pain with hot and cold. The most probable diagnosis is:

A. Exfoliating tooth
B. Acute pulpitis
C. Internal resorption
D. Traumatic occlusion

48. In an 8-year-old child 1st molar is extracted due to caries. The treatment of choice is:

A. RPD
B. Space maintainer
C. Surgical repositioning of 2nd molar
D. Wait for the 2nd molar to drift mesially on its own

49. The stage at which dentinogenesis imperfecta occurs is:

A. Initiation
B. Proliferation
C. Histodifferentiation
D. Morphodifferentiation

50. The permanent anterior tooth which is most commonly atypical is:

A. Maxillary central incisior
B. Maxillary lateral incisor
C. Mandibular central incisior
D. Mandibular 1st premolar

51. 1 part per million fluoride is:
A. 1 mg in 10 L of water
B. 1 mg in 1 L of water
C. 10 mg in 1 L of water
D. 100 mg in 10 L of water

52. Commonly seen changes with nutritional anaemia are:
A. Chilitis
B. Glossodynia
C. Atrophic glossitis
D. Generalised osteolysis

53. Structures passing through the sigmoid notch are:
A. Auriculotemporal nerve
B. Mandibular nerve
C. Masseteric nerve and vessels
D. Chorda tympani

54. Pterygomandibular raphe provide attachment to:
A. Superior constrictor muscle
B. Buccinator
C. Superior constrictor and buccinator muscles
D. Only a ligament with no attachments

55. The intrauterine fusion of the primary palate (lip aveolus and palate anterior to the incisive foramen) occurs at:
A. 2–4 weeks B. 4–8 weeks
C. 9–12 weeks D. 13–17 weeks

56. The major blood supply of hard palate is through:
A. Lesser palatine artery
B. Greater (anterior) palatine
C. Nasopalatine artery
D. Sphenopalatine artery

57. Loss of lamina dura and ground glass appearance indicates:
A. Paget's disease
B. Fibrous dysplasia
C. Caffey's disease
D. Osteomalacia

58. The ingredient of the fixing solution (fixer) of the X-ray is:
A. Hydroquinone B. Elon
C. Sodium bisulphite D. Acetic acid

59. **The major complaint of a patient with Eagle's syndrome is:**
   A. Blood crusted lips
   B. Xerostomia
   C. Dysphagia
   D. Excessive salivation

60. **Hutchinson's triad includes:**
   A. Hypoplasia of incisor and molar, VIII nerve motor paralysis and peg laterals
   B. Hypoplasia of incisor and molar, V nerve motor paralysis interstitial keratitis
   C. Hypoplasia of incisor and molar, VII nerve deafness and interstitial keratitis
   D. None of the above

61. **CREST syndrome includes:**
   A. Calcinosis cutis, Raynaud's phenomenon, esophageal dysfunction, sclerodactyly and telangiectasia
   B. Diabets mellitus, Raynaud's phenomenon and xerostomia
   C. Raynaud's phenomenon, Berger's disease and eosinophilia
   D. Diabetes insipidus, proteinuria

62. **Leafless fruit laden tree or cherry-blossom appearance on a sialogram indicates:**
   A. Mucoepidermoid cell carcinoma
   B. Acinar cell carcinoma
   C. Sjogren's syndrome
   D. Pleomorphic adenoma

63. **Infectious mononucleosis is caused by:**
   A. EB virus
   B. Cytomegalovirus (CMV)
   C. Herpes simplex virus (HSV)
   D. HIV

64. **Features of agranulocytosis includes:**
   A. Gingival haemorrhages
   B. Oral ulcerations
   C. Atrophic glossitis
   D. Keratosis

65. Crater-like lesions on the gingiva are indicative of:
A. Juvenile periodonitis
B. ANUG
C. Periodontitis
D. Herpetic gingivostomatitis

66. The structure which forms of the tooth within ½ hour of brushing and is derived from the saliva is?
A. Plaque
B. Pellicle
C. Material alba
D. Cuticle

67. McCall's festoons are found in:
A. Maxillary incisor region
B. Mandibular incisor region
C. Canine and premolar region
D. Molar region

68. Factor responsible for pregnancy gingivits is:
A. Hormonal imbalance
B. Microorganism associated with plaque
C. Poor oral hygiene
D. Drugs

69. PDL is thinnest at:
A. CEJ
B. Apex
C. Middle
D. None of the above

70. Knife used for gingiventomy is:
A. Kirkland
B. Orbans
C. Merifield
D. Burkitt's

71. Odontoplasty is indicated in:
A. Grade I furcation involvement
B. Grade II furcation involvement
C. Grade III furcation involvement
D. Grade IV furcation involvement

72. Thrush:
A. Occurs only in elderly
B. Is caused by a gram -ve bacteria
C. Is seen clinically as a proliferative lesion
D. Responds to nystatin

73. An iodine test is done on a lesion of the oral mucous membrane. The lesion takes up the dark-blue colour of iodine but the adjacent mucosa does not. The lesion could be:

A. Leukoplakia
B. Erosive licken planus
C. Traumatic ulcer
D. Erythroplakia

74. A disease which only affects the formation and eruption of tooth but does not cause hypoplasia is:

A. Hypoparathyroidism
B. Hyperthyroidism
C. Rickets
D. Syphilis

75. Circumvallate and fungiform papillae are denuded in:

A. Vitamin A deficiency
B. Sprue
C. Severe vitamin B complex deficiency
D. Are not denuded in any glossitis

76. The primay canines erupt:

A. After primary laterals
B. After primary 1st molars
C. After primary 2nd molar
D. Before primary 1st molar

77. The carbohydrate not associated with dental plaque is:

A. Dextrose
B. Levans
C. Glucose
D. Rhamnose

78. The foolproof method to check the success of diet counseling is:

A. Lactobacillus test
B. Snyder test
C. Vinegar test
D. None of the above

79. The percentage of toothpaste expected to be swallowed by a 2–4 years old child is:

A. 50%
B. 20%
C. 30–35%
D. 10%

80. The % reduction in caries to be expected by the application of neutral fluoride solution is:

A. 20%
B. 20–50%
C. Variable
D. 10%

81. **The length of junctional epithelium is:**
   A. 0.25–1.35 mm
   B. 0.5–0.75 mm
   C. 1.0–2.0 mm
   D. 1.0–1.5 mm

82. **The calcified mass found in the PDL are:**
   A. Cementicles
   B. Osteoblastis
   C. Cementoclasts
   D. Osteoclasts

83. **The inorganic component of sub-gingival plaque is derived from:**
   A. Saliva
   B. Crevicular fluid
   C. A and B
   D. Fluids ingested

84. **Gingivitis of pregnancy is called:**
   A. Granuloma pyogenicum
   B. Pyogenic granuloma
   C. Haemangioma
   D. Fibroma

85. **The offset angle of gracey curette between the blade and shank is:**
   A. 60°
   B. 70°
   C. 80°
   D. 90°

86. **The difference between sterilization and disinfection is that:**
   A. Disinfection kills all spores but sterilization does not
   B. Sterilization kill all spores but disinfection does not
   C. Sterilization involves chemicals and disinfection involves physical methods
   D. Sterilization is easier to achieve

87. **The grinding of teeth against each other results in:**
   A. Abrasion
   B. Attrition
   C. Erosion
   D. Cavity

88. **DNA probes:**
   A. Measures periodontal pocket depth
   B. Identify a particular microorganism
   C. Calculate the length of gingival epithelia attachment
   D. None of the above

89. **If the pocket depth is 5 mm and gingival recession is 3 mm then the total loss of attachment is:**
   A. 8 mm
   B. 3 mm
   C. 5 mm
   D. 2 mm

90. Punched-out crater-like deformities on interdental papille are due to:

A. Necrotising ulcerative gingivitis
B. Herpetic stomatitis
C. Syphilis
D. Periodontitis

91. All are the features of lefort II maxillary fractures *except*:

A. CSF rhinorrhoea
B. Malocclusion
C. Upper lip paresthesia
D. Enophthalmos

92. All are features of TMJ dislocation *except*:

A. Deafness
B. Anterior displacement of condyles
C. Anterior open bite
D. Can be reduced by applying pressure on the lower molars

93. All are features of mandibular fracture *except*:

A. Malocclusion
B. Paresthesia of lower lip
C. Fractured ends are prevented from dislocation by masticatory muscles
D. Are usually compound

94. All of the following are true of fracture healing *except*:

A. There is haematoma formation
B. Local acidic pH regulates the amount of bone resorption from fractured ends
C. Haematoma is directly calcified
D. Fibrian connective tissue replaces haematoma

95. In scurvy bone shows:

A. Slow cartilaginous growth
B. Absence of bone remodelling
C. Absence of calcification
D. Defective intercellular matrix formation

96. Battle's sign is:

A. Fracture zygoma
B. Fracture anterior cranial fossa
C. Fracture middle cranial fossa
D. Fracture condyle

97. The graft with maximum osteogenic potential is:

A. Allograft
B. Xenograft
C. Auto cortical
D. Auto cancellous

98. The type of plaque which is the most harmful in causing gingivitis?

A. Supragingival
B. Subgingival tooth attached
C. Subgingival epithelium attached
D. Free subgingival plaque

99. Surgical excision of the parotid gland endangers with of the following structures:

A. Hypoglossal nerve
B. Motor nerve of the muscles of mastication
C. External carotid artery, auriculotemporal nerve, facial nerve
D. Lesser occipital nerve and spinal accessory nerve

100. Which of the following is not hereditary?

A. Amelogenesis imperfecta
B. Cleidocranial dysostosis
C. Regional odontodysplasia
D. Dentinogenesis imperfecta

Answers

1.	B	2.	A	3.	B	4.	B
5.	A	6.	A	7.	B	8.	B
9.	B	10.	D	11.	D	12.	A
13.	B	14.	B	15.	A	16.	B
17.	D	18.	B	19.	C	20.	C
21.	A	22.	B	23.	D	24.	B
25.	A	26.	C	27.	B	28.	A
29.	B	30.	B	31.	A	32.	C
33.	D	34.	B	35.	B	36.	B
37.	A	38.	A	39.	D	40.	C
41.	A	42.	B	43.	B	44.	D
45.	B	46.	B	47.	A	48.	D
49.	C	50.	B	51.	B	52.	C
53.	C	54.	C	55.	C	56.	B
57.	B	58.	B	59.	C	60.	C
61.	A	62.	C	63.	A	64.	A
65.	B	66.	B	67.	C	68.	B
69.	C	70.	A	71.	A	72.	D
73.	C	74.	B	75.	B	76.	B
77.	D	78.	B	79.	C	80.	B
81.	A	82.	A	83.	C	84.	B
85.	B	86.	B	87.	B	88.	B
89.	A	90.	A	91.	D	92.	A
93.	C	94.	C	95.	D	96.	C
97.	D	98.	C	99.	C	100.	C

PGI Paper

1998

1. **External ear cartilage is:**
   A. Hyaline B. Elastic
   C. Fibrous D. All of the above
2. **The nerve supplying submandibular gland is:**
   A. IX B. VII
   C. XII D. V
3. **Foramen ovale transmits:**
   A. Middle meningeal artery
   B. Mandibular nerve
   C. Both of the above
   D. None of the above
4. **Which of the following is/are fan shaped?**
   A. Temporalis B. Middle constrictor
   C. Both of the above D. None of the above
5. **Parathyroid glands are supplied mostly by:**
   A. Thyroidaemia B. Superior thyroid artery
   C. Facial artery D. Inferior thyroid artery
6. **At birth spinal cord extends upto:**
   A. L_1 B. L_2
   C. L_3 D. L_4
7. **The cranial nerves which are part of parasympathetic cord via?**
   A. III, VII, IX, X B. III, VII, VIII, IX
   C. III, IV, V, VII D. VII, IX, X, XI
8. **The ganglion which is associated with the oculomotor nerve is:**
   A. Ciliary ganglion B. Superior cervical ganglion
   C. Optic ganglion D. None of the above

9. **The fat which is esterified with alcohol of high molecular weight are known as:**
   A. Waxes
   B. Oils
   C. Triglycerides
   D. Simple fats

10. **The amount of ATPs generated by glycolytic pathway is:**
   A. 6
   B. 8
   C. 10
   D. 12

11. **Glycogen breakdown leads to formation of:**
   A. Glycoprotein
   B. Lactic acid
   C. Glucose and lactic acid
   D. Glucose

12. **The lipoproteins rich in cholesterol are:**
   A. LDL
   B. HDL
   C. VLDL
   D. Chylomicron

13. **The total blood concentration of ketone bodies in well fed individual is:**
   A. 1 mg%
   B. 5 mg%
   C. 12 mg%
   D. 20 mg%

14. **At the cervical cross-section of the maxillary second premolar has which characteristic shape?**
   A. Dum bell shape
   B. Ovale shape
   C. Kidney shape
   D. Horse-shoe shape

15. **The position of maximum intercuspation of the teeth is referred to as:**
   A. Centric relation
   B. Centric organization
   C. Centric occlusion
   D. Centric position

16. **The permanent posterior tooth which has a pronounced concavity on the mesial surface of its crown is the:**
   A. Mandibular first premolar
   B. Maxillary first premolar
   C. Mandibular second premolar
   D. Maxillary second premolar

17. **The disc of the temporomandibular joint moves forward principally by:**
   A. Stylomandibular ligament
   B. Medial pterygoid muscle
   C. Condyle
   D. Lateral pterygoid muscle

18. Which of the following cement had anti-cariogenic properties?

A. Calcium hydroxide
B. ZnOE cement
C. Zinc phosphate cement
D. Zinc silicophosphate cement

19. When the porcelain is self-glazed by reheating, the best method for reducing voids is:

A. Fused porcelain cooled under process
B. The diffusible gas method
C. Partial vacuum firing method
D. All of the above

20. In method of firing:

A. A long firing period at a very high temperature is preferred
B. A large time period at a lower temperature is preferred
C. A shorter firing period at a higher temperature is considered better
D. A short firing period at a very low temperature is preferred

21. In case of subarachnoid haemorrhage investigation of choice is:

A. MRI
B. CT scan
C. Carotid angiogram
D. MRI angio with MRI imaging

22. The wavelength of electromagnetic radiation is the:

A. Amplitude of the wave
B. Time interval between two successive crests
C. Distance between two successive crests
D. Number of waves per unit of time

23. The conversion of kinetic energy into X-ray energy by the deceleration of a fast-moving electron produces:

A. Characteristic radiation
B. Particulate radiation
C. Orbital radiation
D. Bremsstrahlung radiation

24. The milliamperage (mA) affects the:

A. Cooling of the target
B. Speed at which electrons move from cathode to anode
C. Heating the filament
D. Penetrating ability of X-rays produced

25. Shortest acting local anesthetic is:

A. Bupivacaine B. Chloroprocaine
C. Xylocaine D. Procaine

26. Pre-anesthetic medication is given to:

A. To reduce amnesia
B. Reduction of secretion of saliva
C. Reduce anxiety and fear
D. All of the above

27. In the second stage of anesthesia the pupil is:

A. Normal in size B. Totally dilated
C. Partially dilated D. Constricted

28. The muscle relaxant effect of succinyl choline last for:

A. 1 minute B. 2 minutes
C. 3-5 minutes D. 10 minutes

29. The most efficient respiratory stimulant is:

A. Protheamide B. Doxapram
C. Amiphenazole D. Nikethamide

30. Basal cell carcinoma of the skin:

A. Is almost unknown in blocks
B. Is an important hazard of radiotherapy
C. Accounts for the majority of cancers on the exposed skin
D. Both A and C

31. Lepra cells are:

A. Histiocytes B. Plasma cells
C. Lymphocytes D. Neutrophils

32. Term "Pseudo" used in "Pseudocyst" is due to its:

A. Site B. Course
C. Lining D. Contents

33. Tuberculous infection spreads through following modes except:

A. Nerves B. Lymphatics
C. Direct extension D. Blood stream

34. In Hashimoto's disease, serum antibodies are mainly against:

A. Thyroglobulin B. Iodine
C. Thyroxine D. Thyroid follicles

35. Thyroglossal cyst may occasionally give rise to .... carcinoma.

A. Medullary
B. Anaplastic
C. Follicular
D. Papillary

36. Oedema is caused by fall in plasma proteins below:

A. 5%
B. 0.5%
C. 15%
D. 50%

37. A stitch abscess is usually caused by:

A. Staph aureus
B. Streptococcus
C. Staph albus
D. None of the above

38. The infection with clostridium tetani spreads via:

A. Motor nerves
B. Lymphatics
C. Blood
D. Sensory nerves

39. Tetanus results in muscle rigidity and spasms due to:

A. Simultaneous contraction of both agonists and antagonist muscles
B. Inhibition of agonist muscles and stimulation of antagonists
C. Stimulation of sensory pathways
D. Inhibition of motor pathways

40. The culture medium used for cultivation of mycobacterium tuberculosis is:

A. Ludlum's medium
B. Lowenstein Jensen medium
C. MacConkey's medium
D. None of the above

41. Tuberculosis bacilli can remain alive in sputum for:

A. 20 hours
B. 20 days
C. 2 hours
D. 20 minutes

42. In a patient with AIDS the second most common pathogen isolated is:

A. Mycobacterium tuberculosis
B. Pneumocystic carinii
C. Mycobacterium avium
D. None of the above

43. Pathogenic treponemas can be maintained in:

A. Artificial media
B. Tissue culture
C. Chick embryos
D. Rabbit testis only

44. Which of the following is a slide flocculation test?
- A. Kahn
- B. Vassermann
- C. VDRL
- D. None of the above

45. Drug used in anaphylaxis is:
- A. Antihistaminic
- B. Dopamine
- C. Norepinephrine
- D. Epinephrine

46. Drugs used for accelerated hypertension:
- A. Nitroprusside
- B. Diazoxide
- C. Trimethaphan
- D. All of the above

47. Dapsone is used in:
- A. SLE
- B. Erythema
- C. Dermatitis herpetiformis
- D. Lichen planus

48. Interneurons make up around:
- A. 12% of all neurons of the body
- B. 50% of all neurons of the body
- C. 80% of all neurons of the body
- D. 99% of all neurons of the body

49. The inhibitory neurotransmitter is:
- A. Aspartate
- B. Glutamate
- C. GABA
- D. Acetyl choline

50. Red muscle consists of:
- A. High concentration of myoglobin with oxidative fibres giving it a red colour
- B. High concentration of glycolytic fibres
- C. High concentration of haemoglobin which gives it, the red colour
- D. All of the above

51. The most common plasma protein is:
- A. Keratin
- B. Fibrinogen
- C. Globulin
- D. Albumin

52. Erythropoietin is synthesised in:
- A. Bone marrow
- B. Liver
- C. Lungs
- D. Kidney

53. The best treatment of small notches due to tooth brush abrasion is:

A. Use of dentifrice
B. Cosmetic restoration
C. Amalgam restoration
D. Elimination of the cause

54. Mechanical wear away of teeth due to functional or parafunctional habits is:

A. Ablation
B. Attrition
C. Erosion
D. Abrasion

55. Tooth split syndrome is:

A. Mulberry molars
B. Seen in amelogenesis imperfecta
C. Development of fracture lines resulting in cracking of the tooth
D. Splinting of the tooth due rampant caries

56. In a radiograph proximal caries appears as a triangular radiolucency with its apex towards:

A. Cervical margin
B. Incisal edge
C. Coronal margin
D. Dentino enamel junction

57. X-ray bite wing is used to diagnose all *except*:

A. Overhangs
B. Occlusal pit caries
C. Proximal caries
D. Poorly contoured restorations

58. Using pit and fissure sealant is:

A. Secondary prevention
B. Early diagnosis and treatment
C. Specific protection
D. Limitation of disability

59. Main objective of preventive dentistry is:

A. Secondary prevention
B. Primary prevention
C. Tertiary prevention
D. Limitation of disability

60. Electric pulp test for an immature tooth is:

A. False-positive
B. Negative
C. Positive
D. False-negative

61. In case of an intruded tooth, it is brought to its original position by:

A. Active eruption of tooth and use of ortho appliances
B. Ligation of tooth with composite after active eruption
C. Using extraction forceps and suturing the tooth at appropriate position
D. All of the above

62. A padded blow could cause:

A. Bone fracture
B. Tooth displacement or root fracture
C. Coronal fracture
D. All of the above

63. Several teeth out of alignment indicates:

A. Malocclusion B. Bone fracture
C. TMJ dislocation D. Incompetent lips

64. A patient presenting with a pulp abscess of the finger should be treated in the first instance with:

A. Incision B. Poulticing
C. Penicillin D. Chloramphenicol

65. Madura foot is:

A. An infection caused by a type of actinomyces
B. A swelling due to a stress fracture of the second metatarsal
C. An infection caused by a type of candida
D. A swelling due to an infected perforating ulcer

66. A Brodie's abscess is:

A. A type of breast abscess
B. A chronic abscess of the bone
C. An abscess arising in the inguinal lymph nodes
D. A subperiosteal abscess due to infection of the mastoid air cells

67. Pott's disease is:

A. A neuropathic joint
B. A fracture dislocation about the ankle
C. Tuberculosis of the spine
D. Traumatic osteochondritis of the spine

68. Adrenocorticosteroids administered in excess cause:

A. Osteosclerosis B. Osteoporosis
C. Osteochondritis D. Endochondral ossification

69. Philtrum of upper lip is formed mainly by:

A. Lateral nasal process
B. Maxillary process
C. Medial nasal process
D. Globular process

70. The nerve of the third arch is:

A. Mandibular nerve B. Glossopharyngeal nerve
C. Facial nerve D. Vagus nerve

71. The tongue begins to develop around:

A. 1st week of intrauterine life
B. 2nd week of intrauterine life
C. 4th week of intrauterine life
D. 9th week of intrauterine life

72. The Meckel's cartilage resorbs but its fibrocartilaginous capsule persists as all *except*:

A. Aural cartilages
B. Sphenomandibular ligament
C. Malleus
D. Sphenomalleolar ligament

73. The symphyseal cartilage ossifies:

A. At birth B. Before birth
C. 1 year after birth D. At 21 years of age

74. Which pharyngeal pouches form endocrine tissue?

A. Third pouch only B. First and third pouches
C. First pouch only D. Third and fourth pouches

75. All of the following are characteristics of first arch syndrome (mandibulofacial dysostosis) *except*:

A. Mental retardation
B. Defects in the auricle and external auditory meatus
C. Mandibular hypoplasia
D. Deafness

76. Partitioning of the oral and nasal cavities involves all of the following anatomic structures *except*:

A. The primary palate B. The nasal conchae
C. The nasal septum D. The secondary palate

77. Candida is found as commensal organism in the following *except*:

A. Vagina B. Large bowel
C. Throat D. Stomach

78. HIV patient associated candidiasis is:
A. Chronic atrophic
B. Acute pseudomembranous
C. Chronic hyperplastic
D. Chronic erythematous

79. HIV infection may result to all *except*:
A. Hodgkin's lymphoma
B. Neurological disturbances
C. Atypical ulceration
D. Non-Hodgkin's lymphomas

80. An 8-year-old boy, who has photosensitivity, shows intrinsic brown discoloration of the teeth and skin, which shows red fluorescence? In all probabilities the boy is suffering from:
A. Kwashiorkar
B. Letterer-Siwe disease
C. Porphyria
D. Argyria

81. Which of the following laboratory tests done in a patient with bleeding disordes will not give any specific prediction about platelet functions?
A. Bleeding time
B. Partial thromboplastin time
C. Prothrombin time
D. Platelet count

82. The minimal acceptable platelet count for an oral surgical procedure is:
A. 1,50,000
B. 50,000
C. 1,00,000
D. 2,50,000

83. Radiographically most of the times condensing osteitis can resemble:
A. Odontoma
B. Periapical cemental dysplasia
C. Dentinoma
D. Ameloblastic fibroma

84. Histologically is an odontoma certain cells may be found which are also found in:
A. Primordial cyst
B. Calcifying odontogenic cyst
C. Ameloblastic fibroma
D. None of the above

85. The pathologic entity which cannot be diagnosed on the basis of radiographs alone is:

A. Dentigerous cyst
B. Periapical granuloma
C. Primordial cyst
D. Odontogenic keratocyst

86. In the diagnosis of a lesion which of the diagnostic methods is the best?

A. Differential
B. Clinical examination
C. Surgical
D. History

87. Which of the following is the diagnostic characteristic of peripheral giant cell granuloma?

A. Multinuclear giant cells
B. Epithelium is atrophic in some areas
C. Keloid like enlargement
D. Mass of granulation tissue

88. The histogenesis of pleomorphic adenoma is from which cell?

A. Epithelia cell
B. Intercalated duct cell
C. Myoepithelial cell
D. Neural crest cell

89. The most important clinical sign in the diagnosis of pleomorphic adenoma is:

A. Pointing of the ear
B. Fixation
C. Pain
D. Trismus

90. Warthin's tumor is:

A. Clear cell adenoma
B. Involvement of Wharton's duct
C. Myoepithelioma
D. Papillary cystadenoma lymphomatosum

Answers

1.	B	2.	B	3.	B	4.	C
5.	D	6.	C	7.	A	8.	A
9.	A	10.	C	11.	C	12.	A
13.	A	14.	B	15.	C	16.	B
17.	D	18.	D	19.	B	20.	B
21.	B	22.	C	23.	D	24.	C
25.	B	26.	D	27.	C	28.	C
29.	B	30.	D	31.	A	32.	C
33.	A	34.	A	35.	D	36.	D
37.	C	38.	A	39.	A	40.	B
41.	A	42.	C	43.	D	44.	C
45.	D	46.	D	47.	C	48.	D
49.	C	50.	A	51.	D	52.	D
53.	D	54.	B	55.	C	56.	D
57.	B	58.	B	59.	B	60.	D
61.	A	62.	B	63.	B	64.	A
65.	A	66.	B	67.	C	68.	B
69.	D	70.	B	71.	C	72.	A
73.	C	74.	D	75.	A	76.	B
77.	D	78.	D	79.	A	80.	C
81.	A	82.	B	83.	B	84.	B
85.	B	86.	D	87.	A	88.	B
89.	A	90.	D				

PGI Paper

June 1998

1. **Acrylic resins are used for:**
   A. Anterior restorations
   B. Temporary bridges
   C. Denture bases
   D. All of the above

2. **If dentures are cleaned in boiling water they:**
   A. Become sticky
   B. Warp
   C. Melt
   D. Galvazine

3. **To repair a fractured temporary fixed bridge:**
   A. The bridge is seated in the patient's mouth and small additions of acrylic are brushed on the fractured area
   B. The bridge is seated in the patient's mouth and a large amount of acrylic is mixed and adapted around the entire bridge
   C. The bridge is removed from the patient's mouth, sticky wax is added to hold fractured pieces together and small amounts of acrylic are then added
   D. The bridge is removed from the patient's mouth, the fractured pieces are imbedded in fast setting plaster and small amounts of acrylic are added

4. **What it the main component of composite restorative materials?**
   A. Methyl methacrylate
   B. Zinc oxide
   C. Calcium hydroxide
   D. Inorganic filler

5. **The type of spatula used to mix composite is:**
   A. Plastic
   B. Stainless steel
   C. Iron
   D. None of the above

6. The chemical used to etch enamel is:
A. Zinc oxide
B. Methyl methacrylate
C. Phosphoric acid
D. Eugenol

7. The largest component of amalgam alloy is:
A. Silver
B. Tin
C. Zinc
D. Copper

8. The crushing strength of amalgam is:
A. 15,000 psi
B. 30,000 psi
C. 45,000 psi
D. 60,000 psi

9. First appearance of tooth formation occurs in:
A. 6th week IU
B. 2nd week IU
C. 9th week IU
D. 4th month IU

10. Acellular cementum is typically found in:
A. Coronal half of root
B. Apical half of root
C. Apex of root
D. Entire root

11. Specific disease caused by vitamin B, deficiency:
A. Pellagra
B. Angular cheilitis
C. Megaloblastic anaemia
D. Peripheral polyneuritis

12. Acute pulpitis is treated by:
A. Sedative filling wait and watch
B. Pulpectomy
C. Pulpotomy
D. Pulp capping

13. To prevent porosity in self-cure acrylic resin, curing should be carried in:
A. Cold water
B. Hot water
C. Under tap water
D. Under vacuum pressure

14. Maximum amount of fluoride absorption occurs from:
A. Upper GIT
B. Colon
C. Small intestine
D. Duodenum

15. **Which of the following is the method of treating internal resorption?**
    A. Extirpation of pulp and calcium hydroxide dressing
    B. Extirpation of pulp and formocresol dressing
    C. Pulpotomy
    D. Pulp capping

16. **Porosity in procelain can be prevented by:**
    A. Throroughness of condensation
    B. Rapidity of firing
    C. High firing temperature
    D. All of the above

17. **Accelerator in self-cure composites is:**
    A. Tertiary amines   B. Peroxides
    C. UV light   D. Diketones

18. **Benzoin methyl ether is activated by:**
    A. UV light   B. Visible light
    C. Diketones   D. None of the above

19. **Stepping is a phenomenon used to describe:**
    A. Class-II cavity amalgam preparation
    B. Successive root canal enlargements
    C. Condensation of gold foil
    D. All of the above

20. **Specific contraindication of extraction is:**
    A. Diabetes
    B. Radiation therapy
    C. Adrenal insufficiency
    D. Recent history of myocardial infarction

21. **Antibiotics prophylaxis is specifically indicated for:**
    A. Reflection of mucoperiosteal flap
    B. Slicing of tissue graft
    C. Gingivectomy procedures
    D. None of the above

22. **Kirkland and orbans knife are used for:**
    A. Reflection of mucoperiosteal flap
    B. Slicing of tissue graft
    C. Gingivectomy procedures
    D. None of the above

23. SABE is caused by:

A. Streptococcus mutans
B. Streptococcus viridans
C. Staphylococcus aureus
D. Staphylococcus pyogenes

24. Rectangular wire is used in:

A. Begg's technique
B. Edgewise technique
C. Both of the above
D. Ribbon arch technique

25. Composite resins in comparison to acrylic have:

A. Low compressive strength
B. High abrasive resistance
C. High water resorption
D. High polymerisation shrinkage

26. Primate spaces according to Baume are found in:

A. Mesial to upper deciduous canine and distal to lower deciduous canine
B. Mesial to upper and lower deciduous canines
C. Distal to upper and lower deciduous canines
D. Distal to upper deciduous canine and mesial to lower deciduous canine

27. Which of the following is used in mixed dentition classification of malocclusion?

A. Flush terminal plane
B. Angle's classification
C. Simon's orbital plane
D. All of the above

28. Arch shaped bone loss around maxillary molars occurs in:

A. Gingivitis
B. ANUG
C. Chronic periodontitis
D. Juvenile periodontitis

29. CPITN probe is designed by:

A. WHO
B. Nabers
C. Marques
D. Williams

30. By FDI classification right mandibular permanent canine is represented:

A. PDL
B. Cementum
C. Dentine
D. Alveolar bone

31. The first tissue to react when orthodontic forces are applied is:

A. PDL
B. Cementum
C. Dentine
D. Alveolar bone

32. Cross bite should be treated:

A. Only when result in functional disturbance
B. As early as possible
C. When all permanent teeth erupts
D. No need for correction

33. 18:8 stainless steel contains:

A. 18 percent nickel and 8 percent chromium
B. 18 percent chromium and 8 percent nickel
C. 18 percent chromium and 8 percent titanium
D. 18 percent titanium and 8 percent molybdenum

34. Doubling the cross-section of wire, range of action:

A. Increases
B. Decreases
C. No effect
D. First decreases and then increases

35. Ramfjord index is used on:

A. All permanent teeth
B. Selected six permanent teeth
C. Selected twelve permanent teeth
D. None of the above

36. Floating maxilla is typically found in:

A. Lefort I or Gurein fractures
B. Lefort II or pyramidical fractures
C. Craniomandibular dysjunction
D. All of the above

37. Bevel of the chisel should be facing:

A. Towards the side of the bone removal
B. Opposite to the side of bone removal
C. Direction of bevel is not important
D. Towards cortical plate for easy removal

38. The main aim of obturation is:
A. Fill the canal and prevent apical percolation of fluids
B. Fill the canal and prevent discolouration of teeth
C. Fill the canal to give support to restoration
D. All of the above

39. Main cause of failure of endodontic therapy:
A. Improper biomechanical preparation
B. Improper access cavity peparation
C. Incomplete obturation
D. Over extended filling

40. Material used for pulp capping is:
A. Calcium hydroxide
B. Calcium hydroxide with steroids
C. Formocresol
D. Zinc oxide eugenol

41. Guided tissue regeneration (GTR) is done in:
A. Vestibular deepening procedures
B. Frenectomy
C. Flap surgeries
D. Gingivectomy

42. Drug of given in ANUG:
A. Penicillin
B. Metronidazole
C. Both of the above
D. Tetracycline

43. Scaling is done with:
A. Scaler and files
B. Curette
C. Blade
D. Knife

44. Ankylosis of TMJ can be best viewed in:
A. Lateral oblique view
B. Lateral view
C. Transcranial
D. PA view

45. Most foolproof method of checking person given with previous dietary instruction is:
A. Lactobacillus count
B. Synder test
C. Latest dietary history
D. Patient verbal response

46. **Most common cause of pulp pathology is:**
    A. Microbes
    B. Trauma
    C. Leakage from filling materials
    D. Pressure sensation from condensation of filling materials

47. **Maximum resistance to mastication is given by which of the following?**
    A. Apical fibres
    B. Oblique fibres
    C. Transseptal
    D. Horizontal fibres

48. **Enamel fluorosis without skeletal malformation is seen with:**
    A. 1 ppm of water
    B. 2 ppm of water
    C. 3 ppm of water
    D. 4 ppm of water

49. **Haemophilia is characterised by:**
    A. Decreased bleeding and clotting time
    B. Decreased bleeding and increased clotting time
    C. Increased bleeding time and normal clotting time
    D. Normal bleeding time and increased clotting time

50. **Best way to prevent caries is:**
    A. Systemic fluoridation
    B. Fluoride mouthwash
    C. Fluoride toothpaste
    D. Fluoride prophylaxis

51. **Which of the following tissues have no reparative power?**
    A. Enamel
    B. Dentin
    C. Cementum
    D. Periodontal ligament

52. **Which of the following is the first to appear in newborn?**
    A. Streptococcus sanguis
    B. Streptococcus salivarius
    C. Streptococcus mutans
    D. Streptococcus viridans

53. **Teeth that erupts in the oral cavity within 30 days of birth are called:**
    A. Natal teeth
    B. Neonatal teeth
    C. Supernumerary teeth
    D. Succedaneous teeth

54. Brushing should be ideally started:

A. At the appearance of first tooth
B. At 2 years of age
C. After all primary teeth have erupted
D. After permanent first molars start erupting

55. Content of water in plaque is:

A. 20% B. 40%
C. 60% D. 80%

56. pH of a fully set zinc phosphate:

A. 3–4 B. 4–5
C. 6–7 D. 7–8

57. The best method to prevent initiation of caries in a four-year-old child who no accessibility to community water fluoridation is:

A. Brushing and flossing
B. 2.2% NaF tablet daily
C. 0.05% NaF mouthwash daily
D. 0.5% NaF toothpaste daily

58. Nursing bottle caries results from:

A. Drinking human milk
B. Drinking non-human milk
C. Drinking milk with sweetening additive
D. Improper feeding posture

59. Mouth breathing with enlarged adenoids and tonsils may be best described as:

A. Anatomic B. Obstructive
C. Physiologic D. Habitual

60. Most common curvature of upper lateral incisors in towards:

A. Mesially B. Distally
C. Buccally D. Lingually

61. Recommended time for acid etching before placing a pit and fissure sealant:

A. 30 sec B. 60 sec
C. 90 sec D. 120 sec

62. Child of age 2–3 years living in area of water fluoridation of 0.3 ppm. Recommended dose of fluoride daily is:

A. 1/4 gm B. 1/2 gm
C. 1 gm D. 2 gm

63. Amount of caries reduction achieved by fluoride dentifrices:

A. 20–30% B. 40–50%
C. 50–60% D. 70–80%

64. Palatal abscess most commonly results from infection of:

A. Maxillary centrals
B. Maxillary laterals
C. Maxillary canines
D. Maxillary premolars

65. Paper points are sterilised by:

A. Cold sterilisation with chemical solution
B. Boiling
C. Hot salt/glass bead sterilizer
D. All of the above

66. Candid infection is not seen in:

A. Median rhomboid glossitis
B. Geographic tongue
C. Oral thrush
D. Denture stomatitis

67. Minimum concentration of chlorhexidine needed to inhibit plaque is:

A. 0.2% B. 0.12%
C. 0.3% D. 0.4%

68. Synthesis of antibodies in plasma cells occurs in:

A. Golgi body
B. Endoplasmic reticulum
C. Nucleus
D. Mitochondria

69. All of the following are precancerous conditions *except*:

A. SLE
B. Peutz-Jeghers syndrome
C. Plummer-Vinson syndrome
D. Xeroderma

70. Radiographically 'Sequestrum' formed in osteomyelitis is:

A. More opaque than healthy bone
B. Same opaque than healthy bone

C. Less opaque than healthy bone
D. None of the above

71. The bonding seen in metal ceramics is:
A. Mechanical
B. Chemical
C. Both of the above
D. None of the above

72. Retention for prolonged period is needed in correction of:
A. Rotation
B. Protrusion
C. Retraction
D. Aligning canine into arch

73. Y-axis of Down's analysis describes:
A. The growth of maxilla
B. The growth of mandible
C. The relation maxilla and mandible
D. The relation of incisors to basal bone

74. Frankfort horizontal plane is drawn connecting:
A. Porion and orbitale
B. Orbitale and gonion
C. Gonion and gnathion
D. Nasion and porion

75. Surgical method used for retention of rotated teeth:
A. Supracestal fibrotomy
B. Frenectomy
C. Vestibuloplasty
D. All of the above

76. Dose of epinephrine in 1:20,000 concentration is:
A. 0.0125 mg
B. 0.0250 mg
C. 0.005 mg
D. 0.01 mg

77. The dose of epinephrine given in anaphylaxis:
A. 0.5 mg in 1: 1000 IM
B. 0.5 mg in 1: 10,000 IM
C. 0.5 mg in 1: 500 IM
D. 1 mg in 1:100 IM

78. Immunoglobulin implicated in atopy and anaphylaxis is:
A. IgE B. IgM
C. IgG D. IgA

79. Barbed broach is used for:
A. Extirpation of pulp
B. Enlargement of canal
C. Obturation of canals
D. All of the above

80. Movement of articular disks is controlled by:
A. Temporomandibular ligament
B. Stylomandibular ligament
C. Superior head of lateral pterygoid
D. Inferior head of lateral pterygoid

81. Wide fontenells, slanted eyes, macroglossia and hypoplasia of maxilla are seen in:
A. Down's syndrome
B. Osteopetrosis
C. Treacher Collins syndrome
D. Craniofacial dysostosis

82. Cyclosporine enlargement of gingiva can be classified as:
A. Noninflammatory
B. Inflammatory
C. Developmental
D. Malignant

83. Marked ridge resorption occurs in:
A. Chronic gingivitis
B. Chronic destructive periodontitis
C. Vitamin-B deficiency
D. Vitamin-A deficiency

84. Success of reimplanted avulsed tooth depends on:
A. Proper antibiotic coverage
B. Prevention of dehydration of PD ligament of avulsed tooth
C. Protection of socket
D. All of the above

85. Secondary peripheral seal area in mandible is provided by:
A. Buccal shelf

B. Anterior lingual border
C. Retromolar pad
D. Crest of the ridge

86. Mouth temperature waxes are:
A. Iowa wax
B. Modelling wax
C. Green stick wax
D. None of the above

87. Which of the following is a self correcting anomaly?
A. Ugly duckling stage
B. Deepbite
C. Retrusion
D. Protrusion

88. Most common movement during orthodontic treatment is:
A. Intrusion
B. Tipping
C. Extrusion
D. Bodily movement

89. In a 9-year-old child, caries is commonly seen on:
A. Occlusal surface of lower permanent first molar
B. Occlusal surface of upper permanent first molar
C. Distal surface of lower permanent first molar
D. Mesial surface of upper permanent first molar

90. Space closure is rapid following loss of which primary molars?
A. Maxillary molars; closing within three months
B. Mandibular molars; closing within six months
C. Maxillary molars; closing within six months
D. Mandibular molars; closing within three months

91. According to WHO minimum amount of fluoride that should be present in salt for effective anticaries activity in:
A. 3 mg of F/5 gm of salt
B. 1.5 mg of F/5 gm of salt
C. 10 mg of F/5 gm of salt
D. 100 mg of F/5 gm of salt

92. Which of the following is the nerve of third branchial arch?
A. Facial nerve
B. Trigeminal
C. Vagus
D. Glossopharyngeal

93. The most common cause of amalgam failure is:
A. Poor condensation B. Incorrect mixing
C. Incorrect preparation D. Not polishing the restoration

94. What is the working time of amalgam?
A. One to two minutes B. Three to four minutes
C. Five to six minutes D. Seven to eight minutes

95. The most frequent complaint of patient shortly after amalgam restoration are placed is:
A. Pain on percussion
B. An open contact point
C. Numbness around the gingiva
D. Numbness around the gingiva

96. An advantage of using a gold restoration rather than an amalgam restoration is:
A. The ease of tooth preparation
B. Better adaptation to the walls of the preparation
C. The greater edge strength of cast gold
D. It is less expensive

97. Flux is used during casting to:
A. Remove the oxides formed on the gold alloy
B. Lower the melting point
C. Replace casting wax
D. Speed the burnout process

98. Pickling:
A. Is accomplished by soaking the casting in baking soda
B. Caused porosity in gold
C. Removes surface oxides from gold castings
D. Removes investment from gold castings

99. A problem with a porcelain jacket is it:
A. Is not color stable
B. Is very brittle
C. Has a very high compression strength
D. Is irritating to the gingiva

100. Stainless steel is used most in dentistry:
A. To strengthen amalgam
B. In orthodontic wires
C. To construct clasps for partial dentures
D. To replace internal gold restorations

Answers

1.	D	2.	B	3.	A	4.	D
5.	A	6.	C	7.	A	8.	C
9.	A	10.	A	11.	D	12.	A
13.	D	14.	A	15.	A	16.	A
17.	A	18.	A	19.	C	20.	D
21.	D	22.	C	23.	B	24.	B
25.	B	26.	A	27.	A	28.	D
29.	A	30.	D	31.	A	32.	B
33.	B	34.	B	35.	B	36.	A
37.	A	38.	A	39.	C	40.	A
41.	C	42.	C	43.	A	44.	C
45.	C	46.	A	47.	B	48.	C
49.	D	50.	A	51.	A	52.	A
53.	B	54.	A	55.	D	56.	C
57.	B	58.	C	59.	B	60.	B
61.	B	62.	B	63.	B	64.	B
65.	C	66.	B	67.	B	68.	B
69.	D	70.	A	71.	C	72.	A
73.	B	74.	A	75.	A	76.	C
77.	A	78.	A	79.	A	80.	A
81.	A	82.	A	83.	B	84.	D
85.	B	86.	A	87.	A	88.	B
89.	A	90.	D	91.	B	92.	D
93.	C	94.	B	95.	C	96.	C
97.	A	98.	C	99.	B	100.	B

PGI Paper

1997

1. **In an LA solution of 1:200,00 adrenaline, the amount of latter is:**
   A. 0.5 mg/ml B. 0.05 mg/ml
   C. 0.0005 mg/ml D. 0.005 mg/ml

2. **Barbed broaches are used for:**
   A. Canal preparation B. Pulp extirpation
   C. Canal location D. Obturation

3. **The treatment of internal resorption is:**
   A. Ca $(OH)_2$ pulpotomy
   B. Extraction
   C. Pulp capping
   D. Endodontic therapy

4. **The ingredient which gives glossiness and reduces flow of an inlay wax is:**
   A. Ceresin B. Carnauba wax
   C. Paraffin wax D. Gum dummar

5. **The temperature of the mouth is:**
   A. Variable
   B. Lower than rest of the body
   C. Same as rest of the body
   D. Higher than rest of the body

6. **In anaphylaxis the immunoglobulin commonly involved is:**
   A. IgG B. IgA
   C. IgE D. IgM

7. **Rinsing of the impression is important to:**
   A. Remove saliva
   B. Remove excess impression material
   C. Hydrate the impression
   D. Accelerate the setting

8. **The composite resins are superior to acrylic resins in that composite resins:**
   - A. Have no filler particles
   - B. Have a different method of curing
   - C. Greater resistance to wear
   - D. None of the above

9. **Vitamin B_1 deficiency can lead to:**
   - A. Pernicious anemia
   - B. Glossitis
   - C. Peripheral neuritis
   - D. Dermatitis

10. **Candida infection is involved in:**
    - A. Median rhomboid glossitis
    - B. Migrating geographic tongue
    - C. Prolonged tetracycline therapy
    - D. All of the above

11. **Floating maxilla is found in:**
    - A. Zygomatic fracture
    - B. Guerin fracture
    - C. Craniofacial dysjunction
    - D. Pyramidal fracture

12. **Acellular cementum is found in:**
    - A. Radicular half
    - B. Coronal two-thirds
    - C. Coronal half
    - D. Radicular two-thirds

13. **Response to pulp to stimuli is in the form of:**
    - A. Loss of vitality
    - B. Pain
    - C. Increase in temperature
    - D. Formation of pulp stones

14. **Which of the following cells cannot regenerate?**
    - A. Fibroblasts
    - B. Basal cells of the oral mucous membrane
    - C. Mesenchymal cells
    - D. Ameloblasts

15. **Sequestrum appears in the radiograph:**
    - A. More opaque
    - B. Radiolucent
    - C. Less opaque
    - D. Sun-ray pattern

16. **Ridge resorption increases in:**
   A. Vitamin D deficiency
   B. Parathormone deficiency
   C. Periodontitis
   D. Increase in hormone calcitonin

17. **SABE is caused by:**
   A. Beta hemolytic Streptococci
   B. Alpha hemolytic (viridans) Streptococci
   C. Gamma hemolytic Streptococci
   D. Bacteroides

18. **Which of the following have the capability to produce extracellular polysaccharides?**
   A. Strep. Pyogenes
   B. Strep mutans
   C. Peptostreptococcus
   D. Enterococcus

19. **Cyclosporin is used as an:**
   A. Anti-cancer drug
   B. Anti-arrhythmic
   C. Immunosuppressant
   D. Antibiotic

20. **Child should start brushing at the age of:**
   A. 1 year
   B. 8 months
   C. 2 years
   D. 4 years

21. **Acid-etching is done for:**
   A. 30 seconds
   B. 60 seconds
   C. 90 seconds
   D. 120 seconds

22. **Pit and fissure sealants are contraindicating in:**
   A. Deep pit and fissures
   B. Incipient pit and fissure caries
   C. After fluoride application
   D. Deep pit and fissures of patients with low caries incidence

23. **The most effective method to decrease caries is:**
   A. Use of floss
   B. Tooth brushing after meals
   C. Use of pit and fissure sealants
   D. Regular dental check-ups

24. Systemic water fluoridation reduces caries:
A. By 25"
B. Only on smooth surfaces
C. Is possible only in advanced countries
D. On smooth surfaces and pit and fissures

25. Which of the following silver amalgam alloys have the maximum strength?
A. Lathe cut
B. Spherical
C. Single composition
D. Admixed

26. The obstruction caused due to enlarged adenoids and tonsils results in:
A. Physiologic mouth breathing
B. Anatomic mouth breathing
C. Both A and B
D. None of the above

27. Which of the following is a self-correcting malocclusion?
A. Anterior open-bite
B. Incisor cross-bite
C. Ugly-duckling stage
D. Anterior crowding

28. Primate spaces are found between:
A. Distal to upper deciduous canine
B. Mesial to upper deciduous canine
C. Between upper deciduous canine and deciduous first molar
D. Mesial to lower deciduous canine

29. Which of the following is more prone to osteomyelitis?
A. Zygoma
B. Palatine bone
C. Mandible
D. Maxilla

30. Fluorides are absorbed by the:
A. Colon
B. Jejunum
C. Ileum
D. Stomach

31. The acid in saliva is neutralised by:
A. H_3PO_4
B. Proteins
C. Carbon dioxide
D. HCO_3

32. **pH of the liquid of zinc phosphate cement is:**
A. 4.5 B. 3.4
C. 6.7 D. 8.9

33. **Articular disc of TMJ receives insertion from which muscle?**
A. Masseter B. Temporalis
C. Lateral pterygoid D. Medial pterygoid

34. **Stainless steel contains:**
A. 18% Cr. 8% Ni B. 14% Cr. 7% Ni
C. 8% Cr. 18% Ni D. 16% Cr. 8% Ni

35. **The polymerisation of self-curing resin takes place faster in:**
A. Hot water B. Cold water
C. In vacuum D. Under pressure

36. **The using shrinkage while firing porcelain can be reduced by:**
A. Vacuum firing
B. Increasing the temperature of firing
C. Uniform particle size
D. Decreasing the temperature of firing

37. **The porcelain metal bond is:**
A. Mechanical B. Chemical
C. Both A and B D. None of the above

38. **The GTR technique can be used with:**
A. Frenectomy B. Vestibuloplasty
C. Gingivectomy D. Periodontal flap technique

39. **Generally pulp capping is done with:**
A. ZOE B. Calcium hydroxide
C. Silver amalgam D. Camphorated phenol

40. **The treatment of acute pulpitis is:**
A. Pulpotomy B. Extraction
C. PA curettage D. Pulpectomy

41. **Paper points are sterilised by:**
A. Autoclave
B. Hot-air oven
C. Hot-bead steriliser
D. Incineration

42. The anchorage in a removable appliance is provided by:

A. Pin-head clasp
B. Adam's clasp
C. Teeth and acrylic base
D. Reciprocal

43. The root of maxillary lateral incisor is most commonly curved:

A. No curvature
B. Palataly
C. Mesially
D. Distally

44. Palatal abscess most commonly follows the pulpal necrosis of:

A. Maxillary premolar
B. Maxillary lateral incisor
C. Maxillary third molar
D. Maxillary central incisor

45. Which of the following can reduce a relapse in rotation?

A. Supracrestal fibrotomy
B. Retentive appliance for 3 months
C. Both A and B
D. None of the above

46. Cross-bite should be treated:

A. At the age of 12 years
B. At the age of 8 years
C. When noticed
D. At the age of 6 years

47. The first tooth develops:

A. 4 weeks IU
B. 6 weeks IU
C. 8 weeks IU
D. 10 weeks IU

48. Combinations of deposition and resorption occurring in the different bones of the skull which result in a growth movement towards the deposition surface is termed as:

A. Displacement
B. Physiologic resorption
C. Drift
D. Remodeling

49. Retentive appliance for cross-bite is:

A. Not required
B. Crib
C. Hawley's appliance
D. None of the above

50. The best radiographic view for TMJ is:
A. Water's view B. OPG
C. PA view D. Lateral oblique

51. The incision for drainage in Ludwig's angina extends:
A. Floor of mouth
B. To the angle of the mandible
C. Up to the neck
D. All of the above

52. Clotting time is increased in:
A. Scurvy B. Haemophilia
C. Vascular purpura D. Thrombocytopenic purpura

53. The most abundant group of fibres in the PDL are:
A. Oblique B. Horizontal
C. Transseptal D. Apical

54. Rectangular wire is used in:
A. Begg's technique
B. Edgewise technique
C. Tipping movements
D. None of the above

55. In which orthodontic movement utmost control is required?
A. Tipping B. Rotation
C. Extrusion D. Intrusion

56. Mixed dentition analysis was described by:
A. Tweed B. Moyer's
C. Angle D. Graber

57. Activation of benzoin methyl ether takes place by:
A. UV light B. Hydroquinone
C. Infra-red light D. Visible light

58. The resiliency of an orthodontic wire as regards to its cross-section will:
A. Increase with an increase in the cross-sectional area
B. Remain the same
C. Decrease with an increase in the cross-sectional area
D. Independent of the cross-sectional area

59. The activator in the self-curing resin is:
A. Hydroquinone B. Methyl methacrylate
C. Tertiary amine D. Benzoyl peroxide

60. The term stepping is associated with:

A. Direct gold condensation
B. Silver amalgam condensation
C. Fracture mandible
D. Root canal preparation

61. The factor important in wound irrigation is:

A. Antiseptic content
B. Volume of irrigant
C. Chelating properties
D. Concentration of the irrigant

62. Anterior open fontanelles, slanting eyes, macroglossia, sexual impairment are characteristic seen in:

A. Turner's syndrome
B. Eagle's syndrome
C. Klinefelter's syndrome
D. Down's syndrome

63. The amount of caries reduction achieved by fluoride containing dentifrices is:

A. 20-30% B. 35-50%
C. 40% D. 60%

64. The amount of water in plaque is:

A. 30% B. 40%
C. 60% D. 80%

65. The amount of fluoride required in common salt for caries reduction is:

A. 200 mg/kg B. 350 mg/kg
C. 90 mg/kg D. 100 mg/kg

66. In a patient of RHD, when is it not essential to premedicate with antibiotics?

A. Intraoral fracture reduction
B. Sealing and root planning
C. Extraction
D. Mucogingival surgery

67. The antibiotic most useful in the treatment of ANUG is:

A. Erythromycin
B. Bacitracin
C. Metronidazole
D. Streptomycin

68. In the FDI system, the mandibular right canine is designated as:

A. 13 B. 23
C. 33 D. 43

69. Are-like defects on the radiograph in the first molar area are seen in:

A. Desquamative gingivitis
B. Juvenile periodontitis
C. Chronic gingivitis
D. Chronic periodontitis

70. Minimum therapeutic concentration of chlorhexidine in mouth wash is:

A. 2 mg/ml B. 1.2 mg/ml
C. 0.12 mg/ml D. 0.2 mg/ml

71. Amount of fluoride supplement to a 2-3 years old child in a fluoride deficient area is:

A. 1.0 mg B. 2.0 mg
C. 0.25 mg D. 0.5 mg

72. Elective endodontic treatment is contraindicated in:

A. Diabetes B. Hypertension
C. Recent MI D. Angina patients

73. Kirkland and Orban knives are used for:

A. Gingivectomy B. Flap elevation
C. Oral prophylaxis D. Curettage

74. The teeth present in the oral cavity of a newborn are called:

A. Infantile teeth B. Ghost teeth
C. Neonatal teeth D. Enamel pearls

75. Earliest microorganism to invade an infants oral cavity are:

A. S. salivarus B. S. Mitis
C. S. mutans D. S. Sanguis

76. Secondary peripheral seal of a mandibular complete denture is formed by:

A. Labial flange
B. Retromolar area
C. Distobuccal flange
D. Lingual flange

77. Which of the following is precancerous lesion?

A. Pemphigus B. White sponge nevus
C. Lichen planus D. Erythroplakia

78. The Community Periodontal Index of Treatment Needs uses which probe?

A. CPITN probe B. Russel's probe
C. Both A and B D. None of the above

79. The direction of the bevel of the chisel during bone cutting is:

A. Parallel to stress lines
B. Independent of bone to be sacrified
C. Towards the bone to be sacrificed
D. Away from the bone to be sacrified

80. Most common cause of RCT failure:

A. Large size of PA pathology
B. Incomplete debridement with improper obturation
C. Incomplete removal of PA cyst
D. Non-obturation of accessory canals

81. The function of plasma cell:

A. Opsonisation B. Antibody formation
C. Phagocytosis D. CMI

Answers

1.	D	2.	B	3.	D	4.	B
5.	B	6.	C	7.	A	8.	C
9.	C	10.	C	11.	D	12.	C
13.	B	14.	D	15.	A	16.	C
17.	B	18.	B	19.	C	20.	C
21.	B	22.	C	23.	B	24.	B
25.	C	26.	B	27.	C	28.	B
29.	C	30.	D	31.	D	32.	B
33.	C	34.	A	35.	A	36.	C
37.	C	38.	D	39.	B	40.	D
41.	B	42.	C	43.	D	44.	B
45.	A	46.	C	47.	D	48.	C
49.	A	50.	B	51.	A	52.	B
53.	A	54.	B	55.	D	56.	B
57.	A	58.	A	59.	D	60.	A
61.	B	62.	D	63.	A	64.	D
65.	B	66.	B	67.	C	68.	D
69.	B	70.	C	71.	D	72.	C
73.	A	74.	C	75.	A	76.	C
77.	D	78.	A	79.	C	80.	B
81.	B						

PGI Paper June 1995

1. **Submandibular salivary gland is:**
   A. Purely serous
   B. Purely mucous
   C. Mixed but predominantly serous
   D. Mixed but predominantly mucous
2. **Generalised hypercementosis seen in:**
   A. Paget's disease
   B. Hypothyroidism
   C. Trauma
   D. All of the above
3. **The most common radiopaque mass at root apex of a vital tooth is due to:**
   A. Hypercementosis
   B. Condensing osteitis
   C. Periapical cemental dysplasia
   D. Cementoma
4. **Anterior fontanelle closes at:**
   A. Birth
   B. 18 months – 2 years
   C. 3 – 4 months
   D. 1 year
5. **Flux used in dental ceramics is:**
   A. Alumina B. Silica
   C. Kaolin D. Boric oxide
6. **Mc Kay discovered colorado stain in:**
   A. 1901 B. 1897
   C. 1908 D. 1930

7. Infants acquire adult hemoglobin level at:

A. Birth
B. End of 1st year
C. Puberty
D. 4 years

8. Interocclusal space is:

A. Space between upper and lower teeth
B. Space between maxilla and mandible at rest
C. Space between the jaws when muscles elevate and depress the mandible are in minimum tonic contraction
D. None of the above

9. In nursing bottle syndrome, mandibular incisors are protected from caries because:

A. Lower teeth are resistant to acidogenic bacteria
B. Submandibular secretions are adjacent to lower teeth
C. Lower teeth have more interdental spacing
D. All of the above

10. Bacteria responsible for progression of periodontitis are:

A. Gram +ve and Gram -ve cocci
B. Spirochaetes and Gram -ve aerobes
C. Anaerobes (motile)
D. Gram –ve Bacilli

11. Bacteria responsible for root surface caries:

A. Actinomyces
B. Lactobacillus
C. Streptococcus
D. Spirochaete

12. Bacteria responsible for initiation of caries is:

A. Actinomyces
B. Strep. mutans
C. Lactobacillus
D. Strep. viridans

13. Bacteria which first penetrate pocket wall are:

A. Gram +ve
B. Spirochaetes
C. Gram -ve
D. All of the above

14. Using pit and fissure sealant is:

A. Specific protection
B. Early diagnosis and treatment
C. Secondary prevention
D. Limitation of disability

15. Main objective of preventive dentistry is:

A. Primary prevention
B. Secondary prevention
C. Tertiary prevention
D. All of the above

16. **Meckel's cartilage gives rise to:**
   A. Condylar process
   B. Coronoid process
   C. Rest of ramus
   D. None of the above

17. **1.23% of APF contains:**
   A. 1.23 ppm B. 12.3 ppm
   C. 123 ppm D. 12,300 ppm

18. **Main objective of oral health programme by year 2000 is:**
   A. Caries free mouth
   B. No caries up to 12 years of age
   C. DMF<3, up to 12 years of age
   D. None of the above

19. **Knutson's technique utilizes:**
   A. 1.23% APF
   B. 8% SnF 2
   C. 2% NaF
   D. Any of the above

20. **Colour dry detector is used for:**
   A. Detecting incipient carious lesions
   B. Caries susceptibility
   C. Differentiating between active and arrested carious lesion
   D. All of the above

21. **In acute fluoride toxicity we use:**
   A. Vinegar B. Milk
   C. Water D. $NaHCO_3$

22. **In an ideal restoration, gingival margin should be:**
   A. Below contact point but 1 mm occlusal to gingival crest
   B. Below contact point but at level of gingival crest
   C. Below gingival crest
   D. At contact point

23. **Electric pulp test for an immature tooth is:**
   A. Positive B. Negative
   C. False-positive D. False-negative

24. **In an endodontically treated tooth:**
   A. Resorption is more as compared to a normal tooth
   B. Resorption is less

C. Resorption is same
D. Resorption is more after 2 years

25. As compared to permanent tooth, root formation in primary tooth:
A. Takes less time
B. Takes more time
C. Same time
D. Is complete when tooth erupts in oral cavity

26. In primary tooth intrusion is common because:
A. Alveolar bone is pliable
B. Vertical overlap of teeth
C. Lip protection to max. anterior
D. All of the above

27. Electric pulp test:
A. Requires more current for anterior teeth
B. Requires more current for posterior teeth
C. Same response
D. Better in inflamed teeth

28. A person experiences throbbing pain at night. It is due to:
A. Acute pulpal degeneration
B. Acute periodontal abscess
C. Chronic pulpitis
D. Cellulitis

29. Pain due to acute irreversible pulpitis is:
A. Spontaneous
B. Sharp-shock like
C. Lasting for short time
D. Continuous

30. Local anaesthetic is not effective in an inflamed tissue because:
A. All impulses generated cannot be blocked
B. Myelin sheath is inflamed so it does not absorb the solution
C. pH is more acidic, so LA is ineffective
D. All of the above

31. Lidocaine is metabolised by:

A. Liver
B. Plasma
C. Kidney
D. None of the above

32. First radiological sign:

A. Wedge-shaped radiolucencies
B. Loss of crestal bone
C. No sign
D. Loss of lamina dura

33. Light radiographic film is due to:

A. Overdeveloping
B. Overfixing
C. Directly putting in fixer
D. Exposure to sunlight

34. Diagnosis of bone defect is done accurately by:

A. Clinical examination
B. Radiographs
C. Surgical exposure
D. Probing

35. Diagnosis of dry socket is done by:

A. History
B. Clinical examination
C. Radiographs
D. None of the above

36. Pain of dry socket is experienced on:

A. 1st day after extraction
B. 2nd day after extraction
C. 3rd day after extraction
D. After 7 days

37. Majority of surveyors have following components:

A. Vertical arm
B. Horizontal arm
C. Level platform
D. All of the above

38. In which area of oral cavity, leukoplakia has the greatest malignant potential?

A. Floor of mouth
B. Buccal mucosa

C. Lips
D. Palate

39. Which of the following tell about maxillo-mandibular relationship?

A. SNA
B. SNB
C. IMPA
D. ANB

40. Decreased intrinsical angle indicates:

A. Retrusion of teeth
B. Protrusion of teeth
C. Vertical overlap
D. Horizontal overlap

41. Deep skeletal bite will show which of the following features?

A. High mandibular plane
B. Low mandibular plane
C. Deep palate
D. All of the above

42. In mixed dentition analysis, which tooth is used for classification?

A. Primary 1st molar
B. Primary 2nd molar
C. Permanent 1st molar
D. B or C

43. In Angle's classification for malocclusion, key tooth is:

A. MB cusp of permanent Mx. 1st molar
B. DB cusp of permanent Mx. 1st molar
C. MB cusp of permanent Mx. 2nd molar
D. MB cusp of permanent Md. 1st molar

44. A disease seen in excess of normal in a community results in:

A. Epidemic
B. Endemic
C. Pandemic
D. Endozootic

45. In school water fluoridation, amount of F used is:

A. 0.7–1.2 ppm
B. 1.6–3 ppm
C. 3–4 ppm
D. 12 ppm

46. Most common cancer in India is:

A. Breast
B. Lung
C. Oral
D. Cervix

47. **Cancer which most commonly metastases to jaw bones is:**
A. Breast
B. Prostate
C. Lung
D. Kidney

48. **A 3-year-old child living in area with 0.8 ppm F in water should be given F tablet daily:**
A. 0.25 mg
B. 1 mg
C. 0.5 mg
D. 0.00 mg

49. **In following conditions antibiotic cover should be given prior to any dental procedure:**
A. Ischaemic heart disease
B. Hypertension
C. Congenital heart disease
D. All of the above

50. **Characteristic pathological feature of rheumatic fever is/are:**
A. Joint pains
B. Fever
C. Aschoff Nodules
D. All of the above

51. **Psoriasis is associated with:**
A. Geographic tongue
B. Benign median rhomboid glossitis
C. Lupus erythematosus
D. Lupus vulgaris

52. **Chronic irritation at denture borders results in:**
A. Epulis fissuratum
B. Candidiasis
C. Hyperplasia
D. None of the above

53. **Epstein-Barr virus causes:**
A. Paget's disease
B. Burkitt's lymphoma
C. Osteosarcoma
D. None of the above

54. **Most common cells seen in periodontal ligament is:**
A. Monocyte
B. Melanocyte
C. Fibroblast
D. All of the above

55. During orthodontic tooth movement, periodontal ligament provides:

A. Osteoblasts
B. Osteoclasts
C. Both A and B
D. None of the above

56. Anchorage in removable appliance is provided by:

A. Acrylic base only
B. Teeth
C. Acrylic base and teeth
D. Retentive clasps

57. In FPD, retention is provided by:

A. Cement
B. Parallel walls
C. Grooves
D. Proximal slice

58. Amount of gap required for cement in restoration is:

A. 10–25 µm
B. 2 µm
C. 50–100 µm
D. No gap required

59. Which is the cement with adhesive properties?

A. Zinc oxide eugenol
B. Zinc polycarboxylate
C. Silicate
D. Glass isomer

60. Cement with maximum resistance to disintegration and solubiilty is:

A. Zn phosphate
B. Polycarboxylate
C. Resin
D. GIC

61. Advantage between zinc free and zinc containing amalgam is:

A. Better handling property
B. Dimensional stability
C. Resistance to creep
D. Toxicity to pulp and dentin

62. Cause of expansion in zinc containing amalgam is:

A. Zinc + water
B. Water
C. Hydrogen
D. Nascent oxygen

63. Which substance is used as sealant for obturation of primary teeth?

A. Gutta-percha
B. Silver cones
C. Zinc oxide eugenol
D. Amalgam

64. Maximum development of face takes place in:
A. 1st to 3rd week of IUL
B. 3rd to 8th week of IUL
C. 9th to 12th week of IUL
D. After 12th week of IUL

65. Most commonly retained primary teeth is:
A. Maxillary molar
B. Maxillary anteriors
C. Mandibular molar
D. Mandibular anteriors

66. Turner's hypoplasia most commonly affects:
A. Deciduous maxillary anteriors
B. Deciduous mandibular anteriors
C. Permanent maxillary anteriors
D. Permanent mandibular anteriors

67. Tetracycline staining will occur if child is given the drug in:
A. 1–3 months of IUL
B. 3–6 months of IUL
C. 6–9 months of IUL
D. At birth

68. Immediate swelling after local dental infection is due to:
A. Vascular injection
B. Allergy
C. Infection
D. Paravascular injection

69. Pink tooth is due to:
A. External resorption
B. Inernal resorption
C. Pulpal hyperplasia
D. Pulp stones

70. Histologically proximal caries is seen as:
A. Pyramid shaped lesion with base at extenal surface
B. Pyramid shaped lesion with base facing internally

C. Cone shaped
D. None of the above

71. Chlorhexidine is used in concentration of:
A. 0.2% B. 0.02%
C. 0.4% D. 0.7%

72. In MPDS which muscle goes in spasm:
A. Medial pterygoid
B. Lateral pterygoid
C. Masseter
D. Temporalis

73. Following is derivative of dental lamina:
A. Epithelial rests of Malassez
B. Enamel pearls
C. Rests of serrate
D. All of the above

74. Primary teeth differ from permanent teeth in following aspects:
A. Thickness of enamel and dentin
B. Pulp chambers are longer
C. Roots are flaring
D. All of the above

75. In hot salt steriliser, time and temperature for sterilisation is:
A. 480°F for 10 seconds
B. 425–475°F for 5 seconds
C. 480°F for 5 seconds
D. 425–475°F for 10 seconds

76. Which root canal is most difficult to prepare in maxillary molar?
A. Mesiobuccal
B. Distobuccal
C. Palatal
D. Both A and B

77. Earliest sign of gingivitis is:
A. Mobility
B. Pocket formation
C. Bleeding on probing
D. Change of colour

78. **Main aim of root planing is to remove:**
A. Plaque
B. Calculus
C. Necrotic cementum
D. All of the above

79. **Primary objective for not extracting primary teeth is:**
A. To prevent arch length deficiency
B. Mastication and speech
C. To prevent development of aberrant oral habits
D. All of the above

80. **Amount of reduction in dental caries achieved by denitrifices is:**
A. 20–35%
B. 35–40%
C. 40–50%
D. 50–60%

81. **For obtaining functional impression for RPD:**
A. Teeth are recorded in anatomical form and ridge in functional form
B. Teeth are recorded in functional form and ridge in anatomical form
C. Teeth and ridge are recorded both in anatomical and functional form
D. None of the above

82. **In primary molars when proximal portion of class II cavity preparation extends deep gingivally, a satisfactory gingival seat is not obtained because:**
A. Enamel rods extend occlusally in gingival third
B. Buccal and lingual surfaces cover occlusally
C. Primary teeth have marked cervical constriction
D. All of the above

83. **In primary teeth, gingival seat in a class II preparation is:**
A. Left unbevelled
B. Bevelled so as to remove caries
C. Bevelled so as to remove unsupported enamel rods
D. Bevelled same as permanent tooth

84. **Easy fatigability of muscles seen in:**
A. Epilepsy
B. MPDS
C. Myasthenia gravis
D. Cerebral palsy

85. Most accurate reproducible relationship for recording jaw relations is:
A. Physiologic rest position
B. Centric occlusion
C. Centric relation
D. Both B and C

86. With age, mandibular ridge expands because:
A. No resorption occurs at buccal aspect
B. Resorption occurs at buccal aspect
C. Decreased bone deposition at lingual aspect
D. Both A and C

87. In a newborn child we generally see:
A. Maxillary protrusion
B. Maxillary retrusion
C. Mandibular protrusion
D. Mandibular retrusion

88. For zygomatic arch fracture, best view is:
A. Water's view
B. Towne's projection
C. Submentovertex
D. Lateral oblique view

89. Which of the following cannot be seen radiographically?
A. Interproximal caries
B. Deep caries
C. Root caries
D. None of the above

90. In orthodontic tooth movement which is involved?
A. Osteoblast
B. Osteoclast
C. Both A and B
D. None

91. Fluoride is least effective in which area?
A. Cusp
B. Pits and fissures
C. Buccal areas
D. Palatal area

92. Source of Ca^{++} in dentinal bridge is:
A. Blood
B. $Ca(OH)^{-}$
C. Saliva
D. ICF

Answers

1.	C	2.	A	3.	D	4.	B
5.	D	6.	C	7.	A	8.	A
9.	B	10.	C	11.	A	12.	B
13.	B	14.	B	15.	A	16.	D
17.	D	18.	B	19.	C	20.	A
21.	B	22.	A	23.	D	24.	C
25.	C	26.	A	27.	B	28.	A
29.	A	30.	C	31.	A	32.	D
33.	C	34.	C	35.	A	36.	C
37.	D	38.	A	39.	D	40.	B
41.	A	42.	C	43.	A	44.	B
45.	C	46.	C	47.	A	48.	D
49.	C	50.	C	51.	A	52.	A
53.	B	54.	C	55.	C	56.	C
57.	B	58.	A	59.	B	60.	C
61.	A	62.	C	63.	C	64.	B
65.	C	66.	C	67.	B	68.	A
69.	B	70.	A	71.	A	72.	B
73.	A	74.	D	75.	D	76.	A
77.	C	78.	C	79.	A	80.	A
81.	A	82.	C	83.	A	84.	C
85.	C	86.	D	87.	D	88.	C
89.	D	90.	C	91.	B	92.	A

Golden Points
(Last Minute Revision)

1. A person using vitamin C chewing gum cannot manifest xerostomia.
2. Cariogram was introduced by Brathall in 1994.
3. In normal distribution curve the (SD-/+2) exclude 4.6% of values i.e.100%-95.4% = 4.6%.
4. Caries incidence = caries increment = caries activity = caries attack rate.
5. Prevalence is defined as proportion of population affected by diseases.
6. The effectiveness of systemic fluoridation in caries reduction is 60%.
7. Ideal dentist to patient ratio is 1:2000 according to Bhore committee.
8. According to WHO, the DMF index criteria for 12 years age by year 2012 and 2025 will be 1 and 0.
9. Salt fluoridation is 0.25 mg/kg of salt.
10. Maximum part of Leeway space is provided by primary second molar.
11. A variation of 18-24 months is considered normal during eruption of permanent molar.
12. Deep fascia is the structure which is absent on face.
13. Cases of hemangioma are most commonly associated with head and nek region.
14. Hyperthyroidism is the endocrine disorder which affects eruption timing without causing hypoplasia.
15. APTT is prolonged in case of Haemophilia A.
16. Prothrombin time is used to checkout status of anticoagulant therapy.
17. Glanzmann disease is characterized by normal platelet count but increased bleeding time.
18. Growth of maxilla occurs in downward and forward direction.

19. Anatomical limitations of implant placements:

Buccal cortical plate	1.0 mm
Lingual cortical plate	1.0 mm
Maxillary sinus	1.0 mm
Nasal cavity	1.0 mm
Inter implant distance	3.0 mm
Inferior alveolar canal	2.0 mm
Inferior border of mandible	1 mm
Adjoining natural tooth	0.5 mm
Mental foramen	5.0 mm

20. Infection is the main cause of non-union of fracture.
21. In Turku study, sucrose is replaced by xylitol.
22. Concentration of chlorhexidine used in mouthwash is 0.2%.
23. Primordial prevention is concerned with the prevention of onset of risk factors.
24. A group which is being studied during a study is known as cohort group.
25. An antidote which is used for fluoride toxicity is milk.
26. Case control study is also known as retrospective study.
27. Floating fracture of maxilla is the horizontal fracture of maxilla.
28. Inverted L shaped osteotomy is used to treat mandibular retrognathism.
29. Latency period after mandibular distraction is 5 days.
30. An 18 years old female if comes to dental clinic with pain and swelling in mandibular 3rd molar region most common cause will be pericoronitis.
31. The probing force used during periodontal examination is 25 gms.
32. The type of incision for periodontal surgery mainly depends upon width of attached gingiva.
33. Tooth develops from Ectoderm and mesoderm.
34. All of the muscles of tongue provide attachment from the posterior aspect except Genioglossus.
35. The oropharyngeal isthmus is formed by tongue muscles named Paltoglossus.
36. Space closure is rapid following loss of mandibular primary molars closing within 3 months.

37. A fixed bride is contraindicated if opposing molar extruding 1 mm into the edentulous space.
38. In sutured skin incisions of the face, the edges of the skin should be everted.
39. Least reliable for diagnosis of periodontal diseases is electric test.
40. Ugly duckling stage was described by Broadbent so it is also known as Broadbent phenomenon.
41. Butterfly rash extensions are characteristic of Lupus erythematosus.
42. Charcot's triad includes dysarthrosis, nystagmus, ataxia.
43. Parenterally administered First generation cephalosporins is Cephalothin.
44. Sequence of completion of craniofacial growth is Transverse, Sagittal, vertical.
45. The Art (atraumatic restorative treatment) was inverted by Frecknen.
46. Specific plaque hypothesis was put forward by Loesche.
47. Development of head starts at 21st days after fertilization.
48. Epithelial thickening of the future dental arches occur in 6th week.
49. Anterior and medical displacement of fracture condyle is under the influence of Lateral pterygoid muscle.
50. A fracture of the mandible in the canine region in a 6-year-old child should be managed by Cap splint fixation.
51. During inferior alveolar nerve block the needle is inserted into pterygomandibular space.
52. Infratrochlear nerve does not supply the scalp.
53. The type of nerve cells present in trigeminal ganglion is pseudo-unipolar.
54. The pharyngeal muscle attached to mandible is superior constrictor.
55. Free gingival graft during periodontal surgery is placed on periosteum.
56. Green stains present on the teeth of children are associated with Chromogenic bacteria.
57. Disuse atrophy of periodontium may leads to:
    - Rearrangement of periodontal fibres
    - Thinning of periodontal fibres
    - Alveolar bone becomes porous.
58. Concentration of fluoride in human milk is 6-12 mg/ml.

59. The microorganisms which is increased in pregnant ladies is Prevotella intermedia.
60. Recommended oral dose of midazolam for paediatric patients is 0.25 to 1.0 mg/kg.
61. An advanced diagnostic technique which has been suggested as an alternative to culture methods for detection of fusospirocheates is Phase contrast microscopy.
62. Mineral trioxide aggregate (MTA) is the material of choice in Apexification.
63. The recent modification of MTA used as a root canal irrigant is MTA-D.
64. Flow rate of unstimulated saliva is 0.5-0.6 ml/minute and 60% of the total amount of saliva is secreted by submandibular gland.
65. The most commonly used implants design is/are Endosteal screw implants.
66. The occlusal scheme for implant prosthesis should be Mutually protected occlusion.
67. Before registering face-bow transfer, it is necessary to determine Terminal hinge axis opening.
68. All articulators. *Record jaw relation in horizontal plane.*
69. Materials most commonly used as an implant is Titanium alloys.
70. The best gingival finish line for porcelain jacket crown is Shoulder.
71. Primary relief area in maxillary complete denture is Midpalatine area.
72. For large country surveys the sampling method of choice is Multistage sampling.
73. The kind of sampling which is done in a sample which is easily available is Random sampling.
74. Galagan's formula (given by Galgan and Vermillion) is to calculate the fluoride concentration in drinking water depending on temperature of the area.
75. One tablet of 1.1 mg of NaF contains 0.5 mg of active fluoride.
76. Following is the in office objective caries activity test–Salivary reductase test.
77. The microorganism Streptococcus mutans is chiefly Facultative anaerobes.

78. The following microorganism is the first to colonise in the oral cavity after birth – Streptococcus salivarius.
79. Deltas of accessory canals are most commonly found in anterior teeth at Apical third of root.
80. The concentration of adrenaline given in shock is 0.3-0.5 mg 1: 1000 IM.
81. The recommended concentration of bupivacaine for spinal anaesthesia is 0.75%.
82. Best method to remove gutta-percha in retreatment procedures is Hand instrumentation.
83. True of the Masserann kit technique for removing solid objects. Requires frequent radiographic technique.
84. The increased levels of alkaline phosphate over 200 units indicate most likely in Paget's disease.
85. Endodontic retreatment has a poorer prognosis than original treatment.
86. An endoperio lesion with large bony dehiscence can be classified as Class III.
87. Caridex/Carisolv are alkaline in nature.
88. Fluoride present in fluoride-releasing amalgams is Stannous fluoride.
89. Y axis used to analyse Mandibular growth.
90. Gonial angle can be measured by True lateral Radiograph.
91. Zygomatic arch fractures are best viewed in Submentovertex view.
92. During implant placement the maximum allowed threshold of temperatures rise in centigrade is 47°C.
93. Minimum numbers of implants required for implant denture in mandibular denture are 2.
94. Leucocyte adhesion deficiency I (LAD I) is associated with the chromosome 21.
95. Ecchymosis in the post auricular region (Battle's sign) over the mastoid process indicates Fracture of petrous temporal or Fracture of middle cranial fossa.
96. Cheesy aspirate is seen in OKC.
97. Treatment of odontogenic keratocyte extending into the Mandibular ramus is Enucleation with peripheral osteotomy.
98. The amount of rate of distraction in distraction osteogenesis surgeries is 1 mm/day.
99. Occlusion characterized by proclined maxillary lateral incisors, retroclined central incisors and Disto-occlusion of molars is Class II div 2.

100. Square shaped arch forms with consistent deep bite are found in Class II div 2.
101. BCG vaccine is a–Live attenuated antigen from Mycobacterium bovis.
102. The most frequently performed procedure to correct a skeletal Mandibular prognathism is – Sagittal split osteotomy of the ramus.
103. The Neuro threshold toxicity level of fluoride is 500 nanograms mg F/ml in plasma.
104. Blood is a continuous variable.
105. Positive square root of variance is SD, standard deviation.
106. The treatment needs of a periodontal disease is measured by CPITN.
107. Most common injury to primary dentition is Avulsion.
108. The last tooth to be replaced by a permanent successor is Maxillary canine.
109. The lacrimal gland is located in a groove which is overlapped by Levator palpebrea superioris muscle.
110. The nerve emerges from the two superficial heads of lateral pterygoid muscle is Buccal nerve.
111. Tensor palatine forms a delicate tendon which winds round the pterygoid hamulus and flattens out to form the palatine aponeurosis.
112. Key to occlusion is Maxillary 1st molar.
113. Andrew's 2nd key to occlusion is Crown angulations.
114. Centre of rotation for controlled tipping movement is at Root apex.
115. Edgewise brackets are used with rectangular arch wire.
116. Easiest tooth movement is Extrusion.
117. Facial convexity is determined by Nasion, sup-spinale, pogonion.
118. Anterior cranial base extends between Sella-nasion planes.
119. Maximum permitted distortion in a cephalogram is 5-7%.
120. Non-vital teeth are classified under Ellis-Class IV.
121. Ramu, an 8-year-old child fell on his chin and suffered trauma. When he opens his mouth, it deviates towards left, and then the possible condition is unilateral left TMJ ankylosis.
122. All of the following are features of TMJ dislocation except Deafness.
123. Intraoral vertical ramus osteotomy is done for Mandibular setback.

124. The tear of intracapscular articular disc of TMJ causes Chronic pain.
125. The group of periodontal fibers which resist the masticatory forces Oblique.
126. Calorific value of fat is 9.
127. Most common cleft lip defect is isolated left unilateral deformities.
128. The following is mostly antigenic–Proteins.
129. Most of the metalloproteinase are involved in Dehydrogenases.
130. Purine that is found in relatively high concentrations in saliva is Uric acid.
131. The rate of physiological migration of teeth leading to shortening of the arch. Length is about 0.5 to 0.75 microns per day.
132. Force deflection rate of an orthodontic wire can be increased by increasing lengthening of the wire.
133. Index ages for the pathfinder survey are 5, 12, 15, 35 to 44, 65 to 74 years.
134. Extended/prolonged bleeding after tooth extraction doesn't occur in case of Anti-thrombin III deficiency.
135. All of the following are used as accelerators in zinc oxide eugenol cement expert Bromoglycerine.
136. Distal shoe is indicated when 2nd deciduous molar is lost prior to eruption of mand 1st premolar.
137. Which of the following correctly indicates the infectivity of hepatitis virus in humans – Hbe Ag.
138. The most common oral malignancy of the oral cavity is Squamous cell carcinoma.
139. The most common tumour associated with mandible is Admantinoma.
140. Teratoma is best described as Hamartomous development manifestation consisting of three different layers.
141. The outer Envelope in Ackermann-Proffit classification signifies Alignment.
142. Blue coloured endodontic instrument are 30 and 60 sizes.
143. The low thermal conductivity of impression compound is overcome by placing it in boiling water at 50 °C followed by kneading.
144. Hardening heat treatment of gold alloys decreases Ductility.
145. The inhibitor is added in monomer of self-cure acrylic resin to prolong the shelf life.
146. If a person receives 6 gray of radiation, then he receives 600 rads.

147. Drug contraindicated in infectious mononucleosis is Ampicillin.
148. Maximum absorption of fluoride occurs from Stomach.
149. Best site of absorption of calcium is the Proximal segment of small intestine.
150. In which of the following disease, the cavity lesion of lung act as Clinical manifestation–Wegener's granulomatosis.
151. The best X-ray view to see zygomatic arch fractures is Submentovertex view.
152. Best view to see an unerupted mesiodens is an OPG.
153. All of the following cysts are associated with impacted tooth except Primordial cyst.
154. A 36-year-old female complains of asymptomatic bilateral striation of white lines on buccal mucosa. The histological examination shows hyperkeratosis, degeneration of basal layer of cell and infiltration of T-lymphocytes in papillary layer of connective tissue. The most probable diagnosis is Lichen planus.
155. Not done in mixed dentition period is Distobuccal rotation of laterals.
156. Post auricular ecchymosis in mastoid region is known as Battle's sign.
157. Not a method to increase width of attached gingivals Undisplaced flap.
158. All of the following are protective agents in periodontal disease expert Ochracea.
159. Which of these microorganism is most caries promoting–S. Mutans.
160. Epithelium of the inner surface of the gingival sulcus has no rete pegs.
161. Muscles which are involved in the rotation and protrusion of the mandible are Medial and lateral pterygoid.
162. The secretomotor supply of the parotid gland is through otic ganglion.
163. Streptococcus mutans is implicated in the etiology of dental caries because of its capability to produce 1, 3 alfa glucose extracellular polysaccharide.
164. The change in the colour of traumatic primary incisor is due to diffusion of biliverdin in dentinal tubules.
165. Laboratory test for Anug Dark field examination.

166. Radiographic appearance of the inferior dental canal and roots of the mandibular third molar.
Radiolucent band evident in relation to root of third molar which is grooved tunnelled.
167. A 3 cm squamous cell carcinoma of the retromolar trigone and invading the mandible and the medical pterygoid muscle is at Tnm stage - Stage II.
168. In plummer-vinson syndrome there is strong association with post-cricoid carcinoma.
169. Common oral change seen with nutritional anemia is Atrophic glossitis.
170. The "window period" in HIV infection means the time lapse between the infection and detection of viral antibodies. Opaque porcelain is feldspathic glass.
171. "Brush heap" structure is found in Agar.
172. Score of 8 on the Russel periodontal index shows Beginning destruction periodontal disease.
173. The name of sample group of individuals when followed for successive examinations to evaluate the effect of oral preventive programmes is Cohort group.
174. Highest fluoride con. is found in Tea leaves.
175. 1 part per million F is equal to 1 mg of F in 1 liter of water.
176. The muscle which is resected in classical radical neck dissection is Sternomastoid.
177. The anterior two-third of the tongue is supplied by Chorda tympani nerve.
178. The tongue separated from the epiglottis by both lateral side of vallecula.
179. A high risk dental caries individual is on preventive schedule- the sugar exposure should be reduced to meal times.
180. After diet counselling the foolproof method to monitor diet change is Lactobacillus count.
181. Least cariogenic is Xylitol.
182. Cpitn measure 6 representative teeth.
183. 3D classification of orthodontia was given by Dewey.
184. For large country survey, the sampling method of choice is multistage sampling.
185. Case control studies are also called Retrospective.
186. Dental floss is used to remove interdental plaque.
187. Minimum concentration of chlorhexidine gluconate in mouth wash effective for plaque control is 0.12%.

188. Earliest symptom of gingivitis is increased in gingival fluid exudation.
189. Concentration of fluoride in the drinking water does chronic dental fluorosis occur without skeletal fluorosis 3 ppm.
190. In a 9 years permanent tooth. The surface which will show greatly increased caries incidence is Mesial surface of central incisor.
191. Disclosing solution differentiates between mature and newly formed plaque – Two tone dye solution.
192. Lugol's solution is used to demonstrate Keratinized gingiva.
193. Factor in the Stephan's curve is related to the caries incidence and sugar intake pH of plaque critical PH 5.2.
194. Gracey curettes are area specific instruments because they adapt to specific areas of the tooth or root.
195. While using a periodontal probe to measure the depth of the periodontal pocket the pocket is measured from Base of pocket to the cementoenamel junction.
196. Not a nonabsorbable suture material–Chromic gut.
197. The condition which results from the rubbing of the teeth against each other is called Attrition.
198. Least width of attached gingiva is found on the facial aspect of mandibular premolars.
199. The earliest sign of gingivitis which is of great help for diagnostic and treatment planning bleeding from gingival sulcus on gentle probing.
200. The gingiva in a patient of HIV is similar to the gingiva in ANUG.
201. A radiolucent area between the maxillary central incisors is most probably Nasopalatine cyst.
202. The temperature lag between the gelation temperature and the liquefaction temperature of the gel is known as Hysteresis.
203. After a moisture contamination does zinc containing amalgam alloy starts expanding 2-3 days.
204. A six years molar begins to calcify at birth.
205. The hypoplastic defects of the enamel appear in a radiograph is Radiolucent.
206. The cause of sensation of tissue tearing during local anesthesia administration is due to Barb on the needle.
207. The failure of the calcium hydroxide pulpotomy done on a primary 1st molar is due to internal resorption.
208. Dental age is related to the lost erupted tooth.

209. After the age of six the increase in the size of mandible occurs at Distal to 1st molars.
210. The cranial vault increases rapidly postnatally. By the age of six what % of cranial growth is completed 90%.
211. The stainless steel wires and bands used in orthodontics are composed of 18/8 S.S.
212. Tooth in a mandibular arch is commonly malopposed due to arch space discrepancy 2nd premolars.
213. A canine retractor is best used for moving a buccally placed canine for moving it distally and palatally.
214. For a bodily movement of a small tooth the force required is 150 grams.
215. When an anchor unit is allowed to tip, it is called Stationary anchorage.
216. Down's cephalometric analysis uses FH plane as a reference plane.
217. Tweed's triangle denotes the angle between the mandibular plane and mandibular incisors.
218. Alban's test measures Caries activity.
219. The best sustaining topical effect of fluoride is obtained by varnish.
220. The amount of recommended fluoride in toothpaste is 1000 ppm.
221. The concentration of NaF in a daily mouth rinse is 0.05%.
222. Following is a contraindication for pulp capping and pulpotomy – If there is inflammation of the radicular pulp.
223. Root canal is flooded with antiseptic so as to prevent infection during instrumentation.
224. Caries activity increases in xerostomia.
225. Dark brown lesions present on the labial surfaces of cuspid teeth, not painful to excavation yield few flakes of dry dentin. This type of caries is Arrested carious lesion.
226. Composite restorative material in comparison with acrylic has more abrasive strength.
227. The following does not lie on the mandible- Porion.
228. At which stage of tooth development does an aberration lead to congenital absence of the lateral incisor initiation.
229. Primate spaces occur between Primary maxillary canine and lateral incisor and mandibular primary canine and first molar.
230. Which primary teeth are severely involved in nursing bottle caries Maxillary primary incisors.

231. Green stains which occur frequently in children are due to Chromogenic bacteria.
232. Absorbed-fluoride is eliminated by Kidneys.
233. The reason for localised shrinkage porosity is thin sprue.
234. The relationship between the working edge of the instrument and the tooth surface is Adaptation.
235. Plaque is colonised earliest by Gram positive rods and cocci.
236. The most harmful plaque which penetrates the connective tissue and causes bone destruction is Subgingival tooth unattached plaque.
237. A pocket which is 5 mm in depth and with loss of attachment is 3 mm total loss of attachment is 8 mm.
238. Nerve which hooks around whartons duct is Lingual nerve.
239. Heat hardening is the process done at heating at 750 and then quenching to room temperature.
240. Annealing occurs at Solidus temperature.
241. Si-Cu eutectic alloy has a characteristic property of that fusion temp of the resultant alloy is lesser.
242. Trismus during block anesthesia is as a result of Damage to medial pterygoid.
243. Muscle originating from scaphoid fossa is Tensor palati.
244. Marsupilization is the procedure done in large cyst.
245. Epithelial attachment is derived from Dental papilla.
246. Group of fibers, which resist the masticatory force, is oblique.
247. When probing in gingivitis done, depth is measured from base of pocket to free marginal gingiva.
248. Which of following is a rare occurrence in CE-junction–Both never meet (10%)?
249. Occlusal guards are given to alter the muscle forces.
250. Multiple teeth are splinted in FPD to distribute the load.
251. 8% SnF2 contains how much % of F2- 2%.
252. McCall Festoons are seen in which teeth–Canine and Premolars.
253. Clinical signs of gingivitis appear in early gingivitis.
254. Water irrigating devices are used to alter the plaque and increases gingival health.
255. The lip is supported by relation of lip edge and facial surfaces of teeth.
256. Gracey curretes have characteristic features that they are used for specific area of surface of the tooth root.
257. Bence Jones proteins in urine are found in Multiple myeloma.

258. After PD surgery patient immediate recall is done after 1 week.
259. Objective of scaling and root planning is to improve gingival health.
260. Pregnancy gingivitis is due to plaque (P. intermedia).
261. Crater like punched appearance of gingiva seen in ANUG.
262. Langer's lines on skin are parallel to collagen fibres.
263. Which of the following is true statement of remineralization – Saliva is artificial medium for remineralization.
264. Exarticulation of teeth means Avulsion.
265. Exotoxins are Protein compound.
266. Enzymes involved in degradation of epinephrone epinephrine are Carbamoyl O-transferase.
267. In the edge wise technique, Rectangular wire is used.
268. Anterior mild crowding in mixed dentition. Line of treatment is extraction of all 1st premolars.
269. In tipping of teeth the centre of rotation is at Apical 1/3.
270. Apexification is done with Ca (OH) 2 at the apex 43. If early surgery of cleft palate is done, the facial profile becomes concave.
271. Calcination hormone from parathyroid gland function in Deposition of bone.
272. Trisodium phosphate in alginate acts as retarder.
273. Setting time of ZOE is best controlled by Cooling and glass slab.
274. Setting time of Mercury is best controlled by→Triturtion time.
275. First group of fibers damanged in periodontitis is Dentogingival fibers.
276. The area which is most prone to infection is Interdental col.
277. LA with adrenaline is absolutely contraindicated in Hyperthyroidism.
278. Sterilization and disinfection differ from each other in that sterilization kills spores.
279. Posterior belly of digastrics is derived from First brachial pouch.
280. Total protein content of the body is 6-8 g/100 ml.
281. At birth the following teeth are calcifying–Primary incisors and first 2 molar.
282. Calcification of which tooth starts at birth–Permanent 1st molar.
283. At what age half of 10 and half of 20 teeth are there in the oral cavity – 8 ½ years.
284. Activator in self-cured resins is Tertiary amine.
285. Subsurface porosity is due to Thermal changes.

286. Failure of casting to seat on the cast is overcome by Discard if the discrepancy is more than 0.03 mm.
287. Chances of endodontic failure are maximum with incomplete obturation.
288. Reaming action of the reamer is pushing rotating and regenerating.
289. Fully set $ZnpO_4$ has pH of 3-4.
290. 0.2% NaF mouth rinse is recommended fortnightly.
291. Parent instructions are given to take care of child's oral health since first tooth erupts in the oral cavity.
292. 0.05% of NaF has concentration of F 225 ppm.
293. Repetition of a study in a given group is Panel study.
294. Burkett's lymphoma is associated with E.B. virus.
295. AIDS virus is a retrovirus.
296. The main purpose of sealing the caries in deep cavities is to allow secondary dentine deposition before complete excavation.
297. Acceptable magnification of cephalogram is 5%-7%.
298. Facial plane angle is FHP-N-Pog.
299. Reverse headgear is used mainly to induce growth of maxilla in maxillary retrusion.
300. The usual procedure followed in serial extraction is CD4.
301. The amount of force to be applied by chin cap to stop mandibular growth is 1000-1200 gms.
302. Tipping of anterior tooth requires a force of 50-70 gms.
303. The centre of rotation for bodily movement of a tooth is located at infinity.
304. Apexogenesis of a tooth is closure of apical foramen in developing tooth.
305. The healing of extraction socket is done by secondary intention.
306. The greatest barrier to infection is epithelium.
307. Nalgonda tech is used for deflouridation.
308. PH of Ca(OH)2 is 9-11.
309. In dentifrices concentration of F is 1000 ppm.
310. Non-nutritive sugar is Mannitol.
311. In diet counselling to reduce caries is Sugar is restricted for a period of 21 days.
312. Most effective way to control caries at home is Apf gel.
313. Concentration of Fe 1.23% Apf gel is 12300 ppm.

314. The socket of the permanent first molar should not be curetted after extraction.
315. Odontogenic infections are most commonly caused by mixed bacteria.
316. A mandibular infection which exits through buccal cortical plate above muscle attachment will cause vestibular abscess.
317. RCT does not require prophylaxis for SABE.
318. Pterygomandibular space is not a primary space. It is secondary space.
319. Ranula is most commonly associated with sublingual salivary gland.
320. Supraperiosteal is the preferred technique for LA in haemophilic.
321. Theories of LA: 1. Electrical potential theory 2. Acetylcholine theory 3. Reversible coagulation theory 4. Calcium gate theory 5. Membrane expansion theory 6. Specific receptor theory.
322. Suspension is the hydrocolloid which is used as dental materials.
323. Infectious mononucleosis is also known as kissing disease.
324. Leucopenia is the reduction in the total leucocyte count.
325. Thiamine deficiency leads to beri-beri.
326. Reed-Sternberg cells are found in Hodgkin's disease.
327. Sodium valproate is an anti epileptic agent which causes reversible gingival hyperplasia.
328. The Flash technique of sterilization by autoclave which includes 134 degree/32 lb/3 minutes.
329. On a stained slide clostridium tetani has the appearance of a drum stick.
330. A micrometer is 0.001 mm.
331. Ig G has the maximum serum concentration in human body.
332. The replacement of one type of adult cell by other type of adult cell is known as metaplasia.
333. The volume of pulp cavity of maxillary molar is approximately 0.07 cc.
334. Modifiers are added to the POP to regulate setting time.
335. Maximum carbon content of steel used in dentistryis 1.7%.
336. The most common disadvantage of acrylic resin denture base is shrinkage.
337. Calcium hydroxide is used as a base below restorative resins.
338. Zinc oxide eugenol impression paste harden by chemical reaction i.e. chelation.

339. The enamel of posterior teeth is thickest at the occlusal surface.
340. Malignant neoplasm does not show encapsulation.
341. Absence of pulp chamber i.e. dentinogenesis imperfecta.
342. Hemorrhage and thrombosis of blood vessels is the early sign of TFO.
343. Indomethacin or Indocin is the NSAID which has a tendency to cause blood dyscrasis.
344. The amount of glucose filtered in PCT is 100%.
345. The approximate no. of bacteria one would find in oral cavity is 10,000,000,000.
346. Tyrosine is non essential amino acids.
347. Amoeba, histoplasma and bacteroids are the microorganism found in lung abscess.
348. Spirochetes and Fusobacterium is the microorganism associated with ANUG.
349. Wolf's graft is full thickness graft.
350. At birth cranium is nearest the size it will eventually attain in adulthood.
351. Ostitis fibrosa cystic is associated with hyperparathyroidism.
352. Ameloblastoma most frequently occurs in mandibular posterior or molar region.
353. Warthins' tumour is an adenolymphoma of parotid gland.
354. Extraction or endodontic therapy is the treatment of acute periapical abscess.
355. Dentine is the first formed dental tissue.
356. Antibodies are formed by B lymphocytes.
357. Unmyelinated nerve fibers of pulp supply smooth muscles of blood vessels.
358. ANB is used to determine the relationship of maxilla to mandible.
359. Retention appliance should be retentive and passive.
360. Marginal ridge is the best place for attachment of sprue.
361. Vertical root fracture is having the poorest prognosis.
362. Antidote for fluoride is milk.
363. Trisodium phosphate is added to the resin as stretching agent.
364. Stannous fluoride is the freshly prepared topical fluoride solution.
365. 10% Potassium nitrate is used to treat hypersensitive enamel.
366. Topical application of fluoride is more useful for newly erupted teeth.

367. If fluoride is added to pit and fissure sealants then it will reduce enamel solubility.
368. Arch shaped bone loss is seen around molars in juvenile periodontitis (Localised aggressive periodontitis).
369. Mandibular nerve passes through foramen ovale.
370. During inferior alveolar nerve block the LA is deposited in the pterygomandibular space.
371. Metal ceramic failure occurs most commonly due to improper designing of restoration.
372. Calcium hydroxide is used in weeping canals.
373. The minimum time period lapse after radiographic exposure before surgery is 4-6 weeks.
374. Bite wing X-ray is done to know about incipient caries on proximal surface.
375. Cavity preparation of a tooth is done to prepare a tooth surface to receive restorative material.
376. Tooth paste applied on child's tooth brush should be of pea nut size.
377. The liquid used in tissue conditioner is methyl methacrylate.
378. Intercanine width increases with the eruption of canines.
379. Standard deviation is a measure of variability.
380. Disclosing solution stains dental plaque/microorganisms.
381. The nerve which is hooked around Wharton's duct is lingual nerve.
382. After diet counselling the patient response should be evaluated by latest diet history.
383. Gingival picture of AIDS can be related to ANUG.
384. Infectious mononucleosis in children is characterized by palatal petechiae.
385. Coronoid process of mandible interferes with the thickness of maxillary denture buccal flange.
386. Arch criminal in caries is sucrose.
387. Damage to sublingual duct causes Ranula.
388. Temperature of glass bead sterilizer is 425-475 degree F.
389. Drug induced gingival enlargement is of non-inflammatory type.
390. Mesiobuccal is the most complicated canal to prepare in maxillary 1st molar.
391. Deep bite is associated with low mandibular plane.
392. Generalized cementosis is seen in Paget's disease.
393. Predominant Ig in saliva is IgA.
394. Amyloidosis is associated with multiple myeloma.

395. Best surgical seal is provided by zinc oxide eugenol cement.
396. Dual core resin is the best cement for cementation of porcelain laminates.
397. Occlusal wear of tooth is known as attrition.
398. Removal of contaminated layer of casting is done by pickling.
399. Immediate reaction which occurs below the calcium hydroxide is necrosis of pulp.
400. Odontoplasty is done in Class II embrasures with minimum soft tissue loss.
401. The eye is most sensitive to green and yellow colour and least sensitive to red and blue colour.
402. The object which appears to be of one colour under one source of light may appear different under another light source; this phenomenon is termed as metamerism.
403. The maximum shrinkage during firing process in ceramic occurs in high bisque stage.
404. Microbiology frequently asked in PGI Chandigarh:

First microorganism invading the oral cavity after birth	Streptococcus salivarius
Initiation of smooth surface caries	Streptococcus mutans
Impetigo, carbuncle, fruncle	Staphylococci
Osteomyelitis	Staphylococci
Progression of caries	Lactobacilli
Root surface caries	Actinomyces viscous
Pregnancy gingivitis	Prevotella intermedia
Acute pseudomembranous colitis	Clostridium difficle
Dry socket	Treponema denticola
German measles	Toga virus
Coxsackie group A-10	Acute lymph nodular pharyngitis
Coxsachie group A-16	Hand foot and mouth disease

405. Multiple retained deciduous teeth are associated with Cleidocranial dysostosis.
406. African population is having high incidence of Noma.
407. The first sign which appears after shock is tachycardia.

408. Shore and Barcol test is used to test hardness of rubber based on impression material.
409. Glass transition temperature of impression compound is 39 Degree C and fusion temperature of impression compound is 43.5 degree C.
410. 2% potassium sulphate is used as hardening agent.
411. The term fusion and concrescence were discussed by Levitas.
412. Most eaten appearance is seen in chronic Osteomyelitis.
413. The viral action is differentiated from bacterial action by interferon production.
414. Blood spills in the hospitals are cleaned by sodium hypochlorite.
415. Xi point is the cephalometric point located at the mid of the ramus.
416. Tongue has its effects primarily on palatoglossal arch.
417. Dontrix gauge is used for measurement of force.
418. Lyme disease is transmitted by ticks.
419. Epoxy resin for die preparation cannot be used along with hydrocolloid impression. They can be used with rubber based impression materials.
420. Flow rate of unstimulated saliva is 0.5-0.6 ml/minute.
421. Cartilages differ from bone in that it grows by interstitial growth pattern.
422. Epithelium of nasal and nasopharyngeal mucosa is pseudostratified columnar ciliated epithelium.
423. 24 teeth are present in the radiograph of a newborn.
424. Junctional navus is most likely to turn malignant.
425. The minimum depth of the lesion to be visible on the radiograph is 500 micrometer.
426. The value of prothrombin time is 11-15 seconds.
427. Chemical mediator of orthodontic tooth movement is prostaglandins.
428. Cat gut suture material will lead to maximum tissue response.
429. First step in developing of an X-ray film is stirring of solution.
430. The type of anchorage used in maxillary expansion by quad helix is reciprocal anchorage.
431. Von Ebner's glands are purely serous in nature.
432. Hb molecules consist of 4 heme molecules and 2 alfa and 2 beta chains.
433. Pantograph tracing utilizes 6 styli.
434. Sialography cannot be done in viral parotitis.

435. Slot size most commonly used for orthodontics is 0.018 × 0.028.
436. Hard rays are most penetrating X-rays.
437. 10% formalin is most commonly used fixative in biopsy.
438. ANUG if not treated will lead to an indifferent course.
439. Wit's appraisal AO-BO is the relationship of maxilla to the mandible.
440. Plaque does not have rhamnose moiety.
441. Advance bell stage in tooth development corresponds to the stage of morphodifferentiation.
442. Surface zone is the most remineralized zone in the histology of dental caries.
443. Movement of tooth with digital pressure with hand was proposed by celsius.
444. Demilunes of Guazzini are mucous terminals capped by serous caps in submandibular glands.
445. Combination clasps have retentive arm of wrought gold and a reciprocal arm of cast metal.
446. Interglobular dentine is a hypocalcified dentine.
447. Diet modification is the patients of rampant caries require allow no sugar for 21 days.
448. Activated macrophage secretes IL-1 and TNF-alpha during inflammation.
449. Deep fascia is the structure which is absent on face.
450. Working side contacts from canines to all the posterior teeth without balancing side contacts.
451. Variance is best described as the square of standard deviation.
452. Trans gingival probing is a clinical procedure used to detect underlying bony topography.
453. In blow out fractures enopthalmos is seen.
454. Giant cell lesion of periodontium is most commonly considered as non-neoplastic reactive lesion.
455. Single most reliable criteria for squamous cell carcinoma are invasion. Dental fluorosis with skeletal fluorosis occurs at fluoride conc of 3 ppm.
456. In compound odontoma tooth like denticles are found.
457. Most easiest tooth movement is extrusion while the tooth movement which require least force is intrusion. The type of study involving repetitive examination of a sample is panel study.
458. In a sample of population the maximum observations are concentrated around median.

459. 500 million people of world are using fluoridated tooth paste.
460. FMPA is used to assess mandibular growth pattern.
461. Most posterior point on mandible is gonion.
462. Most common benign neoplasm of oral cavity is fibroma.
463. At 2 months of intrauterine life head: body ratio is 1: 16.
464. Oral health status index was given by Marcus and Greshen in 1980.
465. A splint is defined as an appliance to prevent movement of mobile teeth.
466. The value of condylar inclination is 20-25 degree.
467. Actinobacillus, actinomycetamcommitans attachment with the tooth surface is prevented by Myeloperoxidases.
468. Labiodentals fricatives sounds are most affected in class III malocclusion.
469. Cariogram is given by Brathall (1994).
470. Air sinus which can be used as skeletal maturity indicator is frontal sinus.
471. Granulation tissue is replaced by connective tissue by 21 days.
472. ESR is not the part of complete blood examination (hematocrit, Hb estimation, WBC count).
473. Drug of choice for penicillinase producing infective micro-organism is cloxacillin.
474. Most common occurrence of cleft lip is unilateral left.
475. The type of carcinoma developed in Marjolins' ulcer is basal cell carcinoma.
476. Gingival bleeding index is used to assess state of oral hygiene on the day of examination.
477. Best way to prevent exposure of dehiscence during surgical procedure is to raise partial thickness flap.
478. Type of incision for periodontal surgery depends upon width of attached gingiva.
479. According to WHO dentist to population ratio is 1:4000.
480. Alendronate can cause osteonecrosis of jaw.
481. Pseudo unipolar cells are present in trigeminal ganglion.
482. Sunday bite is present in class II div 1.
483. Latency period after mandibular distraction is 5 days.
484. During jaw relations the protrusive records are used for condylar inclination measurement of both sides.
485. Maximum part of Lee way space is provided by primary second molar.

486. A variation of 18-24 months is considered as normal in eruption of permanent molars.
487. A pier abutment is a single tooth with two adjacent edentulous spaces on either side.
488. In Glanzmann disease there is increase in bleeding time and platelet count remains normal.
489. Prothrombin time is used to check status of anticoagulant therapy.
490. PTT is prolonged in case of Hemophilia A.
491. Sassouni analysis is used to describe skeletal disturbances in vertical plane.
492. Epignathus is teratoma of palate.
493. Pont's index is used for expansion criteria.
494. Gingival cord is kept in the sulcus for a period of 5-10 minutes.
495. Amount of force for trial closure and final closure are 1500 psi and 3500 psi respectively.
496. Minimal dentinal destruction to get evident on the radiograph is 40 microns.
497. Pulp capping and pulpotomy is contraindicated if the pulp is inflamed.
498. ANUG is best visualized in Punched lesions or Crater lesions.
499. Quebec counter in casue activity best is for Lactobacillus colonies.
500. Best method to deflect patient compliance is improvement of oral that likes bleeding on probing.
501. Two or more teeth united by roots is Concrescence.
502. Treatment of mucocele on lower lip is Excision with adjacent glands.
503. Caries activity is increases in Xerostomia.
504. In blow out fracture Enopthalmos is evident.
505. Badges should be worn and replaced by dental technician every 1 month.
506. 1st step in developing film first step is to stirring the solution.
507. Radiographic changes in periodontitis are Lamina dura is damaged.
508. In children radiographic dose should be (that of adults) is 50%.
509. Which of the following are not non-absorbable sutures: Catgut.
510. Purpose of cavity preparation is to receive restorating material.
511. Porcelain, metal bond in PFM is Chemical Mechanical.
512. Functional 1 matrix theory was given by Melvin Moss.

513. HOME is aversive technique.
514. Vitamin K dependent clotting factors are II, VII, IX, X.
515. Thickening agent used in dentifrices is Alginate amylase.
516. Robinson's classification of Ameloblastoma is Unicentric, Nonfunctional, and Intermittent in growth, anatomically benign and clinically persistent.
517. Precocious puberty is most characteristic of Albright syndrome.
518. Main constituent of inlay was is Paraffin wax.
519. Bone at forming stage has Osteoclasts, osteoblasts, osteoid.
520. Organelles contain DNA–Nucleus.
521. Taste sensations from the posterior one third of the tongue are carried by Cranial nerve IX.
522. The muscle arising from the outer surface of the alveolus of the region of the molars is supplied by which nerve – Facial.
523. Secretomotor fibres to the submandibular salivary gland are carried in all of the following except – Mylohyoid.
524. Drugs causing extra pyramidal symptoms – Antibiotics.
525. Developed hyperactivity to a drug is tolerance.
526. Pulp tissue is loose connective.
527. While taking radiographs for children, by what % should X-ray beam exposure should be reduced 50%.
528. The radiographic view of choice for Zygomaticomaxillary complex fracture is Occipitomental.
529. A radiopaque mass continuous with the cementoenamel junction attached to the distal of the first premolar is Calculus.
530. Giant cell lesions of the periodontium are best considered as Non-neoplastic reactive lesions.
531. Most common site of bone destruction in a pathologically involved primary second molar is Bifurcation.
532. Amalgam alloys is least susceptible to creep – Dispersion alloy with high frequency.
533. Properties of dental materials is time dependent–Creep.
534. Function of carnauba wax is to decrease flow at room temperature.
535. Trisodium phosphate is alginate acts as Retarder.
536. Viscoelastic substances may be defined as those which removal of load shows slow recovery.
537. The bilby layer is a synonym for molecular disorganized surface on a highly polished material.
538. Eugenol is not used with zinc oxide in a periodontal dressing as it causes allergic reactions.

539. Most common missing tooth in the permanent dentition is mandibular second premolar.
540. Interdental spacing found in the maxillary arch of the deciduous dentition is 4 mm.
541. Staphylococcal bacteria are found in grapes like clusters.
542. The bacteria associated with root surface caries is Fuso-bacterium.
543. Haemoglobin as four heme molecules, 2 Alpha and 2 Beta chains.
544. S. Mutans is involved in dental caries initiation, other bacteria also involved is S. Sanguis.
545. The organisms that causes infective endocarditis is Streptococcus viridans.
546. Heparin, apart from releasing lipoprotein lipase in the blood exerts its anticoagulant action by inhibiting thrombin synthesis.
547. Retention in a stainless steel crown is achieved primarily by parallel distal and mesial walls.
548. In a 2 years old child due to an accident maxillary deciduous central incisor is intruded by 4 mm treatment is – make patient comfortable and observe.
549. A radiopaque area is seen in the dentine of a 3 months old class- II silver amalgam restoration base is calcium hydroxide.
550. In a Class II division 2, the most typical characteristic seen in lingual inclination of maxillary central incisors.
551. Optimum orthodontic force should not exceed the capillary blood pressure.
552. Helix in a finger spring for mesial movement lies on the distal side.
553. The best time to treat cross-bite is as and when detected.
554. Dolichocephalic facial type is long and narrow dental arches.
555. Most common malocclusion found in people is Class I with incisor crowing.
556. Chin cap therapy is used for Skeletal Class III deformity.
557. Four canals are seen in upper 1st molars.
558. Desirable root canal filling material in deciduous teeth is Zinc oxide and eugenol.
559. Pulp horn exposure occurs most commonly with Mesiobuccal horn of the 1st molars.
560. Moisture contamination of amalgam can lead to delayed expansion.

561. Stain of yeast is found in the root canal – Candida albicans.
562. The most effective and least objectionable topical fluoride is APF gel.
563. Tooth arch relieved with cold water indicates irreversible pulpitis.
564. Increased bleeding during pulp amputation indicates arterial hyperaemia.
565. A small radiolucent area at the periapical region of a non-vital root. Canal treated tooth is observed Treatment is Periapical curettage with apiectomy.
566. Benzoin methyl ether in a polymer indicates that they may be cured in the presence of UV light.
567. Plaque is most harmful and causes spread of inflammation to the connective tissue leading to bone destruction, subgingival epithelial attached.
568. Severely crowded mandibular incisors are due to tooth size-arch length discrepancy.
569. Adult face is formed by fusion of first and second branchial arches and tissues surrounding the developing forebrain.
570. Highest point on the concavity posterior to the occipital condyles is Bolton's point.
571. Not an example of intermaxillary anchorage–Retraction of the upper incisors by tipping them lingually and using lower molars as anchorage.
572. If the pocket depth is 5 mm and the gingival recession is 3 mm, the total loss of attachment is 8 mm.
573. Genes involved in craniofacial development are – MSX-1, MSX-2 Indian hedgenog, Oxi (Orthodontical TXN family).
574. Concept of Canalization of growth given by–Waddlington.
575. Pioneer work on Infant orthopaedics was given by–Lathem.
576. Apert Syndrome is caued by – FG-GR.
577. Fusion of Palatal shelves starts at age of 60 days.
578. APNEA-HYPONEA INDEX (AHI) is number of apneas and/or hypoapneas per hour of sleep (or study time).
   –Reflects the severity of sleep apnea
   AH= 0-5—Normal range
   AHi = 5-15 – Mild sleep apnea
   AHi = 15-30—Moderate sleep apnea
   AHi > 30 – Severe sleep apnea
579. Carpel bones are arranged in 2 rows – Proximal and distal.

580. Adductor sesamoid appears is—No. 4 Indicator in Fishman Skeletal maturity Index.
581. Primary stability of Micro Implant is by – Cortical bone.
582. Index for Complexity Outcome and need (Icon).

Complexity Grade	**Score Range**
Easy	< 29
Mild	29-50
Moderate	51-63
Difficult	64-777
Very difficult	> 77

583. Nd : YAG Laser used in Periodontal surgery with a tendency of absorption in pigmented tissue is – Soft tissue laser.
584. On debonding speed of micromotor with TC burr—30 K.
585. Goslon evaluation is done in which planes – Sagittal, Vertical and Transverse.
586. Acid etching was done for first time in – 1955.
587. Negative Growth is given by – Thymus.
588. Day to day variations in growth are known as – Diurnal variations.
589. Lamella of ulna grows and joins around – Pubertal Growth Spurt.
590. Fusion of two palatal shelves starts at – Anterior to Posterior.
591. Bite registered with more vertical and less horizontal component in – Vertical gromer.
592. Incidence of C2-C3 fusion is –0.3-0.7%.
593. Enamel surface dissolute after demineralization – 3-9 mm.
594. Friction during sliding of urine is – Kinetic friction.
595. BAKERS ANCHORAGE is – Intermaxillary Anchorage.
596. Most common complication of Bilateral Sagittal Split osteotomy—Damage to Inferior Alveolar Nerve.
597. Collagen is secreted from Pulp fibroblast—Type I and III.
598. In retention classical experiment in dogs days taken by gingival fibers – 232 days.
599. Flutes in Microimplant helps in – Primary stability.
600. In standard edgewise system torque values for bracket is – Zero.
601. Primary palate derived from – MNP (Median Nasal Process).

602. If a V bend is place in between wire in canine and molar then – Anticlockwise momentum is generated due to intrusion on molar with short arm.
603. Phenomenon of faster eruption of teeth around 11-12 years of age is due to – Juvenile thyrotoxicosis.
604. Most likely reason for the mandibular incisor crowding in late twenties is – Late maxillary growth.
605. Chi-square test cannot be applied if – any expected cell frequency is less than one.
606. For ruling out disease in a patient, you would use a – Test with high Negative predictivity.
607. Incidence rate of disease refers to – New cases.
608. Indicator of severity of disease is – Case fatality rate.
609. Maximum force a Microimplant can bear is — 500 grams.
610. Centre of resistance during intrusion—At middle third of root.
611. Relapse in orthodontics due to – Supracrestal fibers.
612. Centre of rotation during Intrusion – Outside the tooth.
613. In a 15 years patient with unrepaired cleft, the P.A. Ceph shows — Decreased Transverse diameter of maxilla.
614. According to Registration of Births and Deaths Act 1969 the birth and the death respectively are to be registered within – 21 days.
615. Scatter diagram shows – Relationship between two variables.
616. Longitudinal studies can provide – Incidence of disease.
617. Matching in case-control studies is done to control uncertainities due to – Bias arising from confounders.
618. In an epidemiological study, the first case which comes to attention on investigator is – Index Case.
619. The principal cells of gingival epithelium are – Keratinocytes.
620. Probing depth of clinically healthy gingivalis – 2-3 mm.
621. COL is – Valley like depression of Inter dental gingiva.
622. Normal width of marginal gingiva is – 1 mm.
623. Markel cells are – Tactile receptors.
624. Stratum granulosum is Absent in – Parakeratinised epithelium.
625. Length of junctional epithelium is – 0.25-1.35 mm.
626. Width of attached gingiva increases with age and supraeruption of teeth and decreases with pocket formation.
627. Earliest sign of gingival inflammation is – Bleeding on Gentle probing.
628. Group of Periodontal fibres not attached to the bone are – Transseptal group.

629. The principal fiber group that gets reconstructed even after destruction of alveolar bone – Transseptal group.
630. Passive eruption divided into – 4 stages.
631. Largest group of Principal fibres is – Oblique group.
632. The principle fibre group that prevents extrusion of the tooth and resists lateral tooth movement is – Alveolar crest group.
633. The principal connective tissue cells present in Periodontal ligament are – Fibroblast.
634. Acellular Cementum commonly in – Cervical Third of root.
635. Cellular cementum commonly seen in – Apical Third of root.
636. Total inorganic content of cementum is – 45-50%.
637. Cementum overlaps the enamel at cementoenamel junction at about – 60-65% cases.
638. Thickness of Acellular cementum – 30-230 m.
639. Sulcular epithelium can be penetrated by a substance with molecular weight – One million.
640. Sulcular fluid is an – Inflammatory exudates.
641. Most important buffer system in Saliva is – Bicarbonate-Carbonic and buffers.
642. One gram of plaque (wet weight) contains – 2 x 1011 bacteria.
643. Content of which element increases with depth of periodontal pockets – Na+ (Sodium).
644. Hard deposit that forms by mineralisation of dental plaque – Calculus.
645. Attrition is a problem with – Cohort Study.
646. Chi-Square test is used to measure degree of – Association between two variables.
647. Method of presenting Data of geographic distribution is – Cartogram.
648. Continuous age specific, area distribution of incidence of cancer can be represented by – Stem and Leaf diagram.
649. Zirconium and Zinc is added to b-TMA arch wires to Increases formability by decreasing a phase formation.
650. The cantilever system configuration is produced by An off-center V-Bend located at the "one third" position on the interbracket span.
651. To produce bodily movement of a tooth in an adult patient, with bone loss, condition which is desirable is Lighter forces and higher countervailing moment.
652. To determine the effect of headgear being applied, the most important is Line of action of force, Point of application of force and Direction of force.

653. Recommended procedure for conditioning deciduous teeth is sandblasting with 50 mm Al2O3 for 3 second.
654. Survival time of brackets bonded with self-etching primer in comparison to conventional two stage bonding group is less.
655. Stobies extraction is a procedure in which 2 premolars are extracted at the same time.
656. Chromium oxide in stainless steel prevents tarnish and corrosion by Passivating effect.
657. In group C space closure with a segmented T loop, the spring is positioned closer to anterior segment.
658. In 0.018 inch slot, the brackets could be ranked in order from highest to lowest friction as Polycrystalline ceramic, ceramic reinforced composite with metal slot, Stainless.
659. Treatment for an ankylosed primary tooth with no permanent successor is Retain in mouth as long as possible.
660. In distraction osteogenesis, the segments are separated at a rate of 0.5-1.5 mm per day.
661. Ricketts utility arches from Two-couple system.
662. Interleukin-1 helps in osteoclast activation.
663. Most of the adhesives used in orthodontics has the bond strength in the range of 15-20 Mpa.
664. Ceramic brackets were introduced by Michael I. Swartz in 1987.
665. Functional occlusal plane was given by Jarvinen in 1985.
666. In type-A growth trend the growth of middle face is more as compared to the lower face.
667. The correct sequence for distraction osteogenesis is: Osteotomy – Latency period – Distraction – Consolidation – Remodeling.
668. The most effective method for preventing the transfer of infection between health care personnel and patients within the hospital is hand washing.
669. The latency period for alveolar distraction is usually 1 week.
670. When the strength of agreement between two examiners is very good, the kappa (K) value is 1.
671. Spearman's coefficient test is used for Correlation.
672. Finite element analysis is used to determine stress distribution on a material.
673. Nickel allergy is Type-IV sensitivity.
674. Maxillary lateral incisor is most susceptible to root resorption during premolar extraction treatment.

675. Disinfection used for alginate impression is Glutaraldehyde.
676. The diagnostic method commonly used for the diagnosis of obstructive sleep apnoea is Polysomnography.
677. Frankel appliance is a tissue-borne functional appliance.
678. Broussard bracket has both horizontal and vertical slots.
679. During distraction osteogenesis, the adaptive changes in the surrounding soft tissue are known as Distraction histogenesis.
680. Cephalometric parameter which is used for the diagnosis of vertical jaw Dysplasia is Jaraback ratio.
681. Normal facial index is 80%-85%.
682. Class I molar relationship is not a key related to the functional occlusion as suggested by Roth.
683. In centric occlusion, the clearance between the anterior teeth is 0.005".
684. Class II elastics is not an anchorage saver.
685. Situation which need long term retention is Expansion of palate in a repaired cleft palate patient at the age of 12 years.
686. Human mandibular osteodistraction procedure was first performed by Mc Carthy.
687. Conventional nickel-titanium wire is an arch wire which is not superelastic.
688. The property of an orthodontic arch wire that represents the stress value at which a small amount (0.1% or 0.2%) of plastic deformation occurs is known as Yield strength.
689. Excessive collum angle is a characteristic of Class II Division-2 malocclusion.
690. X-occlusion is common among Australian arborigines.
691. Isolated cleft palate is more common in female.
692. In matrix rotation of the mandible, centre of rotation is at Condyle.
693. Lip strain is a characteristic feature of Class II division-1 malocclusion with deep bite.
694. GOSLON index is used for the assessment of maxillary growth in cleft patients.
695. The most common site for enamel demineralization during fixed orthodontic treatment is Labiogingival area of maxillary lateral incisor.
696. MPA is not a fixed functional appliance.
697. Recently diagnosed case of acute leukemia is an absolute contraindication of orthodontic treatment.
698. Achondroplasia results Mandibular excess.

699. Andrews was the pioneer of straight wire appliance.
700. Moment to force ratio for translation is 8-10.
701. The recommended force magnitude for the forward movement of maxilla is 12 oz/side.
702. Thc concept of "overcorrection" is recommended in Roth philosophy.
703. Differential force concept was introduced by Begg.
704. Pendulum appliance is used for Molar distalization.
705. Straight wire appliances are MBT appliance, Vari-simplex discipline and Andrew's straight wire appliance.
706. Speech sound problems which are related to skeletal Class III malocclusion is Labiodental fricatives.
707. All patient activated orthodontic appliances produce intermittent force.
708. Short Class II elastics were recommended by Roth.
709. The choice of wire used in fabrication of pendulum appliance .036 Elgiloy.
710. Orthognathic surgical procedures will have more amount of relapse tendencies are Lefort I with inferior positioning of maxilla, Sagittal split with mandibular advancement and Augmentation Genioplasty.
711. The anterior face height in Horn's facial height index is measured from N to Me.